J. Inher. Metab. Dis. 14 (1991) 405–406

Preface

THE 28th ANNUAL SYMPOSIUM OF THE SSIEM – BIRMINGHAM, 1990

The 3rd Annual Symposium of the SSIEM was held in Birmingham in 1965 and it was to this same City that the Society returned 25 years later. It was particularly fitting that the programme be based on the theme of the Liver and Inherited Metabolic Disorders in view of the major interest in this field in Birmingham.

As usual, members of the Society contributed to the success of the meeting with submission of over 120 posters and 10 oral presentations.

As a preamble to the main meeting the organizers had planned a half-day symposium on "Cost–effectiveness of the Diagnosis and Management of Inherited Metabolic Disorders". Professor Charles Scriver introduced and chaired the session, with presentations from a health economist, several professionals and finally a view from the UK Government given by Dame Jill Knight, DBE, MP.

The main symposium had plenary sessions covering Metabolic Functions of the Liver, Bile Acids, α_1-Antitrypsin Deficiency, and reviews on Tyrosinaemia type I, Crigler–Najjar type I and Niemann–Pick C. These sessions provided updates on a wide range of metabolic disorders and illustrated the importance of the complementary contributions from the professionals in different disciplines.

The Society has always striven to promote interest from paediatricians and it was with this as the objective that a half-day symposium on the Diagnosis of Inherited Metabolic Disorders presenting as Liver Disease was organized. Papers covering a practical approach to clinical, laboratory and radiological investigation were discussed.

Liver transplantation for the treatment of several inborn errors of metabolism is now a realistic possibility. Mr Buckles presented a 'state-of-the-art' overview of transplantation with more specific information on inborn errors by Dr Burdelski. The exciting possibilities for fetal liver transplantation presented by Professor Touraine were a fitting end to an interesting and stimulating meeting for both clinicians and biochemists.

Many organizations contributed financially towards the success for the meeting. The National Reye's Syndrome Foundation of the United Kingdom funded part of the plenary session on Metabolic Functions of the Liver. The Children's Liver Disease Foundation generously supported the half-day symposium on Diagnosis of Inherited Metabolic Disorders presenting as Liver Disease. The Society also wishes to express their appreciation to Mr Brian Gill for the continuing support from Scientific Hospital Supplies Ltd. of Liverpool.

The meeting was organized by Anne Green with unstinting support and hard work from the Birmingham Children's Hospital team of George Gray, Edith Green, Kate Hall, Ann Insley, Robert Leeming, Stuart Mann, Mary Anne Preece and Registration Secretary Ian Sewell. Although this same team are not anxious to take on a repeat performance immediately, Birmingham hopes it won't be another 25 years before the city plays host again to the SSIEM.

G. M. Addison
G. T. N. Besley
A. Green (*Guest Editor*)
R. A. Harkness
R. J. Pollitt
(*Editors*)

SOCIETY FOR THE STUDY OF INBORN ERRORS OF METABOLISM

The SSIEM was founded in 1963 by a small group in the North of England but now has more than 70% of its members outside the UK. The aim of the Society is to promote the exchange of ideas between professional workers in different disciplines who are interested in inherited metabolic disorders. This aim is pursued in scientific meetings and publications.

The Society holds an annual symposium concentrating on different topics each year with facilities for poster presentations. There is always a clinical aspect as well as a laboratory component. The meeting is organized so that there is ample time for informal discussion; this feature has allowed the formation of a network of contacts throughout the world. The international and multidisciplinary approach is also reflected in the *Journal of Inherited Metabolic Disease*.

If you are interested in joining the SSIEM then contact the Treasurer: Dr. D. Isherwood, Department of Clinical Biochemistry, Royal Liverpool Children's Hospital, Alder Hey, Liverpool, L12 2AP, UK. The current subscription is £30 per year payable January 1st each year. This subscription includes the 6 issues of the *Journal of Inherited Metabolic Disease* as well as the regular circulation of a newsletter.

Journal of Inherited Metabolic Disease

Copyright © 1991 Springer Science+Business Media Dordrecht
Originally published by Kluwer Academic Publishers in 1991

ISBN 978-0-7923-8982-8   ISBN 978-94-011-9749-6 (eBook)
DOI 10.1007/ 978-94-011-9749-6

Journal of Inherited Metabolic Disease

EDITORS

R. A. Harkness (London), R. J. Pollitt (Sheffield) and
J. M. Addison (Manchester)

EDITORIAL BOARD

[publisher and subscription information text — illegible]

J. Inher. Metab. Dis. 14 (1991) 407–420
© SSIEM and Kluwer Academic Publishers.

The Role of the Liver in Metabolic Homeostasis: Implications for Inborn Errors of Metabolism

G. VAN DEN BERGHE

Laboratory of Physiological Chemistry, International Institute of Cellular and Molecular Pathology, Avenue Hippocrate 75, B-1200 Brussels, Belgium

Summary: The mechanisms by which the liver maintains a constant supply of oxidizable substrates, which provide energy to the body as a whole, are reviewed. During feeding, the liver builds up energy stores in the form of glycogen and triglyceride, the latter being exported to adipose tissue. During fasting, it releases glucose and ketone bodies. Glucose is formed by degradation of glycogen and by gluconeogenesis from gluconeogenic amino acids provided by muscle. Ketone bodies are produced from fatty acids, released by adipose tissue, and from ketogenic amino acids. The major signals which control the transition between the fed and the fasted state are glucose, insulin and glucagon. These influence directly or indirectly the enzymes which regulate liver carbohydrate and fatty acid metabolism and thereby orient metabolic fluxes towards either energy storage or substrate release. In the fed state, the liver utilizes the energy generated by glucose oxidation to synthesize triglycerides. In the fasted state it utilizes that produced by β-oxidation of fatty acids to synthesize glucose. The mechanisms whereby a number of inborn errors of glycogen metabolism, of gluconeogenesis and of ketogenesis cause hypoglycaemia are also briefly overviewed.

Metabolic homeostasis, restrictively defined in this paper as the maintenance of a constant supply of substrates which can be oxidized to provide energy, requires both the capacity to build up reserves during feeding and the ability to break down these stores while fasting. The main metabolic fuels of the human body are glucose, fatty acids and ketone bodies. Its principal energy stores are liver glycogen, adipose tissue triglyceride and muscle protein. In the metabolic homeostasis of the body as a whole, the liver occupies a central position. Indeed, besides building up glycogen in its own cells, the liver plays an essential rôle in the synthesis of adipose tissue triglyceride, by producing very-low-density lipoproteins, and of muscle protein, by synthesizing non-essential amino acids. Furthermore, the liver furnishes oxidizable substrates, not only to meet its own needs, but also to cover those of other tissues. Glucose, the only fuel which red blood cells can use and nearly the only one which the brain utilizes, is only synthesized by liver and, to a lesser extent, by kidney cortex. Ketone bodies which during prolonged fasting are a major fuel for heart and muscle, and also for brain, are exclusively formed by the liver.

In this review the hepatic pathways involved in the synthesis and degradation of energy stores and fuels will first be outlined. Some recent advances in the field will also be briefly described. Thereafter the main regulatory mechanisms whereby the liver switches from the build-up of reserves during feeding to the production of oxidizable substrates during fasting will be reviewed. A description of the energy requirements for metabolic homeostasis will be followed by a brief discussion of its implications for the pathophysiology of a number of inborn errors of metabolism.

HEPATIC PATHWAYS INVOLVED IN THE SYNTHESIS AND DEGRADATION OF ENERGY STORES AND FUELS

Metabolic homeostasis by the liver involves mainly carbohydrate, fatty acid and amino acid metabolism. These pathways are depicted schematically in Figure 1, and will be briefly reviewed in the following paragraphs. For more details, the reader is referred to biochemistry handbooks or to reviews of the subject in textbooks of hepatology (Seifter and Englard, 1988; Zakim, 1990). An extensive discussion of the mechanisms whereby the liver controls blood glucose homeostasis has been recently published in this journal (Hers, 1990).

Carbohydrate metabolism

The first step of the hepatic metabolism of glucose is phosphorylation into glucose 6-phosphate by glucokinase. Glucokinase is an isozyme of hexokinase, which is only found in hepatocytes and in pancreatic islets. It differs from the other hexokinases in its specificity for glucose, high V_{max} (approximately $3\,\mu mol/min$ per g of liver) and low affinity for glucose (K_m is around $10\,mmol/L$, as compared to $0.1\,mmol/L$ or less for the other isoenzymes). Glucose 6-phosphate can be further metabolized in three directions: synthesis of glycogen, the pentose phosphate pathway, and glycolysis. Synthesis and degradation of glycogen occur by different pathways, of which the rate-limiting steps are, respectively, glycogen synthase and glycogen phosphorylase. Both enzymes may exist in an active and in an inactive form, which are interconvertible by cAMP-dependent phosphorylation and dephosphorylation. The active form of glycogen synthase is dephosphorylated, whereas the active form of glycogen phosphorylase is phosphorylated. The pentose phosphate pathway provides NADPH, most of which is utilized for the synthesis of fatty acids by fatty acid synthetase, and pentose phosphates, from which nucleotides are formed.

Glycolysis produces pyruvate and lactate via a sequence of enzymes, among which phosphofructokinase 1, which catalyses the conversion of fructose 6-phosphate into fructose 1,6-bisphosphate and pyruvate kinase, which converts phospho-enol-pyruvate into pyruvate, are rate-limiting. Phosphofructokinase 1 is only active in the presence of fructose 2,6-bisphosphate. Pyruvate kinase is interconvertible by cAMP-dependent phosphorylation/dephosphorylation, the active form being dephosphorylated.

Gluconeogenesis involves conversion of lactate and pyruvate and of other substrates which are converted into intermediates of the glycolytic-gluconeogenic pathway into

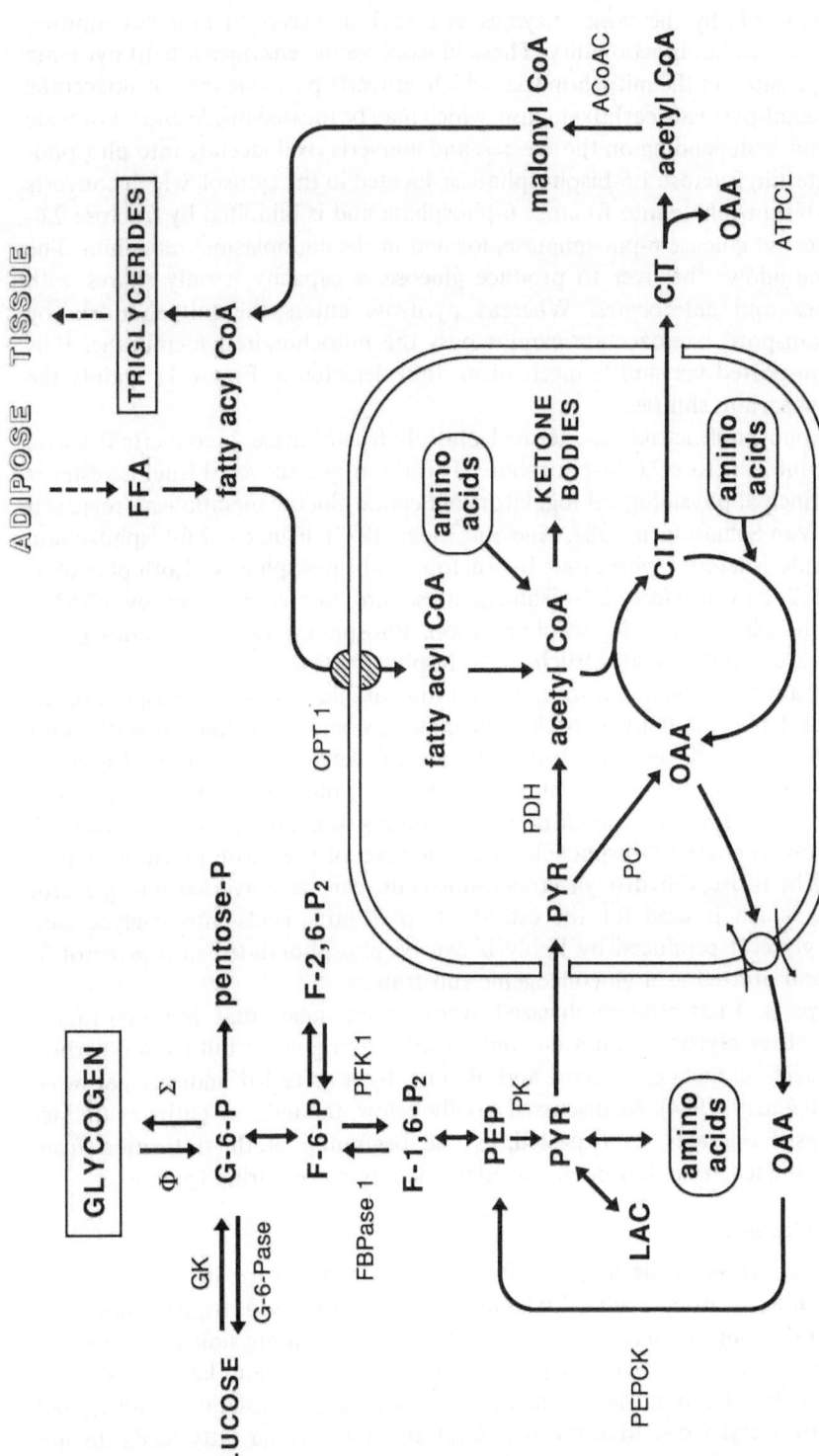

Figure 1 Schematic representation of the pathways of glucose, fatty acid and amino acid metabolism in the liver. ACoAC, acetyl CoA carboxylase; ATPCL, ATP citrate lyase; CIT, citrate; CPT, carnitine palmitoyl transferase; F, fructose; FBPase 1, fructose-1,6-bisphosphatase; FFA, free (non-esterified) fatty acids; G, glucose; GK, glucokinase; G-6-Pase, glucose 6-phosphatase; LAC, lactate; OAA, oxaloacetate; PC, pyruvate carboxylase; PDH, pyruvate dehydrogenase; PEPCK, phospho-enol-pyruvate carboxykinase; PFK 1, phosphofructokinase 1; PK, pyruvate kinase; PYR, pyruvate; Φ, glycogen phosphorylase; Σ, glycogen synthase

glucose. It proceeds by the same enzymes as glycolysis except at four key limiting steps, which ensure unidirectionality. These gluconeogenic enzymes are: (i) pyruvate carboxylase, located in the mitochondria, which converts pyruvate into oxaloacetate; (ii) phospho-enol-pyruvate carboxykinase, which may be located inside and/or outside the mitochondria depending on the species, and converts oxaloacetate into phospho-enol-pyruvate; (iii) fructose 1,6-bisphosphatase, located in the cytosol, which converts fructose 1,6-bisphosphate into fructose 6-phosphate and is inhibited by fructose 2,6-bisphosphate; (iv) glucose 6-phosphatase, located in the endoplasmic reticulum. The latter enzyme allows the liver to produce glucose, a capacity it only shares with kidney cortex and enterocytes. Whereas pyruvate enters the mitochondria by facilitated transport, oxaloacetate cannot pass the mitochondrial membrane. It is therefore transported via shuttle mechanisms (not depicted in Figure 1), mainly the malate and aspartate shuttles.

A second phosphofructokinase, termed phosphofructokinase 2, converts fructose 6-phosphate into fructose 2,6-bisphosphate. This recently discovered fructose ester is one of the principal physiological regulators of hepatic glucose metabolism (reviewed in Hers and Van Schaftingen, 1982; Hue and Rider, 1987). Fructose 2,6-bisphosphate is degraded into fructose 6-phosphate by fructose 2,6-bisphosphatase. Both phosphofructokinase 2 and fructose 2,6-bisphosphatase are interconvertible by cAMP-dependent phosphorylation/dephosphorylation. Phosphorylation inactivates phosphofructokinase 2 and activates fructose 2,6-bisphosphatase.

Galactose, a major constituent of milk and thus of infant food, is phosphorylated into galactose 1-phosphate by a specific galactokinase and thereafter converted into glucose 6-phosphate via glucose 1-phosphate (not shown in Figure 1). Fructose, which is also an important constituent of normal diets, is phosphorylated into fructose 1-phosphate by a specific fructokinase, and enters the glycolytic-gluconeogenic pathway below fructose 1,6-bisphosphate, at the level of the triose phosphates (not illustrated). The triose, dihydroxyacetone-phosphate, can be converted into glycerol 3-phosphate, which is used for the esterification of fatty acids into triglycerides. Conversely, glycerol produced by lipolysis can be phosphorylated into glycerol 3-phosphate, and utilized as a gluconeogenic substrate.

In recent years, it has been emphasized over and over again that, in fasted rats, a major part of liver glycogen is not derived directly from glucose but from 3-carbon compounds such as lactate, glycerol and alanine, by a so-called 'indirect pathway' (Katz and McGarry, 1984). As discussed briefly below, the indirect pathway (in fact gluconeogenesis) operates, as expected, at the beginning of the transition from starvation to the fed state, but does not intervene any more during feeding.

Fatty acid metabolism

Fatty acid metabolism in the liver involves three main pathways: catabolism by β-oxidation, synthesis from acetyl CoA, and esterification into triglycerides. The catabolism of the long chain (C_{12}–C_{20}) free fatty acids, which physiologically are the most abundant, involves successively, activation to long-chain fatty acyl CoA, transport into the mitochondria via the carnitine palmitoyl transferase I and II, and β-oxidation to acetyl CoA. Medium (C_6–C_{10}) and short chain fatty acids do not require the carnitine palmitoyl transferases to be transported into the mitochondria, and are activated in the mitochondrial matrix.

β-Oxidation proceeds inside the mitochondria by cyclic repetition of four reactions (Figure 2): (i) a first dehydrogenation by FAD-dependent acyl CoA dehydrogenases, of which three types are known with specificities for long, medium and short chain fatty acids; (ii) hydration by enoyl CoA hydratase; (iii) a second dehydrogenation by NAD-dependent 3-hydroxyacyl CoA dehydrogenase; and (iv) splitting off of acetyl CoA by 3-ketoacyl CoA thiolase. Reoxidation of NADH proceeds in the respiratory chain through an ordered series of coenzymes. A specific carrier system, composed of electron transfer protein (ETF) and the enzyme ETF dehydrogenase, transfers the electrons from $FADH_2$ to the respiratory chain.

Mitochondrial acetyl CoA can be metabolized in two main directions: (i) condensation with oxaloacetate to citrate, a reaction catalysed by citrate synthase, the first enzyme of the Krebs cycle; and (ii) conversion into the ketone bodies, acetoacetate and 3-hydroxybutyrate. Production of the latter only occurs when acetyl CoA is formed in excess of the capacity of citrate synthase. The formation of ketone bodies involves four enzymes (Figure 3), which constitute the so-called hydroxymethylglutaryl CoA cycle: acetoacetyl CoA thiolase, hydroxymethylglutaryl CoA synthase, hydroxymethylglutaryl CoA lyase, and 3-hydroxybutyrate dehydrogenase. That ketone body formation is restricted to the liver is explained by the fact that only this tissue possesses hydroxymethylglutaryl CoA synthase. That liver, in contrast with peripheral tissues, cannot utilize ketone bodies is due to the absence of the transferase which utilizes succinyl CoA to reconvert acetoacetate into acetoacetyl CoA.

Synthesis of fatty acids occurs in the cytosol (Figure 1) and requires first export of citrate from the mitochondria, followed by the splitting of citrate into acetyl CoA and oxaloacetate by ATP citrate lyase. The first and rate-limiting step of fatty acid

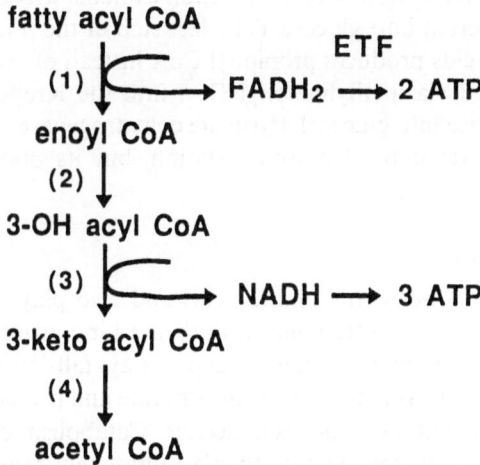

Figure 2 β-Oxidation of fatty acids. 1, acyl CoA dehydrogenase; 2, enoyl CoA hydratase; 3, 3-hydroxyacyl CoA dehydrogenase; 4, 3-ketoacyl CoA thiolase. ETF, electron transfer protein and dehydrogenase

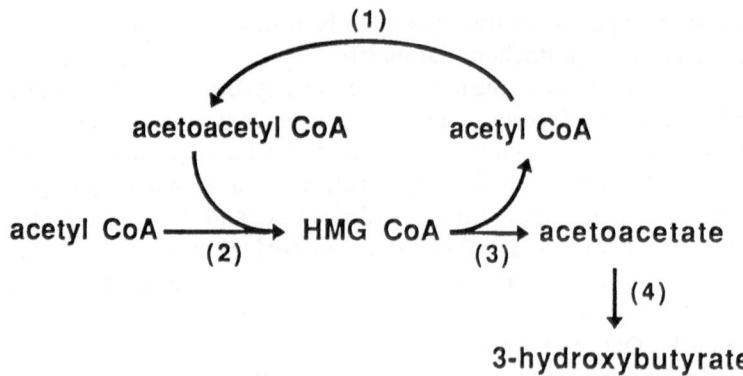

Figure 3 Formation of ketone bodies. 1, acetoacetyl CoA thiolase; 2, HMG CoA synthase; 3, HMG CoA lyase; 4, 3-hydroxybutyrate dehydrogenase. HMG, hydroxymethylglutaryl

synthesis is the ATP-dependent carboxylation of acetyl CoA into malonyl CoA, catalysed by acetyl CoA carboxylase. This enzyme is also interconvertible by cAMP-dependent phosphorylation/dephosphorylation, and is activated by dephosphorylation. Conversion of malonyl CoA into fatty acyl CoA is catalysed by fatty acid synthetase. This multi-enzyme complex includes 3-ketoacyl synthase, NADPH-dependent 3-ketoacyl reductase, 3-hydroxyacyl dehydrase, and NADPH-dependent enoyl reductase (not illustrated). It also acts in a cyclic repetitious manner, which results in the elongation of acetyl CoA to long-chain fatty acyl CoA. Fatty acyl CoA is esterified into triglyceride, with glycerol 3-phosphate provided by glycolysis. Triglycerides are exported towards adipose tissue in the form of very-light-density lipoproteins (VLDL).

Pyruvate dehydrogenase converts pyruvate into acetyl CoA, and thereby carbo-hydrate into fat. The irreversibility of the reaction explains why even-numbered fatty acids cannot be converted into glucose. (The last step of the β-oxidation of the rare odd-numbered fatty acids produces propionyl CoA instead of acetyl CoA. Propionyl CoA can be converted via methylmalonyl CoA into the Krebs cycle intermediate, succinyl CoA, and hence into glucose). Pyruvate dehydrogenase is an interconvertible enzyme which is activated by dephosphorylation, but its phosphorylation is not cAMP-dependent.

Amino acid metabolism

The liver synthesizes non-essential amino acids and also plays a major rôle in the catabolism of all amino acids after removal of their amino group through the action of transaminases. Description of the individual pathways falls outside the scope of this review. Biosynthetic pathways originate from pyruvate and from two intermediates of the Krebs cycle, α-ketoglutarate and oxaloacetate. Catabolism of the gluconeogenic amino acids (or of their gluconeogenic moieties) ultimately results in the formation of pyruvate and/or of various intermediates of the Krebs cycle (α-ketoglutarate, succinyl CoA, fumarate and oxaloacetate), which can be converted into glucose. Catabolism of the ketogenic amino acids (or of their ketogenic moieties) involves formation of CoA derivatives, and ultimately of acetyl CoA, which can be converted into ketone bodies. The catabolism of the branched-chain amino acids, leucine, isoleucine and valine, which starts in muscle by deamination to α-keto acids, is followed by formation of CoA derivatives in the liver. Further catabolism of the latter involves FAD-dependent dehydrogenases which, similarly to the FAD-dependent fatty acyl CoA dehydrogenases, transfer electrons to the respiratory chain via ETF and ETF dehydrogenase. The further catabolism of leucine requires hydroxymethylglutaryl CoA lyase, which also functions in the synthesis of the ketone bodies.

Zonation of liver metabolism

In recent years, the fact that liver metabolism is quantitatively and even qualitatively different in the periportal inflown zone, as compared to the perivenous outflow area, has been extensively documented (Jungermann, 1987; Quistorff, 1990). Several studies have revealed hepatocyte heterogeneity with respect to various metabolic functions. Gluconeogenesis and consequently glycogen synthesis by the indirect pathway, glutamine hydrolysis and urea synthesis and possibly fatty acid oxidation and ketogenesis predominate in the periportal hepatocytes. Glycolysis and glycogen synthesis from glucose, glutamine synthesis, drug detoxication and maybe fatty acid synthesis preponderate in the perivenous cells. Zonation can be based on several factors, including gradients of enzyme activity but also of hormones, substrates, oxygen, etc. One of the best documented zonations by enzyme gradients is that of ammonia and glutamate metabolism (Häussinger, 1990). Zonation of carbohydrate metabolism seems to be mainly determined by hormonal gradients, namely a lower insulin/glucagon ratio in the periportal as compared to the perivenous cells.

REGULATORY MECHANISMS IN METABOLIC HOMEOSTASIS

In the fed state the liver receives, by way of the portal vein, a variety of small molecular weight substrates, which result from intestinal digestion of food. These substrates are monosaccharides (mainly glucose but also fructose and galactose), amino acids and limited amounts of short chain fatty acids. In addition the liver receives some long chain fatty acids provided by processing of chylomicrons by endothelial lipoprotein lipase. These substrates are utilized for the synthesis of glycogen, non-essential amino-acids, triglycerides and phospholipids.

In the fasted state, the liver degrades glycogen into glucose. In addition it receives glucogenic amino acids (mainly alanine) from muscle, and glycerol from adipose tissue. Both are utilized for the production of glucose by gluconeogenesis. The fasting liver also receives non-esterified fatty acids (mainly long chain fatty acids), released from adipose tissue triglycerides, and ketogenic amino acids, derived from muscle. Both can be converted into ketone bodies.

All these changes require reversal of the fluxes through the pathways depicted in Figure 1. The major signals which command this reversal are glucose, insulin and glucagon. Glucose and glucagon are the principle short-term regulators of hepatic energy metabolism. Acute effects of insulin on the liver are notoriously difficult to demonstrate but long-term effects are well documented. The effects of insulin on adipose tissue also markedly influence hepatic metabolism but in an indirect way.

Regulation by glucose

The concentration of glucose in the portal vein increases during feeding and decreases during fasting. Owing to the very rapid hepatic transport of glucose, changes in its portal concentration are immediately reflected inside the hepatocytes. In the liver cell an increase in glucose exerts, both directly and indirectly, a series of effects which result in the orientation of its metabolism towards glycogen synthesis, glycolysis, and formation of fatty acids. A first direct effect of glucose is to stimulate its hepatic uptake. This is explained by the kinetic characteristics of glucokinase; since its K_m for glucose is about 10 mmol/L, a postprandial increase in glucose above its basal concentration of around 5 mmol/L, nearly proportionally increases the formation of glucose 6-phosphate. Recent studies of the phosphorylation of glucose by isolated rat hepatocytes (Van Schaftingen, 1989), have shown that it is stimulated by low concentrations of fructose. At 200 μmol/L concentration, fructose stimulates the phosphorylation of physiological concentrations of glucose 2- to 4-fold. Fructose acts by increasing the affinity of glucokinase for glucose, without modifying its V_{max}. Further studies (Van Schaftingen and Vandercammen, 1989) have led to the discovery of a protein regulator of glucokinase which inhibits the enzyme in the presence of micromolar concentrations of fructose 6-phosphate. The inhibitory effect is, however, antagonized by similar concentrations of fructose 1-phosphate. These findings may explain the long-standing observation that fructose stimulates the utilization of glucose and the deposition of glycogen (Van den Berghe, 1986).

Glucose also directly stimulates the synthesis of glycogen by causing the sequential inactivation of glycogen phosphorylase and activation of glycogen synthase, both by dephosphorylation (Stalmans, 1976). This effect results from the binding of glucose to the active form of phosphorylase, which renders the enzyme a better substrate for phosphorylase phosphatase. When active phosphorylase has decreased below a threshold level (about 10% of its total activity), the inhibition it exerts on glycogen synthase phosphatase is suppressed, allowing its activation to proceed.

Increased phosphorylation of glucose also results in elevated concentrations of derivatives and intermediates of the glycolytic pathway, among them fructose 2,6-bisphosphate and fructose 1,6-bisphosphate. Fructose 2,6-bisphosphate stimulates phosphofructokinase 1, the main regulatory enzyme of glycolysis, and inhibits fructose 1,6-bisphosphatase thereby preventing futile recycling of fructose 1,6-bisphosphate (Hers and Van Schaftingen, 1982; Hue and Rider, 1987). Increased concentrations of fructose 1,6-bisphosphate result in forward stimulation of pyruvate kinase, the third limiting enzyme of glycolysis.

The increase in the glycolytic flux brought about by the changes listed results in an increase in the supply of pyruvate and hence of mitochondrial acetyl CoA and oxaloacetate (Lane and Mooney, 1981). This in turn results in an enhanced formation of citrate, which is re-exported out of the mitochondria. In the cytosol, citrate exerts a forward stimulation on acetyl CoA carboxylase; its activation by dephosphorylation might also be directly stimulated by glucose. The increase in the concentration of malonyl CoA results in an enhancement of the synthesis of fatty acids and subsequently of the formation of triglycerides. In addition, elevated levels of malonyl CoA inhibit carnitine palmitoyl transferase I, and thereby limit the entry of long chain fatty acyl CoA in the mitochondria (McGarry and Foster, 1980). This results in a decrease in the rate of β-oxidation and hence of the production of NADH and of acetyl CoA. The latter metabolites are both inhibitors and inactivators of pyruvate dehydrogenase. Their decrease therefore results in a diminished inhibition and in an activation of pyruvate dehydrogenase, which promote the formation of acetyl CoA from pyruvate and thereby from glucose.

Insulin

Insulin increases during feeding and decreases on fasting. Its principal effect is to stimulate the uptake of glucose by muscle and adipose tissue. In addition, insulin favours the hepatic utilization of glucose and conversion into fatty acids, mainly by enhancing the synthesis of several rate-limiting enzymes involved in these processes. Glucokinase, phosphofructokinase 1, pyruvate kinase, pyruvate dehydrogenase and acetyl CoA carboxylase are induced by insulin. Accordingly, the amounts of these enzymes increase on refeeding and/or administration of insulin. Conversely, their activities decrease during prolonged fasting, even more so in the diabetic state. Unlike those provoked by glucose, however, these changes occur over hours to days, rather than over minutes. Nevertheless, some studies suggest that insulin might also rapidly stimulate the protein phosphatases which activate a number of the key enzymes involved in glycogen synthesis and glycolysis, namely glycogen synthase (Toth *et al.*, 1988) and pyruvate kinase (Feliu *et al.*, 1986).

Besides its direct effects on the liver, insulin also influences liver metabolism by way of its action on adipose tissue. In the fed state, the antilipolytic effect of insulin decreases the supply of long chain fatty acids which is offered to the liver, whereas in the fasted state the decrease in insulin results in an increase in this supply.

Glucagon

Glucagon increases during fasting and is the principal signal which reverses the matabolic fluxes in the liver from the build-up of energy stores to the release of fuels. Other hormones, namely catecholamines, vasopressin and angiotensin II, also provoke this reversal, although their effects are less potent. Glucagon and β-adrenergic agents stimulate adenylate cyclase, and thereby increase the concentration of cAMP. This results in a stimulation of protein kinase and in the subsequent phosphorylation of a series of interconvertible enzymes. Phosphorylation of phosphorylase kinase, glycogen phosphorylase and fructose 2,6-bisphosphatase results in their activation, whereas glycogen synthase, phosphofructokinase 2, pyruvate kinase and acetyl CoA carboxylase are inactivated. α-Adrenergic agents, vasopressin and angiotensin II, activate phosphorylase via a cAMP-independent, Ca^{2+} mediated stimulation of phosphorylase kinase. It should be mentioned that glucagon does not directly influence the phosphorylation and hence the activation state of pyruvate dehydrogenase.

The activation of phosphorylase results in the degradation of glycogen into glucose. The simultaneous inactivation of glycogen synthase turns off glycogen synthesis. Inactivation of phosphofructokinase 2 and activation of fructose 2,6-bisphosphatase provoke arrest of synthesis, and degradation of fructose 2,6-bisphosphate respectively. This results in a disappearance of the stimulatory effect of fructose 2,6-bisphosphate on phosphofructokinase 1, which leads to arrest of glycolysis and to relief of the inhibition exerted on fructose 1,6-bisphosphatase, which allows gluconeogenesis to proceed. Inactivation of pyruvate kinase contributes markedly to the arrest of glycolysis and to the reorientation of metabolic flux in the direction of gluconeogenesis. Inactivation of acetyl CoA carboxylase results in a decrease in the formation of malonyl CoA and the synthesis of fatty acids. The decrease in the concentration of malonyl CoA suppresses the inhibition which it exerts on carnitine palmitoyl transferase 1 and thereby allows entry of long chain fatty acyl CoA into the mitochondria. Since glucagon also activates adipose tissue hormone-sensitive lipase, and thereby increases the supply of free fatty acids to the liver, β-oxidation is strongly enhanced. This leads to a marked increase in the supply of NADH and acetyl CoA, which results in both inhibition and inactivation of pyruvate dehydrogenase, and thus in suppression of the transformation of carbohydrate into fat. On the other hand, the elevation of acetyl CoA increases the activity of pyruvate carboxylase, of which it is an obligatory stimulator. Pyruvate, formed from lactate and by transamination of alanine, is therefore not converted any more into acetyl CoA but is chanelled exclusively into the gluconeogenic pathway. Concomitantly the supply of acetyl CoA provided by β-oxidation surpasses the capacity of the Krebs cycle, which leads to the formation of ketone bodies.

The starved-to-fed transition

The transition from the fasted to the fed state requires a reversal of the metabolic responses to starvation described in the previous paragraph. The available experimental evidence indicates that refeeding provokes an immediate arrest of hepatic glycogenolysis and of adipose tissue lipolysis, but that other adaptations of the liver to prolonged starvation may persist for variable periods of time (Sugden *et al.*, 1989). One of these adaptations is the high rate of utilization of 3-carbon compounds by gluconeogenesis. This high rate accounts for the observation that, following starvation, a major part of liver glycogen is not derived directly from glucose, but from lactate, glycerol and alanine by the so-called indirect pathway (Katz and McGarry, 1984). During the postprandial state, however, the direct pathway accounts for almost all the hepatic glycogen synthesized (Huang and Veech, 1988).

ENERGY REQUIREMENTS FOR METABOLIC HOMEOSTASIS

All cellular functions, including metabolic homeostasis, require energy. In the fed state the liver utilizes the energy generated by glucose oxidation to synthesize glycogen and fatty acids. In the fasted state it uses that derived from the β-oxidation of fatty acids to synthesize glucose. Cells preserve the energy derived from oxidation of substrates in the form of high energy phosphate bonds, mainly the pyrophosphate bond between the β and γ phosphate of ATP. In the fed state metabolic flux through both glycolysis and the Krebs cycle generates substantial amounts of energy. This occurs in part by phosphorylation at the level of the substrate but mainly by the production of reduced $FADH_2$ and NADH, reoxidation of which in the mitochondrial respiratory chain generates two and three molecules of ATP respectively. One molecule of glucose yields eight molecules of ATP along the glycolytic pathway, taking into account the ATP generated from NADH, and each molecule of pyruvate yields 15 molecules of ATP in the Krebs cycle. This energy is utilized in part in the form of UDPGlucose for the synthesis of glycogen and in the form of ATP for the synthesis of fatty acids. The latter requires two molecules of ATP per molecule of acetyl CoA, together with two molecules of NADPH which are provided by the utilization of glucose in the pentose phosphate pathway. Synthesis of one molecule of palmitoyl CoA from mitochondrial acetyl CoA therefore requires 14 molecules of ATP.

During fasting mitochondrial oxidation of fatty acids generates both $FADH_2$ and NADH (Figure 2). One molecule of palmitate therefore yields 35 molecules of ATP at the level of β-oxidation. Each molecule of acetyl CoA, which is not converted into ketone bodies but oxidized in the Krebs cycle, yields 12 additional molecules of ATP. This production of ATP is utilized for the formation of glucose by gluconeogenesis. The latter requires 6 molecules of ATP per molecule of glucose formed from pyruvate.

The close relationship between glucose and fatty acid metabolism in the liver thus extends beyond the metabolic pathways and their regulation to the exchange of energy. This close relationship also has implications for the pathophysiology of a number of inborn errors of metabolism which will be discussed in the next section.

IMPLICATIONS FOR INBORN ERRORS OF METABOLISM

A series of inborn errors of metabolism disturb the mechanisms whereby the liver ensures metabolic homeostasis. Whereas only two enzyme deficiencies are known which influence the formation of glycogen, several impair its degradation. Other enzyme defects impede the synthesis of the metabolic fuels, glucose and ketone bodies. These inborn errors will be briefly reviewed, with particular emphasis on their consequences for the mechanisms whereby the liver maintains blood glucose, For more details, the reader is referred to appropriate chapters in textbooks (Scriver *et al.*, 1989; Fernandes *et al.*, 1990).

Disturbances in the synthesis of glycogen

Two very rare enzyme defects disturb the formation of liver glycogen: glycogen synthase deficiency and branching enzyme deficiency or glycogen storage disease type IV. In glycogen synthase deficiency, the synthesis of liver glycogen is profoundly, although not completely, impaired. The defect provokes severe morning hypoglycaemia with hyperketonaemia, which appear in early infancy with cessation of nocturnal feeding. Branching enzyme deficiency results in the formation of normal amounts of structurally abnormal glycogen molecules which resemble amylopectin. The defect provokes cirrhosis owing to poor solubility of the abnormal glycogen. It does not cause hypoglycaemia because it only partially disturbs the degradation of glycogen by phosphorylase.

Disturbances in the degradation of glycogen

Several enzyme defects located on the glycogenolytic pathway impair the degradation of liver glycogen. Profound hypoglycaemia is the hallmark of glucose 6-phosphatase deficiency (glycogen storage disease type I) because the enzyme defect not only suppresses the release of glucose from glycogen but also the formation of glucose by the gluconeogenic pathway. In acid α-glucosidase deficiency (glycogen storage disease type II), patients do not become hypoglycaemic because the block in the degradation of glycogen is restricted to the lysosomes and does not affect glycogen in the cytosol. In amylo-1,6-glucosidase deficiency (glycogen storage disease type III) hypoglycaemia is usually mild, because degradation of glycogen by phosphorylase remains possible. Hypoglycaemia is rare in phosphorylase kinase deficiency (glycogen storage disease type IX) because other mechanisms, besides activation by phosphorylase kinase, can increase the activity of phosphorylase.

Glycogenolysis can also be impaired by enzyme defects located in other metabolic pathways which result in the accumulation and/or depletion of metabolites which influence the activity of glycogenolytic enzymes. In hereditary fructose intolerance, the profound hypoglycaemia provoked by the ingestion of fructose is explained by an inhibition of the activity of phosphorylase, owing to the ensuing accumulation of fructose 1-phosphate and depletion of inorganic phosphate.

Impairment of gluconeogenesis

In addition to glucose 6-phosphatase deficiency, several enzyme defects disturb the formation of glucose by the gluconeogenic pathway, namely the deficiencies of fructose 1,6-bisphosphatase, phospho-enol-pyruvate carboxykinase, and pyruvate carboxylase. The latter can be either isolated or part of multiple carboxylase deficiency, which results from a defect in biotin metabolism, either holocarboxylase synthetase or biotinidase deficiency. All these deficiencies can cause fasting hypoglycaemia which, as a rule, is more pronounced when the enzyme defect is located closer to glucose 6-phosphate on the pathway leading from pyruvate to glucose. Whereas hypoglycaemia is a major feature in fructose 1,6-bisphosphatase deficiency and also in phospho-enol-pyruvate carboxykinase deficiency, it is only occasionally mentioned in pyruvate carboxylase deficiency. This may be explained by the fact that the latter defect does not hinder the entrance of a number of substrates, such as glycerol and serine, into the gluconeogenic pathway.

Gluconeogenesis can also be impeded by enzyme defects located in other metabolic pathways which provoke the accumulation of inhibitors of gluconeogenic enzymes. In hereditary fructose intolerance, gluconeogenesis is impaired owing to inhibition of aldolase, acting on dihydroxyacetone phosphate and glyceraldehyde 3-phosphate, by fructose 1-phosphate. In maple syrup urine disease, the accumulation of branched chain ketoacids inhibits the branched chain amino transferase which leads to the formation of glutamate and hence of alanine, the principal gluconeogenic amino acid. In methylmalonic acidaemia, the accumulation of methylmalonyl CoA in the mitochondria inhibits pyruvate carboxylase and the malate shuttle.

Impairment of the formation of ketone bodies

Several enzyme defects hinder the formation of ketone bodies. These consist mainly of the disturbances of carnitine metabolism, the various defects of fatty acid oxidation, and hydroxymethylglutaryl CoA lyase deficiency. The rare deficiencies of carnitine synthesis and of carnitine transferase impede the entrance of long chain fatty acids into the mitochondria and their subsequent β-oxidation. Deficiencies of long, medium and short chain acyl CoA dehydrogenase and multiple acyl CoA dehydrogenase deficiency have been identified. The latter results from defects in either ETF or ETF dehydrogenase. Since ETF and ETF dehydrogenase also function in the catabolism of the branched chain amino acids, leucine, isoleucine and valine, the breakdown of their CoA intermediates is also blocked in multiple acyl CoA dehydrogenase deficiency. Profound deficiencies of ETF or ETF dehydrogenase cause glutaric aciduria type II, whereas less pronounced defects result in ethylmalonic-adipic aciduria. Recently, patients with 3-hydroxyacyl CoA dehydrogenase deficiency have also been identified (Hagenfeldt *et al.*, 1990). Impaired β-oxidation of fatty acids can also be caused by defects in oxidative phosphorylation. HMG CoA lyase deficiency blocks both ketogenesis and the catabolism of leucine.

In the disorders listed, the prominent clinical feature is often non-ketotic hypoglycaemia, accompanied by urinary excretion of organic acids and of their carnitine esters, which reflect the enzyme defect. The hypoglycaemia most likely results from several mechanisms. The pronounced deficiency in the formation of ketone bodies leads to a compensatory overutilization of glucose. In addition, the formation of glucose by gluconeogenesis may be impaired by several mechanisms: (i) insufficient provision of free CoA, required for continuing β-oxidation, owing to the accumulation of CoA intermediates proximally from the enzyme defect; (ii) insufficient production of ATP, required to drive the conversion of pyruvate and of other gluconeogenic precursors into glucose; (iii) decrease in the concentration of acetyl CoA, which is an obligatory stimulator of the gluconeogenic enzyme pyruvate carboxylase; (iv) inhibition of gluconeogenic enzymes by the accumulation of organic acids and of their CoA derivatives.

Maintenance of a normal concentration of blood glucose is thus essential in several inborn errors of metabolism. This can be accomplished by various means, including the administration of frequent carbohydrate-rich meals, of oral glucose as such over day and night and of glucose infusions when hypoglycaemia becomes manifest. Patients with glucose 6-phosphatase deficiency should be fed carbohydrate polymers such as starch, which release glucose over a long period of time. In defects of fatty acid oxidation, excessive fat intake, medium chain triglycerides and drugs which interfere with β-oxidation (for example, valproate) should also be avoided.

REFERENCES

Feliu, J. E., Mojena, M. and Lopez-Alarcon, L. Modulation of hepatic pyruvate kinase phosphatase activity. *Adv. Prot. Phosphatases* 3 (1986) 163–186

Fernandes, J., Saudubray, J.-M. and Tada, K. (eds.), *Inborn Metabolic Diseases. Diagnosis and Treatment*, Springer-Verlag, Berlin, 1990, 655 pp.

Hagenfeldt, L., von Döbeln, U., Holme, E., Alm, J., Brandberg, G., Enocksson, E. and Lindeberg, L. 3-Hydroxydicarboxylic aciduria – a fatty acid oxidation defect with severe prognosis. *J. Pediatr.* 116 (1990) 387–392

Häussinger, D. Nitrogen metabolism in liver: structural and functional organization and physiological relevance. *Biochem. J.* 267 (1990) 281–290

Hers, H. G. Mechanisms of blood glucose homeostasis. *J. Inher. Metab. Dis.* 13 (1990) 395–410

Hers, H. G. and Van Schaftingen, E. Fructose 2,6-bisphosphate two years after its discovery. *Biochem. J.* 206 (1982) 1–12

Huang, M.-T. and Veech, R. L. Role of the direct and indirect pathways for glycogen synthesis in rat liver in the postprandial state. *J. Clin. Invest.* 81 (1988) 872–878

Hue, L. and Rider, M. H. Role of fructose 2,6-bisphosphate in the control of glycolysis in mammalian tissues. *Biochem. J.* 245 (1987) 313–324

Jungermann, K. Metabolic zonation of liver parenchyma: significance for the regulation of glycogen metabolism, gluconeogenesis and glycolysis. *Diabetes/Metab. Rev.* 3 (1987) 269–293

Katz, J. and McGarry, J. D. The glucose paradox. Is glucose a substrate for liver metabolism? *J. Clin. Invest.* 74 (1984) 1901–1909

Lane, M. D. and Mooney, R. A. Tricarboxylic acid cycle intermediates and the control of fatty acid synthesis and ketogenesis. *Curr. Top. Cell. Regul.* 18 (1981) 221–242

McGarry, J. D. and Foster, D. W. Regulation of hepatic fatty acid oxidation and ketone body production. *Annu. Rev. Biochem.* 49 (1980) 395–420

Quistorff, B. Metabolic heterogeneity of liver parenchymal cells. *Essays in Biochemistry* 25 (1990) 83–136

Scriver, C. R., Beaudet, A. L., Sly, W. S. and Valle, D. (eds.), *The Metabolic Basis of Inherited Disease*, 6th ed., McGraw-Hill, New York, 1989, 3006 pp.

Seifter, S. and England, S. Energy metabolism. In: Arias, I. M., Jakoby, W. B., Popper, H. Schachter, D. and Shafritz, D. A. (eds.), *The Liver: Biology and Pathobiology*, 2nd ed., Raven Press, New York, 1988, pp. 279–315

Stalmans, W. The role of the liver in the homeostasis of blood glucose. *Curr. Top. Cell. Regul.* 11 (1976) 51–97

Sugden, M. C., Holness, M. J. and Palmer, T. N. Fuel selection and carbon flux during the starved-to-fed transition. *Biochem. J.* 263 (1989) 313–323

Toth, B., Bollen, M. and Stalmans, W. Acute regulation of hepatic protein phosphatases by glucagon, insulin, and glucose. *J. Biol. Chem.* 263 (1988) 14061–14066

Van den Berghe, G. Fructose: metabolism and short-term effects on carbohydrate and purine metabolic pathways. *Prog. Biochem. Pharmacol.* 21 (1986) 1–32

Van Schaftingen, E. A protein from rat liver confers to glucokinase the property of being antagonistically regulated by fructose 6-phosphate and fructose 1-phosphate. *Eur. J. Biochem.* 179 (1989) 179–184

Van Schaftingen, E. and Vandercammen, A. Stimulation of glucose phosphorylation by fructose in isolated rat hepatocytes. *Eur. J. Biochem.* 179 (1989) 173–177

Zakim, D. Metabolism of glucose and fatty acids by the liver. In: Zakim, D. and Boyer, T. D. (eds)., *Hepatology: A Textbook of Liver Disease*, 2nd Edn., W. B. Saunders, Philadelphia, 1900, pp. 65–96

J. Inher. Metab. Dis. 14 (1991) 421–430
© SSIEM and Kluwer Academic Publishers.

Detoxification Pathways in the Liver

D. M. GRANT

Division of Clinical Pharmacology and Toxicology, Research Institute, Hospital for Sick Children, 555 University Avenue, Toronto, Ontario M5G 1X8, Canada

Summary: The liver plays an important rôle in protecting the organism from potentially toxic chemical insults through its capacity to convert lipophiles into more water-soluble metabolites which can be efficiently eliminated from the body via the urine. This protective ability of the liver stems from the expression of a wide variety of xenobiotic biotransforming enzymes whose common underlying feature is their ability to catalyse the oxidation, reduction and hydrolysis (Phase I) and/or conjugation (Phase II) of functional groups on drug and chemical molecules. The broad substrate specificity, isoenzyme multiplicity and inducibility of many of these enzyme systems make them particularly well adapted to handling the vast array of different chemical structures in the environment to which we are exposed daily. However, some chemicals may also be converted to more toxic metabolites by certain of these enzymes, implying that variations in the latter may be important predisposing factors for toxicity. Pharmacogenetic defects of xenobiotic biotransformation enzymes, a subclass of inborn errors of metabolism which are manifested only upon drug challenge, introduce marked variation into human populations for the pharmacokinetics and pharmacodynamics of therapeutic and toxic agents, and thus may have important clinical consequences for drug efficacy and toxicity.

One of the most vital roles of the liver is in defence. Every day the human organism may be exposed, either intentionally or otherwise, to hundreds of exogenous chemical substances in food and water, in the air, or in purified formulations intended to elicit a specific therapeutic response. Many of these compounds, however, tend to be highly lipophilic and therefore to remain in the body for long periods of time. This would have drastic consequences for drug therapy and xenobiotic toxicity. Fortunately, a multitude of enzyme systems exist, many present in highest amounts in the liver, which are uniquely equipped for converting lipophilic substances into more water-soluble derivatives which can then be efficiently excreted by the kidney. This article presents an introductory discussion of the concepts and pathways of xenobiotic biotransformation by liver enzymes, an overview of some inherited pharmacogenetic defects affecting the activity of these enzymes and their potential clinical consequences, and finally an example of one such defect, the acetylation polymorphism.

DRUG BIOTRANSFORMATION REACTIONS

Depending on its structure, a drug may be subjected to two types of enzymatic manipulation which have been classified under the general headings of Phase I and Phase II reactions (Figure 1 and Table 1; Jakoby, 1988; Ziegler, 1988). Phase I reactions, which include oxidation, reduction and hydrolysis by a number of enzyme classes, tend to introduce or expose functional groups (often hydroxyl groups) on the drug molecule which may either directly improve its hydrophilicity for subsequent excretion, or allow it to be further acted upon by enzymes of the Phase II class. The latter reactions are conjugative or synthetic, that is, water-soluble side groups are added to enhance excretability. From Table 1 it can be seen that a number of the enzymes capable of biotransforming certain xenobiotics (e.g. xanthine dehydrogenase, catechol O-methyltransferase) also play an important rôle in the intermediary metabolism of endogenous substrates. However, some of the enzymes (e.g. arylamine N-acetyltransferase) possess no presently known endogenous substrates, implying that they may have evolved specifically for the purpose of protecting the organism from environmental chemical insults.

Although the title of this review suggests that the endpoint of drug biotransformation is detoxication, this is certainly not always the case. Indeed, it is important to emphasize that the only common underlying feature of biotransformation processes is that they attempt to convert chemicals from lipophiles to hydrophiles. As shown in Table 2, this process may have a number of biological consequences. A drug may lose its pharmacological activity as a result of biotransformation or be more rapidly eliminated so as to significantly decrease its duration of action. On the other hand, inactive prodrugs may be converted to active metabolites, or a drug may attain an altered pharmacological specificity due to the changes introduced into its structure.

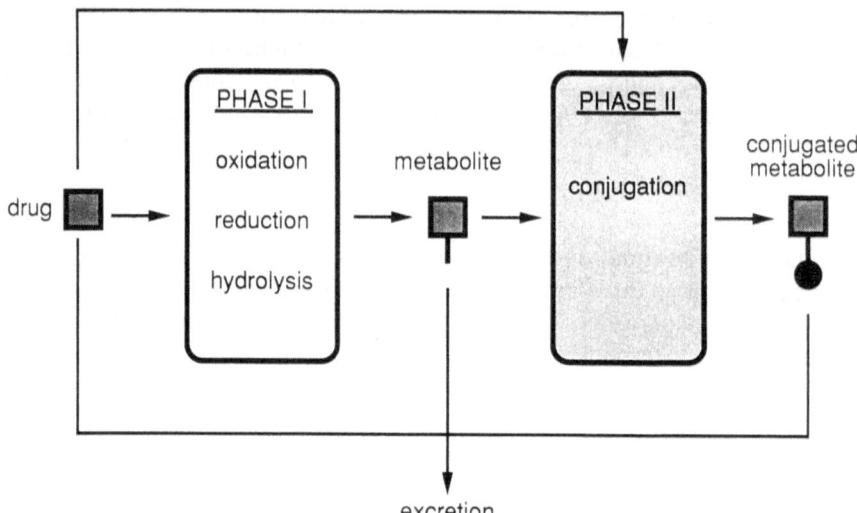

Figure 1 Potential routes of drug and xenobiotic biotransformation. Phase I and Phase II enzymes are generally present in the highest concentrations in the liver, but may also be found in significant amounts in many other tissues

Table 1   Enzymes of xenobiotic biotransformation

Phase I	*Phase II*
Dehydrogenases	Conjugation reactions
Alcohol dehydrogenase	UDP-glucuronyltransferase
Aldehyde dehydrogenase	Alcohol sulphotransferase
Dihydrodiol dehydrogenase	Amine O-sulphotransferase
Xanthine dehydrogenase	Phenol sulphotransferase
Reductases	Glutathione transferase
Ketoreductase	Phenol O-methyltransferase
Nitroreductase	Catechol O-methyltransferase
Azoreductase	Amine N-methyltransferase
N-oxide reductase	Histamine N-methyltransferase
Sulphoxide reductase	Thiol S-methyltransferase
Oxidases	Glycine acyltransferase
Aldehyde oxidase	Glutamate acyltransferase
Monoamine oxidase	Arylamine N-acetyltransferase
Mono-oxygenases	Cysteine N-acetyltransferase
Cytochromes P450	Cysteine conjugate β-lyase
Flavin-containing mono-oxygenase	Thioltransferase
Hydrolases	Rhodanese
Esterases and amidases	
Epoxide hydrolase	

Table 2   Biological consequences of drug biotransformation

Production of stable metabolites with:
  Decreased pharmacological activity – inactivation
  Increased pharmacological activity – prodrug activation
  Altered pharmacological specificity

Production of chemically reactive metabolites:
  Covalent binding with cellular macromolecules
  Toxic consequences – hepatotoxicity, carcinogenicity, teratogenicity

Moreover, biotransformation may even produce an increase in chemical toxicity by formation of chemically reactive electrophiles with the potential to bind covalently to intracellular macromolecules and result in cell death, immune responses and mutational events.

A number of important features of xenobiotic metabolizing enzymes makes them particularly suited for the conversion of thousands of potential substrates in the environment to metabolites which will hopefully be eliminated from the body. Firstly, in contrast to many enzymes of intermediary metabolism which have a restricted substrate specificity for a particular endogenous compound, most drug-metabolizing enzymes have evolved to have an extremely broad substrate specificity, allowing them in some cases to biotransform hundreds of potential chemical compounds, albeit with varying degrees of success. Secondly, isozyme multiplicity is a common feature of these enzyme systems. Again, evolution has ensured, by the production of

J. Inher. Metab. Dis. 14 (1991)

many closely related enzyme isoforms with distinct but often overlapping substrate specificities, that chemicals with widely divergent structures are unlikely to escape biotransformation. Thirdly, the activity of many drug biotransforming enzymes may be induced, at the level of transcriptional activation, by exposure to certain drugs and environmental substances which are themselves often substrates for metabolism. These points are well illustrated by the microsomal cytochrome P450 mono-oxygenase enzyme superfamily, probably the most important and widely studied drug biotransformation enzyme system (Gonzalez, 1989; Okey, 1990). Not only are individual cytochrome P450 isozymes usually capable of adding hydroxyl groups to a wide variety of chemical structures, but the number of related isozymes with the potential to catalyse such reactions may number as many as 50–100 proteins produced from at least 14 different gene families (Nebert *et al.*, 1989).

A further extension from these points and from the existence of a variety of biotransforming enzyme systems (Table 1) is the fact that a given drug may undergo a wide variety of competing biotransformation reactions to produce multiple metabolites, each with its own potential for pharmacological activity or for toxicity. There are many examples of xenobiotics with relatively simple chemical structures which undergo a remarkably complex series of metabolic conversions. Examples of such compounds include the most widely used drug in the world, caffeine (Arnaud, 1984), and the potent experimental carcinogen 2-aminofluorene (Miller, 1978). The latter compound in fact requires metabolic activation for its carcinogenic potential to be manifested. Thus the balance of competing biotransformation pathways, each with the potential for variations in activity due to environmental (i.e. enzyme induction) and genetic factors, may ultimately determine the efficacy or toxicity of drugs and environmental chemicals.

INHERITED DEFECTS OF DRUG BIOTRANSFORMATION

It is well recognized that the response to drugs and toxic substances varies widely among individuals in a given population. The discipline termed pharmacogenetics aims to assess the rôle of inheritance in producing such variation, most prominently in recent years with respect to genetic defects in the enzymes of drug biotransformation (Meyer *et al.*, 1990). Numerous pharmacogenetic variants affecting drug disposition have been detected (Table 3), encompassing both polymorphisms and rare defects. The most important feature which distinguishes these pharmacogenetic defects from other inborn errors of metabolism is that they are manifested only upon drug challenge. Consequently they are not in themselves life threatening, eliminating any discussion of prenatal diagnosis and genetic counselling. However, because of their potential clinical consequences for affecting drug action and chemical toxicity (Table 4), it is often important to identify affected individuals before or during exposure to substances whose biotransformation leads to alterations in their potential for efficacy or toxicity.

The detection and study of pharmacogenetic defects can be approached from two different directions. One is the classical, event-based approach where affected probands are identified and family pedigrees are then investigated in detail for the presence of

Table 3 Genetic variations affecting the pharmacokinetics of drugs and xenobiotics

Polymorphisms	McKusick no.	Rare defects	McKusick no.
Arylamine N-acetyltransferase	24340	Pseudocholinesterase	17740
Alcohol dehydrogenase	10370	Catalase	11150
Aldehyde dehydrogenase	10064	Xanthine dehydrogenase	27830
Paraoxonase	16882	Glucuronyltransferase	21880
Glutathione transferase	13834	Trimethylamine N-oxidase	27570
Glucosyltransferase	20480		
Thiopurine methyltransferase	18768		
Catechol O-methyltransferase	11679		
Carboxymethylcysteine S-oxidase			
Cytochromes P450:		Cytochromes P450:	
Debrisoquine 4-hydroxylase	12403	Phenacetin O-de-ethylase	20030
S-Mephenytoin oxidase	12402	Phenytoin oxidase	22275
Antipyrine oxidase	10729	Coumarin hyroxylase	12272
Theophylline oxidase (?)	18765		
Nifedipine oxidase (?)	12401		
Tolbutamide oxidase (?)			

Table 4   Clinical consequences of genetically defective drug metabolizing enzymes

Functional overdose due to inefficient elimination of active drug
Lack of efficacy due to inefficient prodrug activation
Idiosyncratic toxicity unrelated to the intended drug effect
Associations with apparently spontaneous diseases

defective gene products. The second approach, which is unique to pharmacogenetics and is likely to become increasingly popular in the pharmaceutical industry for new drug development, is drug-based. Starting with a specific chemical structure, *in vitro* studies with human tissues or cell culture systems expressing specific xenobiotic-metabolizing enzymes can predict the occurrence of pharmacogenetic variation *in vivo*. At this stage, experimental methodologies for the two approaches converge. Since these defects are silent in the absence of a drug, patient testing methods often involve the administration of a specified dose of a so-called 'probe' drug whose disposition (1) is affected by the genetic defect, and (2) may be conveniently monitored by measurement of plasma elimination kinetics or urinary metabolite profiles. However, such screening approaches may present a risk of producing toxicity from the probe drug itself if genetically predisposed individuals exist in the population studied. For this reason, testing methods which minimize or avoid toxic drug exposures continue to be developed. These include the development of safer probe drugs without toxic potential, such as caffeine for the determination of acetylator phenotype (see below), the use of peripheral blood lymphocytes expressing xenobiotic-metabolizing enzymes for *in vitro* toxicology testing (Spielberg, 1984), and the use of molecular genetic tests for the direct diagnosis of mutations in the genes encoding drug-metabolizing enzymes (Meyer, 1990).

THE ACETYLATION POLYMORPHISM

This example, reviewed in depth recently (Evans, 1989), illustrates some of the features unique to pharmacogenetic defects as a subset of inborn errors of metabolism. It was in the mid-1950s, before the term pharmacogenetics was even devised, that a significant incidence of unwanted side effects associated with the use of the antitubercular drug isoniazid led to a closer examination of its disposition in healthy human subjects. Population frequency histograms of plasma ioniazid concentrations after a single oral dose were distinctly bimodal, allowing for segregation of roughly equal numbers of 'slow' and 'rapid' eliminators of the drug in unrelated Caucasian subjects. The inherited nature of this phenomenon was first suggested by twin studies and by the observation of a marked interethnic difference in the proportions of the two isoniazid elimination subgroups, with a number of Oriental populations displaying a much lower frequency of the slow eliminator phenotype. Pedigree analysis verfied the genetic hypothesis and suggested that the ability to eliminate isoniazid was controlled by the action of two alleles at a single autosomal gene locus, with rapid elimination as the apparently dominant trait.

The biochemical basis of these population variations was soon found to be related to differences in the rate of isoniazid N-acetylation taking place predominantly in the liver. The reaction is catalysed by the soluble enzyme arylamine N-acetyltransferase (EC 2.3.1.5), which mediates the transfer of an acetyl group from the essential cofactor acetyl coenzyme A to aromatic amines or hydrazines, producing an acetamide. Many investigations have established that the acetylation of a large number of arylamine and hydrazine xenobiotics is under the same genetic control.

Evans (1989) has critically assessed the large body of literature documenting the possible clinical and toxicological consequences of the acetylation polymorphism (Tables 5 and 6). The first studies of isoniazid showed that neurological side effects were indeed more frequent among genetically slow acetylators due to functional overdose on standardized drug administration schedules. Dose-related phenomena have also been reported with numerous other drug therapies (Table 5). It could be argued that such toxicities or therapeutic failures could be avoided by individualizing drug dosing, by therapeutic drug monitoring in patients taking these medications, or by using related drugs whose disposition is unaffected by the genetic defect. These alternatives, however, are often not possible or practical. In addition, there exist several associations of acetylator phenotype with apparently spontaneous disorders (Table 6) where exposure to causative agents is either undocumented or uncontrolled.

Table 5 Adverse reactions related to the acetylation polymorphism

Drug	Phenotype	Effect observed
Isoniazid	Slow	Peripheral neuropathy
		Phenytoin adverse effects
	Rapid	Therapeutic failure with 1x weekly doses
Hydralazine	Slow	Development of antinuclear antibodies and SLE-like syndrome
	Rapid	Higher dose required to treat hypertension
Salicylazosulphapyridine	Slow	More adverse reactions to sulphapyridine
	Rapid	Methaemoglobinaemia
Procainamide	Slow	More prone to SLE-like syndrome
	Rapid	More ventricular premature beats in cardiac patients

Table 6 Associations of acetylator phenotype with certain disorders

Disorder	Phenotype
Bladder cancer in workers exposed to aromatic amines	Slow
Colorectal cancer	Rapid
Laryngeal cancer	Slow
Advanced cancer of the breast	Rapid
Diabetes (Caucasians)	Rapid
Gilbert's disease	Slow
Leprosy (Chinese patients)	Slow

For these reasons and for basic mechanistic studies it is often of value to know the acetylator phenotype of individuals in a population. Until very recently, phenotyping tests have made use of probe drugs which are themselves polymorphically acetylated. Among the drugs which have been used for this purpose are isoniazid itself, the antibacterial agents sulphamethazine and dapsone, and the antiarrhythmic procainamide. Analytical methods such as colorimetric, fluorimetric or high perform-ance liquid chromatographic (HPLC) assays are then employed to quantify the amount of parent drug and/or its acetylated metabolite in plasma or urine samples at a specified time after drug intake. These tests suffer from two significant shortcomings: firstly, the drugs are potentially toxic, especially to genetically defective subjects; and secondly, the test parameters are generally not sensitive enough to distinguish between the three acetylation genotypes, even though detailed kinetic analyses have established that significant activity differences exist between heterozy-gous and homozygous rapid individuals, implying an additive gene dosage effect. It has been observed more recently, however, that the excretion of a caffeine metabolite is related to the acetylation polymorphism, leading to the development of a caffeine test for acetylator phenotype (Grant *et al.*, 1984). The test is safe, analytically simple and rapid, and sensitive enough to discriminate between the three genotypes of acetylation capacity, a feature that allows for the assessment of differential suscepti-bility of heterozygous and homozygous individuals to toxicity from certain drugs and xenobiotics.

Until only a few years ago, the low liver content and *in vitro* instability of human N-acetyltransferase enzyme protein(s) had hindered studies of the biochemical and molecular mechanisms leading to the occurrence of the slow acetylator phenotype in man. This situation has changed with recent technical improvements in analytical methods coupled with the use of recombinant DNA technologies to clone and express mutant alleles at the polymorphic gene locus. Using a specific polyclonal antiserum raised against a purified human arylamine N-acetyltransferase protein (Grant *et al.*, 1989) and with access to liver tissue from individuals whose *in vivo* acetylator phenotype could often be determined with the caffeine test, we were able to demonstrate that at the protein level, the slow acetylator phenotype is associated with a decrease in the quantity of functional enzyme present in human liver rather than a change in the substrate kinetics of a variant gene product (Grant *et al.*, 1990).

To study the molecular basis of the defect, a full-length cDNA encoding rabbit arylamine N-acetyltransferase (Blum *et al.*, 1989) was used to screen a human genomic DNA library, resulting in the isolation of two independently regulated N-acetyltransferase genes, designated *NAT*1 and *NAT*2, at separate loci on chromosome 8, pter-q11 (Blum *et al.*, 1990a). These genes both encode functional acetylating enzymes upon transient expression in mammalian (COS-1) cell culture. The recombi-nant *NAT*2 gene product shows protein immunoreactivity and enzyme kinetic characteristics identical to those of the human liver enzyme whose content is decreased in slow acetylators, suggesting that the *NAT*2 gene locus is the site of the acetylation polymorphism (Grant *et al.*, 1991). To date, four mutant alleles at the *NAT*2 gene locus have been identified; fortuitously, the three most common of these may be detected by RFLP analysis on Southern blots even though each contains only a small number of nucleotide substitutions relative to the wild-type allele. Of the two most common mutant alleles, accounting for roughly 95% of those present in a Caucasian population, one contains point mutations which may impair mRNA translation efficiency, while the other contains a point mutation which appears to decrease enzyme stability (Blum *et al.*, 1991). The third mutant allele, identified by cloning and expression of its cDNA (Ohsako and Deguchi, 1990), is much less frequently observed both in Caucasian and Oriental populations, and a fourth mutant has been detected only once so far.

Interestingly, the *NAT*1 gene produces an acetylating enzyme with kinetic characteristics different from any that we had observed in human liver until quite recently. *NAT*1 is indeed expressed in human liver and probably also in many other tissues, but is unrelated to the acetylation polymorphism (Grant *et al.*, 1991; Ohsako and Deguchi, 1990). However, the existence of *NAT*1 has provided the solution to one of the puzzling clinical aspects related to the acetylation polymorphism, namely the existence of so-called 'monomorphic' arylamine substrates such as *p*-aminosalicylic acid, which are very efficiently acetylated *in vivo* but do not correlate with acetylator phenotype. It is now clear that such substrates are selectively metabolized by *NAT*1. This gene multiplicity, although certainly not as extensive as that displayed by many other drug biotransformation enzyme systems, nevertheless imparts upon the organism the capability to metabolize and thereby hopefully to detoxify a wider diversity of xenobiotics.

CONCLUSION

The purpose of this review has been to illustrate the importance of hepatic xenobiotic biotransforming enzymes in the conversion of drugs and environmental chemicals to metabolic products with altered potential for toxicity. It is clear that pharmacogenetic defects affecting many of these enzymes may be significant predisposing factors for the occurrence of toxic events associated with chemical exposures, and the mechanisms underlying these defects continue to be very active areas of research in pharmacology.

REFERENCES

Arnaud, M. J. Products of metabolism of caffeine. In: Dews, P. B. (ed.), *Caffeine*, Springer-Verlag, Berlin, 1984, pp. 3–38

Blum, M., Grant, D. M., Demierre, A. and Meyer, U. A. N-acetylation pharmacogenetics: a gene deletion causes absence of arylamine N-acetyltransferase in liver of slow acetylator rabbits. *Proc. Natl. Acad. Sci. USA* 86 (1989) 9554–9557

Blum, M., Grant, D. M., McBride, W., Heim, M. and Meyer, U. A. Human arylamine N-acetyltransferase genes: isolation, chromosomal localization, and functional expression. *DNA Cell Biol.* 9 (1990) 193–203

Blum, M., Demierre, A., Grant, D. M., Heim, M. and Meyer, U. A. Molecular mechanism of slow acetylation of drugs and carcinogens in man. *Proc. Natl. Acad. Sci. USA* (1991) (in press)

Evans, D. A. P. N-acetyltransferase. *Pharmacol. Ther.* 42 (1989) 157–234

Gonzalez, F. J. The molecular biology of cytochrome P450s. *Pharmacol. Rev.* 40 (1989) 243–288

Grant, D. M., Tang, B. K. and Kalow, W. A simple test for acetylator phenotype using caffeine. *Br. J. Clin. Pharmacol.* 17 (1984) 459–464

Grant, D. M., Lottspeich, F. and Meyer, U. A. Evidence for two closely related isozymes of arylamine N-acetyltransferase in human liver. *FEBS Lett.* 244 (1989) 203–207

Grant, D. M., Moerike, K., Eichelbaum, M. and Meyer, U. A. Acetylation pharmacogenetics: the slow acetylator phenotype is caused by decreased or absent arylamine N-acetyltransferase in human liver. *J. Clin. Invest.* 85 (1990) 968–972

Grant, D. M., Blum, M., Beer, M. and Meyer, U. A. Monomorphic and polymorphic human arylamine N-acetyltransferases: a comparison of liver isoenzymes and expressed products of two cloned genes. *Mol. Pharmacol.* 39 (1991) 184–191

Jakoby, W. B. Detoxication: conjugation and hydrolysis. In Arias, I. M., Jakoby, W. B., Popper, H., Schacter, D. and Shafritz, D. A. (eds.), *The Liver: Biology and Pathobiology*, Raven Press, New York, 1988, pp. 375–388

Meyer, U. A. Molecular genetics and the future of pharmacogenetics. *Pharmacol. Ther.* 46 (1990) 349–355

Meyer, U. A., Zanger, U. M., Grant, D. M. and Blum, M. Genetic polymorphisms of drug metabolism. *Adv. Drug Res.* 19 (1990) 197–241

Miller, E. C. Some current perspectives on chemical carcinogenesis in humans and experimental animals. *Cancer Res.* 38 (1978) 1479–1496

Nebert, D. W., Nelson, D. R. and Feyereisen, R. Evolution of the cytochrome P450 genes. *Xenobiotica* 19 (1989) 1149–1160

Ohsako, S. and Deguchi, T. Cloning and expression of cDNAs for polymorphic and monomorphic arylamine N-acetyltransferases from human liver. *J. Biol. Chem.* 265 (1990) 4630–4634

Okey, A. B. Enzyme induction in the cytochrome P450 system. *Pharmacol. Ther.* 45 (1990) 241–298

Spielberg, S. P. *In vitro* assessment of pharmacogenetic susceptibility to toxic drug metabolites in humans. *Fed. Proc.* 43 (1984) 2308–2313

Ziegler, D. M. Detoxication: oxidation and reduction. In Arias, I. M., Jakoby, W. B., Popper, H., Schacter, D. and Shafritz, D. A. (eds.), *The Liver: Biology and Pathobiology*, Raven Press, New York, 1988, pp. 363–374

J. Inher. Metab. Dis. 14 (1991) 431–435

Hereditary Variation of Liver Enzymes involved with Detoxification and Neurodegenerative Disease

A. C. WILLIAMS, G. B. STEVENTON, S. STURMAN and R. H. WARING

University Departments of Neurology and Biochemistry, University of Birmingham, Edgbaston, Birmingham B15 2TT, UK

Summary: Enzymes involved with the metabolic transformation of xenobiotics have recently been studied in patients with the neurodegenerative diseases, Alzheimer's disease, Parkinson's disease and motor neurone disease. Defects were detected in sulphur pathways and also, in the case of Parkinson's disease, in monoamine oxidase B. The possibility exists that the ability to cope safely with endogenous and exogenous substances which have neurotoxic properties is important in the pathogenesis of these diseases. Potentially such individuals could be identified preclinically and these diseases postponed by reduction in the load of toxin or modification of the relevant enzymic activity.

A considerable body of evidence suggests that the late onset neurodegenerative diseases, Parkinson's disease, Alzheimer's disease and motor neurone disease (amyotrophic lateral sclerosis), could be caused by slow chemical poisoning over much of a lifetime. In the story of MPTP (1-methyl-4-phenyl-1,2,3,6-tetrahydropyridine) we have a simple compound causing a syndrome almost identical to idiopathic parkinsonism (Davis *et al.*, 1979; Langston *et al.*, 1983). There is a considerable overlap at many levels between each of these neurodegenerative diseases. If MPTP can cause parkinsonism then it is at least possible that other toxins exist which are capable of causing the selective neuronal death necessary to cause other syndromes like amyotrophic lateral sclerosis and Alzheimer's disease. Amyotrophic lateral sclerosis has, for instance, been associated with pyrethrum poisoning (Steventon *et al.*, 1990d).

Alzheimer's disease and Parkinson's disease have a large subclinical component suggesting that the disease process consists of steadily accumulating damage compatible with the finding at a clinical level that these diseases occur in the young adult but increase markedly in incidence with advancing age. The brain has several defence mechanisms against chemical damage. Intracellular antioxidant defences are in place against attack by radicals, as are conjugation reactions usually involving glutathione against other forms of chemical attack. Glia have a protective rôle against damage from ammonium. Close control of the release of excitatory neurotransmitters such as glutamate is important. Naturally the blood/brain barrier forms an important physical and enzymatic hurdle.

In addition, some potentially toxic compounds will not be absorbed from the gut. Also man will have learnt by experience to avoid some compounds in the environment, although this can only happen if an immediate unpleasant symptom develops and will not be a protection against slow, asymptomatic poisoning over many years. However, several cytochrome P-450 and linked xenobiotic enzymes have been identified in olfactory tissue. These are often eventually damaged in neurodegenerative disease, suggesting a possible feedback mechanism whereby the individual avoids, via an unpleasant taste or smell, reactive metabolites which are also being formed at other sites where they could cause more serious damage to neurones over the long term. Enzymic activity in the liver is likely to be important, converting many foreign chemicals (xenobiotics) to hydrophilic metabolites which are more likely to be excreted and less capable of crossing the blood/brain barrier.

Once a foreign compound of no nutritional value has entered the system, perhaps from the diet or after the action of indigenous microbiotica in the intestinal canal, it is likely that metabolism – predominantly in the liver – will take place. This usually converts such a substance into a less toxic compound, although on occasion transformation to a more toxic metabolite may occur. Failure of the detoxifying metabolism taking place on a chronic basis could damage other organs, and neurones are most at risk in this scenario as their capacity for regeneration is limited. In the case of MPTP poisoning the rôle of the liver may have been underestimated as in both the drug addicts and the laboratory animal the compound was given parenterally, thus avoiding first pass metabolism. MPTP is a protoxin which, after conversion by the enzyme monoamine oxidase-B (MAO-B), is converted to MPP^+ (1-methyl-4-phenylpyridinium) (Chiba *et al.*, 1984). If this transformation occurs in the brain toxicity results, but if it occurs before crossing the blood/brain barrier toxicity does not result, because MPP^+ as a charged ion cannot cross the blood/brain barrier. Conversion to MPP^+ was shown to occur avidly in liver tissue and hence no MPTP or MPP^+ crossed into the brain (Fuller *et al.*, 1987). A recent study in the mouse showed that oral MPTP was absorbed almost as well as after a subcutaneous injection (Fuller *et al.*, 1987). No natural source of MPTP is known, although suggestions as to how it could be formed from tryptamine metabolism have been made (Ramsden and Williams, 1985). Endogenously produced MPP^+-like compounds could also be produced by overproduction of N-methylated derivatives of pyridines. If MPTP or similar compounds are in the environment the diet is the most likely source, so it is clear that in this situation (and one would expect this to be the case for most potential toxins) liver metabolism is crucial.

We have looked at unmedicated patients with these neurodegenerative diseases and have used either probe drugs or measured enzyme activity *in vitro* using easily accessible tissue such as red cell membranes or platelets.

PROBE DRUGS

Others had looked at Parkinson's disease and debrisoquine metabolism. Initially positive reports were, however, retracted and our own experience using debrisoquine, a carbon oxidation reaction, is that there is no abnormality of metabolism in Parkinson's disease, Alzheimer's disease or amyotrophic lateral sclerosis (Steventon *et al.*, 1989a).

We have also looked at N-acetylation using sulphadimidine as a probe (unpublished). We have not found any substantial derangement although there was a tendency for Parkinson's disease and amyotrophic lateral sclerosis patients to be slow acetylators. These changes were slight so we doubt whether they are of biological significance.

More positive results came when we started to look at sulphur metabolism using a probe drug, S-carboxymethylcysteine, and measured the production of sulphoxides. This is an S-oxidation reaction with high hereditability which involves the enzyme cysteine dioxygenase which converts cysteine to sulphate. Parkinson's disease, Alzheimer's disease and amyotrophic lateral sclerosis patients were all poor at this reaction, with Alzheimer's disease patients being by far the worst (Steventon *et al.*, 1988, 1989b, 1990a). Differences compared with normal controls, including very elderly controls, were striking. We then measured the ratio of plasma cysteine/sulphate and as we predicted found differences, with the patient groups having relatively high cysteine and low sulphate, confirming that this enzyme system was underactive (Heafield *et al.*, 1990). Using another probe, paracetamol, the degree of sulphate and glucuronide conjugation was determined. The low amount of sulphate was reflected in diminished sulphate conjugation in all of these diseases (Steventon *et al.*, 1990b). Intriguingly, Parkinson's disease and amyotrophic lateral sclerosis patients did not compensate by increasing glucuronidation but the Alzheimer's disease patients did. Recently we have observed that individuals with Trisomy 21 who are all destined to get an Alzheimer's disease-like syndrome have abnormalities very similar to those seen in Alzheimer's disease (unpublished observations).

These studies demonstrated that there was a marked defect in sulphur metabolism in these neurodegenerative diseases. If cysteine dioxygenase is underactive and there is accumulation of cysteine in the nervous system, this could be toxic. Cysteine is a known neurotoxin acting on glutamate receptors and both it, in the presence of bicarbonate ion, and other sulphur-containing amino acids which may well be increased from this block in the sulphur cycle, are potent excitotoxins. Additionally, cysteine could disturb metal metabolism by its chelating capacity and thus affect free radical reactions. There is an interesting link with Hallervorden–Spatz disease in which this same enzyme is deficient in the brain; in patients suffering from this disease there is marked accumulation of iron as there is in Parkinson's disease. Disturbed metal metabolism has also been claimed in both Alzheimer's disease and amyotrophic lateral sclerosis.

Another mechanism involves the ability to handle safely xenobiotics from our environment. Poor sulphoxidisers may, for instance, handle sulphur-containing compounds (perhaps from vegetables) differently and allow toxins to accumulate. Failure to conjugate with sulphate or the increased glucuronidation permitting entry into the enterohepatic circulation in the cases of Alzheimer's disease and Trisomy 21 may increase the half-life of some substances.

IN VITRO ENZYMATIC STUDIES

Monoamine oxidase B: We have looked at this enzyme in the platelets of untreated Parkinson's disease patients. The importance of monoamine oxidase B to MPTP toxicity has already been mentioned and interest in it is substantial as it has recently been demonstrated that inhibition of this enzyme by selegiline slows the progression of Parkinson's disease. We have found with one substrate (phenylethylamine) that activity appears to be increased (Steventon *et al.*, 1989c). We have recently used another substrate (dopamine) and have found the activity to be markedly reduced (Steventon *et al.*, 1990c); thus substrate specificities appear to differ in the disease group. Increasing the number of hydroxyl groups on the aromatic ring from 0 to 2 appears to alter activity radically, which suggests a structural defect at the binding site rather than dysregulation. It is conceivable that this is genetically determined, and like ecogenetic illnesses such as glucose-6-phosphate dehydrogenase deficiency, an individual with an isoform of monoamine oxidase B which was poor at converting MPTP or similar molecules to MPP$^+$ during first pass metabolism could be at risk of getting Parkinson's disease provided his environmental exposure to such substances was significant. Initial unpublished studies by our group using MPTP as substrate on platelet monoamine oxidase B suggest that this is, however, not the case.

Thiolmethyltransferase: We have studied this enzyme which is known to be important in detoxification, particularly of hydrogen sulphide in the red blood cells of patients with neurodegenerative disease. Mercaptoethanol was used as substrate and the results were strikingly different in the disease groups compared with the controls. With Alzheimer's disease and Parkinson's disease, activity was very low but with amyotrophic lateral sclerosis it was very high (Waring *et al.*, 1989). This enzyme is known to have high hereditability. It is possible that individuals with low activity determined by genetic factors have throughout their lifetimes been exposed to toxicity from substances such as hydrogen sulphide, which is in the environment and is also produced in significant quantities in the bowel by the action of gut bacteria as well as endogenously. Hydrogen sulphide is toxic and is similar to cyanide in its mechanisms of toxicity, and so like MPTP is a mitochondrial poison which is of relevance in the light of present reports of a variety of mitochondrial defects which are likely to be acquired in neurodegenerative disease. It is a known neurotoxin causing an encephalopathy with electrophysiological features identical to those seen in Alzheimer's disease.

CONCLUSION

We have demonstrated significant abnormalities in enzymes concentrated in the liver which are concerned with detoxification of xenobiotics and are also important in endogenous metabolism. The activity of these enzyme systems is largely determined by genetic factors although may well be induced or repressed on occasion by environmental or endogenous factors. Dysregulation or polymorphisms of these enzymes may be involved. Interracial differences in the frequencies of certain polymorphisms could explain some of the differences in incidence of these diseases, and differences between the sexes could be explained by hormonal influences in relevant enzymes. Simple measures such as eating a diet which is broadly based may turn out to be healthy in part due to a reduction in the dose of particular toxins from any given source; eating at regular intervals at normal times of the day may be important for the same reason, as well as avoiding chronotoxicity since many of these enzymes demonstrate large diurnal variation in activity. This line of research could lead to the identification of individuals at risk of toxicity. Further research to confirm this is required, but the exciting prospect of modification of enzyme activity or reduction in environmental load of certain toxins once identified exists. These approaches could lead to the postponement or avoidance of these increasingly important diseases.

REFERENCES

Chiba, K., Trevor, A. and Castagnoli, N. Metabolism of the neurotoxic tertiary amine, MPTP, by brain monoamine oxidase. *Biochem. Biophys. Res. Commun.* 120 (1984) 574–578

Davis, G. C., Williams, A. C., Markey, S. P., Ebert, M. H., Caine, E. D., Reichart, C. M. and Kopin, I. J. Chronic parkinsonism secondary to intravenous injection of meperidine analogues. *Psychiatr. Res.* 1 (1979) 249–254

Fuller, R. W. and Hemrick-Luecke, S. K. Oral versus parental efficacy of 1-methyl-4-phenyl-1,2,3,6-tetrahydropyridine (MPTP): Differential effects on depletion of heart norepinephrine and striatal dopamine in mice. *Biochem. Pharmacol.* 36 (1987) 789–792

Heafield, M. T. E., Fearn, S., Steventon, G. B., Waring, R. H., Williams, A. C. and Sturman, S. G. Plasma cysteine and sulphate levels in patients with Motor Neurone, Parkinson's and Alzheimer's disease. *Neurosci. Lett.* 110 (1990) 216–220

Langston, J. W., Ballard, P., Tetrud, J. W. and Irwin, I. Chronic Parkinsonism in humans due to a product of meperidine-analog synthesis. *Science* (New York) 219 (1983) 979–980

Ramsden, D. B. and Williams, A. C. Production in nature of compound resembling methylphenyltetrahydropyridine, a possible cause of Parkinson's disease. *Lancet 1* (1985) 215–216

Steventon, G. B., Williams, A. C., Waring, R. H., Pall, H. S. and Adams, D. Xenobiotic metabolism in Motor Neurone disease. *Lancet* 2 (1988) 644–647

Steventon, G., Heafield, M. T. E., Sturman, S. G., Waring, R. H., Williams, A. C. and Ellingham, J. Degenerative neurological disease and debrisoquine-4-hydroxylation capacity. *Med. Sci. Res.* 17 (1989a) 163–164

Steventon, G., Heafield, M. T. E., Waring, R. H. and Williams, A. C. (1989b). Xenobiotic metabolism in Parkinson's disease. *Neurology* 39 (1989b) 883–887

Steventon, G., Sturman, S. G., Heafield, M. T. E., Waring, R. H., Napier, J. and Williams, A. C. Platelet monoamine oxidase-B activity in Parkinson's disease. *J. Neural Transmission* (Parkinson's disease Section) 1 (1989c) 255–261

Steventon, G. B., Heafield, M. T. E., Sturman, S., Waring, R. H. and Williams, A. C. Xenobiotic metabolism in Alzheimer's disease. *Neurology* 40 (1990a) 1095–1098

Steventon, G., Heafield, M. T. E., Waring, R. H., Williams, A. C., Sturman, S. G. and Green, M. Metabolism of low dose paracetamol in patients with chronic neurological disease. *Xenobiotica* 20 (1990b) 117–122

Steventon, G., Humfrey, C., Sturman, S., Waring, R. H., Williams, A. C. MAO-B and Parkinson's disease. *Lancet* 335 (1990c) 180

Steventon, G. B., Waring, R. H. and Williams, A. C. (1990d). Pesticide toxicity and Motor Neurone disease. *Neurol. Neurosurg. Psychiatry* 53 (1990d) 621–622

Waring, R. H., Steventon, G., Heafield, M. T. E., Sturman, S. G., Williams, A. C. and Smith, M. S-Methylation in Parkinson's disease and Motor Neurone disease. *Lancet* 2 (1989) 356–357

J. Inher. Metab. Dis. 14 (1991) 436–458
© SSIEM and Kluwer Academic Publishers.

Interrelationships of Liver and Brain with Special Reference to Reye Syndrome

J. K. BROWN and H. IMAM

Department of Paediatric Neurology, Royal Hospital for Sick Children, Edinburgh, Scotland

Summary: Reye syndrome is an acute non-inflammatory encephalopathy that can be precipitated by toxic, infective, metabolic or hypoxic upsets. The biochemical changes point to mitochondrial dysfunction and this is substantiated by structural changes in mitochondria on electron microscopy. The toxic metabolites that accumulate are similar to those incriminated in hepatic encephalopathy and other metabolic diseases. These metabolites exert their deleterious effects by direct neuronal damage, neurotransmitter blockade, vascular damage, cerebral oedema, hypoxic ischaemic damage, demyelination, retardation of brain growth and neuronal storage. Brain capillary endothelial cells are very rich in mitochondria and mitochondrial disorders can effect the central nervous system primarily, and not just as a consequence of systemic metabolic upset.

REYE SYNDROME

A non-inflammatory encephalopathy of childhood has been recognized for a long time (Brain *et al.*, 1929). It was the description of the association of this encephalopathy with fatty degeneration of the viscera (Reye *et al.*, 1963) that drew world attention to the disease. It has been defined by the American Center for Disease Control (1980) as 'acute non-inflammatory encephalopathy associated with coma. No evidence of cerebral inflammation as shown by a CSF containing less than 8 leukocytes per microlitre, together with evidence of cerebral oedema. There is fatty metamorphosis of   or a greater than 3-fold increase in the level of serum glutamic oxaloacetic t   se or pyruvic transaminase or a rise in serum ammonia.' (Glasgow *et al.*, 1   er, 1989).

Incidence

Reye syndrome has an incidence of 1 : 100 000 in children of less than 18 years of age in the United States but in the United Kingdom only 1 : 300 000. Part of the definition in some of the epidemiological surveys is that there must be no alternative reasonable explanation for cerebral/hepatic abnormalities. Difficulty comes when paraviral cases are regarded as primary Reye syndrome, whilst toxic and metabolic cases are regarded as secondary Reye syndrome. This is an artificial definition as all cases of Reye syndrome are the result of acute mitochondrial dysfunction (Hurwitz *et al.*, 1982; Hall and Bellman, 1984).

CLINICAL FEATURES OF REYE SYNDROME

Reye syndrome can occur at any age including the neonatal period but is rare in the adult. It appears to peak round about 2 years of age. In a typical case the child appears to be recovering from a non-specific virus infection when there is onset of intractable vomiting. Vomiting is much more the hallmark of Reye syndrome than fits, which are relatively uncommon. The child changes in behaviour, becomes overactive, irritable, resents interference and becomes combative. He may appear tremulous and clumsy. The child may remain irritable, delirious, drowsy, with disturbance of higher cortical function and then recover or progress to deeper coma.

Progression appears to depend on the development of cerebral oedema, when coma deepens, pupils dilate, decerebrate postures appear and progressive brain-stem failure (fixed heart rate, apnoea and dopamine-dependent vasoparalytic shock) may herald a fatal outcome (Brown, 1991b). In small infants the presentation can be very acute as a cot death syndrome (Bonnell and Beckwith, 1986; Roe *et al.*, 1986).

Respiration is initially deep and regular, either due to the hyperammonaemia, due to central neurogenic hyperventilation from cerebral oedema, or as a result of metabolic acidosis. Reflexes are brisk. The plantar responses are often extensor. Occasionally the findings are asymmetrical. Asymmetrical neurological signs or a frank hemiplegia do not negate the possibility of an underlying metabolic disease. The liver is usually easily palpable in the very young child; jaundice should not be present, or the syndrome of haemorrhagic shock encephalopathy, fructose intolerance, Weil disease, poisoning with paracetamol, etc., should be suspected (Levin *et al.*, 1983).

Lovejoy and colleagues (1974) suggested five grades of coma staging. This is not particularly helpful as grades 3, 4 and 5 relate essentially to the development of cerebral oedema progressing to brain-stem failure. Any child who enters these phases from any cause, has a poor prognosis (Brown, 1991b). The child who does not develop signs of tentorial herniation has a better prognosis.

Electroencephalogram

The EEG at first shows slow waves in the delta frequency, usually $1–3\,\text{s}^{-1}$ in the frontal area. As coma deepens this spreads posteriorly and becomes generalized, sometimes (20% of cases) with the typical triphasic wave (Bickford and Butt, 1955). In children with metabolic encephalopathy the slow waves are often posterior rather than anterior at the start. The EEG abnormalities are not specific to hepatic coma; they may appear before the clinical symptoms appear and persist after consciousness has returned. Continuous triphasic waves suggest a poor prognosis. EEG abnormalities correlate with cerebral spinal fluid glutamine concentration in hepatic coma (Rothstein and Herlong, 1989).

If raised intracranial pressure occurs with resultant cerebral hypoxia the fast activity on the EEG disappears; the EEG flattens and eventually becomes isoelectric, indicating brain death (Laidlaw and Read, 1963).

Evoked responses

Abnormal visual evoked responses have been found in preclinical hepatic encephalopathy and the latency of the evoked response increases with the severity of the encephalopathy. Again electrical recovery may be delayed after clinical recovery. The late components of the sensory evoked potential (p3, N3) appear to be particularly sensitive to hepatic encephalopathy. They can be made to reappear by the administration of benzodiazepine antagonist drugs — e.g. Flumazenil (Grimm et al., 1988).

Pathology

Visceral changes: The liver shows pallor and yellow discoloration from the presence of fat when seen macroscopically. On microscopic examination the fat is found to be microvesicular, although some macrovesicular fat does not exclude the diagnosis. In mild cases the fat is deposited in the periphery of the lobules and in severe cases there is fat distribution of the whole lobule. There should not be extensive hepatocyte destruction. The composition of the lipid deposited is mainly triglyceride. There should be no evidence of inflammation, bile duct stasis or other abnormalities of the duct system (Brown and Madge, 1972). Fat is also deposited in other tissues and in particular in the heart and kidney.

Electron microscopy at biopsy shows that the mitochondria are enlarged (Bove *et al.*, 1975). In mild cases the matrix is electron-lucent with fewer dense bodies; in more severe cases cristae are disrupted; and in very severe cases the external membrane is also disrupted, often with adherent lysosomes (Partin *et al.*, 1975). Liver peroxisomes may show a compensatory increase. Histochemical examination shows complete absence of succinate dehydrogenase and an elevation of glutamate dehydrogenase (Filipe and Lake, 1983). Glycogen stores are either depleted or reduced.

Brain pathology: The brain is swollen; the gyri are flattened with evidence of tentorial or foramen magnum herniation. There may be evidence of laminar necrosis of neurones consistent with the degree of cerebral hypoxia.

On histological examination of *post mortem* or biopsy specimens there should be no evidence of inflammation, no perivascular cuffing, no primary necrotic encephalitis, no demyelination, no neuronal storage material and no evidence of a primary vasculitis.

Examination of brain biopsy material shows that the astrocytes are swollen and there are blebs of fluid in the myelin consistent with a toxic myelinoclastic oedema. Alteration in mitochondria appears in astrocytes and neurones with enlargement of the matrix together with reduction in electron density. The mitochondria may show electron-dense inclusions (Partin *et al.*, 1975). *Post mortem* studies have shown that there are also abnormalities in the endothelial cells. There are thus abnormalities in the endothelial cells, astrocytes, neurones and myelin consistent with a toxic or primary metabolic abnormality rather than an inflammatory cause. In hepatic failure, from primary liver disease, portocaval anastomosis or genetic hyperammonaemias, the neuropathology is the same, with enlargement of the protoplasmic astrocytes to form Alzheimer type 2 cells (Bruton *et al.*, 1970). These are the hallmarks of hepatic encephalopathy and are found throughout the brain in cortex, basal ganglia, thalamus, cerebellum and pontine nuclei. The astrocyte is thought to be important in the metabolism of brain ammonia (Cavanagh and Kyu, 1971) and to convert plasma ammonia to glutamine. The astrocytes also show accumulation of glycogen, proliferation of endoplasmic reticulum with prominent nucleoli and a lobulated nucleus (Adams and Foley, 1953; Norenberg and Lapham, 1974). The endothelial cells can be regarded as a 'cerebral glomerulus' and filter, whilst the astrocyte is a 'cerebral hepatocyte' and detoxifies.

AETIOLOGY OF REYE SYNDROME

The causes of Reye syndrome can be considered to arise from four main groups (Table 1).

Table 1   Causes of Reye syndrome

Infection
Chickenpox
Influenza B
Influenza A

Toxic
Salicylate
Sodium valproate
Aflatoxin (*Aspergillus flavum*)
Hypoglycin (unripe akee fruit)
Insecticide
Bacterial endotoxin

Inborn errors of metabolism
Ornithine transcarbamylase deficiency
Carbamyl phosphate synthetase deficiency
Medium-chain acyl dehydrogenase deficiency
Long-chain acyl dehydrogenase deficiency
Glutaric aciduria type 2
Biotinidase deficiency
Carnitine deficiency
Carnitine palmitoyl transferase deficiency
Isovaleric acidaemia
3-Hydroxyl, 3-methylglutaryl-CoA lyase deficiency
Late onset citrullinaemia

Hypoxia
Status epilepticus

Infective causes: Reye syndrome classically follows a few days after a clinical virus infection. It may appear in epidemics associated with epidemics of influenza B. Influenza A has also been implicated. The other common virus implicated as a cause of Reye syndrome is the varicella zoster (chickenpox) virus (Hurwitz and Goodman, 1982).

Toxic causes: The two drugs associated with Reye syndrome are sodium valproate and aspirin. Sodium valproate is thought to act by forming valproyl carnitine, which is lost in the urine. Some of the cases of severe hepatopathy caused by sodium valproate have been due to the precipitation of inborn errors of metabolism such as ornithine transcarbamylase deficiency (Kay *et al.*, 1986; Brown, 1988). Hyperammonaemia is quite frequent during the treatment of children with sodium valproate and this may be reduced by the administration of carnitine. Valproate toxicity is thought to affect 1 in 500 children under 3 years of age while the risk to older children is in the order of 1 in 30 000 (Brown, 1988). There has been a reduction in the incidence of Reye syndrome over recent years and it is not certain whether this is due to the restricted use of salicylates in children. Aspirin was withdrawn from general use in 1986 (Hall, 1986). The liver histology at post-mortem in children dying from aspirin overdose resembles that of Reye syndrome (Starko and Mullick, 1983). Children suffering from rheumatic fever and rheumatoid arthritis who have taken large doses of salicylates have also been reported as dying from Reye syndrome (Rennebohm *et al.*, 1985). Aspirin given to animals can also be shown to produce a Reye-type syndrome particularly if combined with virus infection. Aspirin, like valproate, can precipitate pre-existing metabolic disease (Editorial, 1987). Sixty-six per cent of normal people receiving salicylates in high dosage have raised transaminases.

Other toxins include aflatoxin, which may be produced from the effects of the fungus *Aspergillus flavum*, particularly found in peanut products and in corn kept for long periods in warm countries to make 'mealies'. Jamaican vomiting sickness is known to be due to ingestion of the substance hypoglycin that is found in the unripe Akee fruit. This is known to be an inhibitor of certain acyl Coenzyme A dehydrogenases required for fatty and amino-acid metabolism (Tanaka, 1976). Insecticides or their propellants used in Newfoundland have been thought to act as mitochondrial poisons. Margosa oil is a further toxin that has been incriminated as a cause of Reye syndrome and also the toxin in hornet stings (Sinniah and Baskaran, 1981; Weizman *et al.*, 1985).

Inborn errors of metabolism: Mitochondria require a supply of pyruvate from glucose or fatty acids from lipid stores. They also require oxygen. Reye syndrome can theoretically therefore occur whenever there is a failure of (1) primary substrate, (2) glycolysis, (3) incorporation of pyruvate or fatty acid into the mitochondria, (4) Krebs cycle or (5) urea cycle abnormalities, (6) electron-transfer chain failure, (7) failure of oxygen supply.

Some of the inborn errors of metabolism known to be associated with Reye syndrome (Glasgow *et al.*, 1980; Coates *et al.*, 1984; Bougeneres *et al.*, 1985; Pollit, 1987) are given in Table 1.

Differentiation also may be difficult clinically from acute exacerbations of other organic acidaemias such as proprionic acidemia and methyl malonic acidemia. The differential diagnosis essentially is of a child arriving in coma with either a metabolic acidosis and or hyperammonaemia. Mitochondrial enzymes such as ornithine transcarbamylase, carbamylphosphate synthetase, succinate dehydrogenase and cytochromeoxidase are all depressed in Reye syndrome secondary to a mitochondropathy of any type. Dicarboxylic acids also appear in the urine so that it is not easy in the acute stage to differentiate a toxic or infective mitochondropathy from an inborn error of metabolism. The child may be metabolically normal between exacerbations even though suffering from an inborn error of metabolism. Table 2 shows some factors precipitating decompensation of some of these disorders.

Table 2   Factors precipitating metabolic disease

Hypoxia
Starvation
Infection/pyrexia
    (hypercatabolism, mitochondropathy)
Exercise
Diet
    Overload: protein
    Deficiency: biotin, B6, carnitine
Specific toxin
    (H_2S, Cu, valproate)

Hypoxic causes: Respiratory failure has been defined as a PO_2 of less than 8 mm Hg in the mitochondrion. Prolonged hypoxia can result in changes reminiscent of Reye syndrome with hypoglycaemia, a rise in plasma ammonia, marked rise in serum transaminases, coagulation defects, cerebral oedema with mitochondrial change on electron microscopy and accumulation of intracellular glycogen. Difficulty often arises in that when the child is found convulsing, in the morning by his parents, one is not certain whether he has convulsed during the whole night and developed severe secondary asphyxia, or whether the fits are secondary to a metabolic disease such as ornithine transcarbamylase deficiency that has been precipitated by a virus infection (e.g. Singapore disease).

BIOCHEMICAL DISTURBANCES IN REYE SYNDROME

Biochemical abnormalities in Reye syndrome include:

Hypoglycaemia
Raised plasma lactate
Raised plasma alanine
Raised plasma triglyceride
Raised plasma free fatty acids
Raised plasma ammonia (greater than $100\,\mu mol/L$)
Raised plasma alanine amino transferase (greater than 100 IU/L)

Metabolic acidosis
Increased dicarboxylic acid excretion in urine
Increase in plasma and urinary ketones (apart from those diseases that are specifically hypoketotic)
Raised creatine phosphokinase
Prolonged prothrombin time

The results are as are to be expected if adequate energy cannot be provided by total oxidation of glucose. Glucose is converted to lactate with exhaustion of the carbohydrate stores. A switch to fatty acids from lipolysis then occurs. Lipolysis is continuously stimulated, but the resulting fatty acids and triglyceride produced from the fat stores of the body are not removed by the mitochondria, resulting in an acute lipid storage disease with elevated plasma free fatty acids and triglyceride storage within the cells as microvacuoles of lipid. ω-Oxidation and peroxisomal oxidation cause an increase in urinary dicarboxylic acids, the β-oxidation produces peroxide and accumulation of short chain C_5 and C_6 fatty acids as peroxisomes can metabolize long chains down to C_5 only. One of the main reasons for the immediate administration of glucose is to try to switch off this uncontrolled lipolysis (Ansevin, 1980). There is nothing specific about the metabolic abnormalities in Reye syndrome that may not also be produced by prolonged hypoxia or starvation. Apart from hyperlipidaemia, the other major metabolic upset is hyperammonaemia (Huttenlocher *et al.*, 1969).

MECHANISMS OF BRAIN DAMAGE IN HEPATIC AND METABOLIC DISEASE

We have considered Reye syndrome in some detail as an example of the clinical presentation of an acute mitochondropathy. Organelles may suffer damage as a result of multiple pathologies in the same way that organs may present a stereotyped clinical picture of organ failure due to many causes. Hepatic failure itself tends to be the end result of different diseases — inflammatory, toxic, autoimmune or neoplastic. The end result of hepatic failure is the same no matter what the actual cause. The clinical picture of Reye syndrome is identical whether due to chickenpox or medium-chain acyl dehydrogenase deficiency. Mitochondria in different organs, e.g. heart, muscle, liver or brain, need not be affected to the same degree in different diseases of mitochondria (Alberts *et al.*, 1989). There are several ways in which the brain itself is affected by mitochondrial disease so that the presentation may be:

(1) Acute Reye syndrome
(2) Leigh encephalopathy
(3) Stroke (MELAS syndrome)
(4) Epilepsy (myoclonus epilepsy, ragged red fibre syndrome)
(5) Increased susceptibility to hypoxia
(6) Cerebellar ataxia (continuous or intermittent)
(7) Blindness and dementia (e.g. complex 3 disease, Leber's optic atrophy)
(8) Basal ganglia degeneration with calcification
(9) Alpers disease.

In addition to these 'central' nervous system presentations there are a whole range of metabolic myopathies involving abnormal mitochondrial function.

The rest of this paper will consider how disordered mitochondrial function in the liver may affect brain and how disordered mitochondrial function in the brain may present with neurological syndrome independently of the liver disease. We can consider the pathophysiology under the following headings: (1) direct neuronal toxicity, (2) neurotransmitter blockade, (3) vascular damage, (4) cerebral oedema, (5) hypoxic ischaemic damage, (6) demyelination, (7) retardation of brain growth, (8) neuronal storage.

Direct neuronal toxicity

The encephalopathy in hepatic coma is potentially reversible and fluctuates from hour to hour and day to day. The changing EEG pattern together with the reversible changes in evoked responses, the neuropathology (i.e. the formation of Alzheimer type 2 cells) all suggest that the brain is being 'anaesthetized' by some circulating compound that should normally be detoxified by the liver. This is also supported when one studies the factors that precipitate or aggravate hepatic encephalopathy, which include an increase in the protein load to be detoxified by the liver or colonic toxins bypassing the liver and entering the systemic circulation.

Factors precipitating and aggravating hepatic encephalopathy include:

(1) Gastrointestinal bleeding causing increased intestinal protein load.
(2) Increase in dietary protein.
(3) Infection causing catabolic muscle breakdown increasing protein load from endogenous protein.
(4) Hypokalaemia, e.g. from diuretics or as part of hepatic failure, causes increased renal ammonia production.
(5) Portocaval anastamosis.
(6) Uraemia — gut ureases change urea back to ammonia, which is then absorbed into the bloodstream.
(7) Metabolic alkalosis — NH_4 is changed in ionization to NH_3, increasing brain penetrance.
(8) Halothane anaesthesia.
(9) Sedative drugs, in particular benzodiazepines and barbiturates (?increased GABA inhibition in the brain).

There are several possible toxic substances that may be responsible for the encephalopathy (Table 3). We shall consider ammonia, mercaptans, fatty acids, amino acids and bilirubin in detail.

Ammonia: Ammonia arises from the deamination of proteins and is normally converted to urea. The muscles produce ammonia on exercise and the rise in plasma ammonia is proportionate to the amount of exercise. Ischaemic forearm exercise also results in the liberation of ammonia, i.e. anaerobic metabolism. It is thought that the ammonia in skeletal muscle is produced by the hydrolytic deamination of AMP. This increases as the muscle approaches exhaustion and AMP concentration therefore

Table 3   Possible neurotoxic substances in liver failure

Ammonia
Hypoglycaemia
Bilirubin

Amino acids
Free tryptophan
Decreased branched-chain amino acids
Mercaptans (thiols)

Fatty acids
Octanoic acid
Long-chain fatty acids

Neurotransmitter substances
Octopamine (dopa)
Tyramine
Noradrenaline (3-methoxy-4OH-phenylethylene glycol)
GABA
Leucine encephalin
Serotonin
Propionylcholine

rises. Resting muscle takes up ammonia from plasma (Bessman and Bradley, 1955). The kidney also produces ammonia, particularly in the presence of a hypokalaemic alkalosis (Weber, 1984).

The gut produces ammonia from the bacterial effects of urea and glutamine. Ureases cause release of ammonia and this is reabsorbed back into the bloodstream. Protein in the diet is a very potent source of ammonia as a result of bacterial action. Even a sterile gut, however, will produce ammonia from glutamine and urea. Vegetable protein produces less ammonia than animal protein or blood. Portal blood contains five times the concentration found in systemic venous blood (Lockwood, 1985). The brain itself also produces ammonia and this is metabolized in the small glutamate pool in the astrocytes. Ammonia is an excitant and a convulsant, not a depressor. Glutamine levels in CSF are reduced after prolonged fits when cerebral ammonia is raised and CSF glutamine may be raised by anticonvulsant therapy (Perry *et al.*, 1975).

Elevation of blood ammonia is most characteristic of hepatic failure or portacaval anastomosis. High ammonia concentrations are seen in mitochondrial diseases, both inborn errors of metabolism and Reye syndrome. There is not, however, a constant relationship between depth of coma and level of blood ammonia. Deep coma may be associated with relatively low concentrations of ammonia. Extremely high levels of ammonia may occur in children with inborn errors of metabolism, e.g. argininosuccinic aminoaciduria, who are fully conscious. Venous ammonia concentration is usually 50% lower than arterial ammonia as the muscles remove ammonia when not exercising (Stahl, 1963).

Brain tissue ammonia is raised in hepatic coma. Infusion of ammonia will cause Alzheimer changes in the astrocytes and an encephalopathy; the astrocytes show mitochondrial degeneration and lobulation of nuclei (Norenberg, 1977). The CSF glutamine and its precursor α-ketoglutaramate (Vergara *et al.*, 1974) are raised in the CSF and show a very good correlation between the level of coma, the EEG abnormality, and CSF glutamine concentration (Glion *et al.*, 1959; Hourani *et al.*, 1971). Glutamine synthetase in brain is localized in astrocytes and its concentration is increased in chronic hyperammonaemia (Martinez-Hernandez *et al.*, 1977). If however, one, blocks this enzyme, and hence cerebral glutamine formation, so that brain ammonia rises, this does not cause an encephalopathy (Warren and Schenker, 1964). The brain can extract un-ionized ammonia from the blood (the amount being proportional to cerebral blood flow) (Phelps *et al.*, 1977) and this is changed to glutamine in the small glutamate pool of the astrocyte. This reaction requires ATP and so asphyxia could theoretically make things worse by preventing the astrocyte from detoxifying the ammonia. The pH of blood influences ammonia penetration of brain as normally 97% is carried as NH_4^+ and only 3% as free NH_3. The un-ionized free form penetrates the blood–brain barrier very freely and the NH_4^+ not at all (Lockwood, 1985). The glutamine formed in the astrocyte is then returned to the brain ECF and so to the CSF (brain lymph). CSF concentrations of glutamine are high in hepatic coma and the concentrations closely parallel the degree of coma much better than does blood ammonia concentration.

Feeding of animal protein or ammonium salts to cirrhotic patients certainly precipitates hepatic encephalopathy. Glutamine, threonine, serine and glycine cause the greatest rise in ammonia (Rudman *et al.*, 1973). It would appear, however, that the ammonia either must act synergistically with some other compound (Zieve, 1980) or represent an epiphenomenon paralleling the degree of mitochondrial metabolic dysfunction, including brain mitochondria. The effect of ammonia depends upon pH, free ammonia concentration, glutamate supply, adequate ATP, the removal of glutamine into CSF and phosphate, as well as glutamine synthetase concentrations (Benjamin, 1981). In addition to affecting the cells' energy supply, NH_4^+ can substitute for Na^+ or K^+ and influence neuronal excitability and also acts on the chloride ionophore, i.e. the same as GABA (see below). NH_3 has a selective effect on regional brain glucose metabolism (Lockwood *et al.*, 1982).

Mercaptans: Historically, all illness was attributed to the absorption of toxins such as indoles and skatoles from the bowel, so that purging was the answer to most diseases. We are now returning to the idea of toxins from the gut as a possible cause for diseases such as the haemolytic uraemic syndrome and haemorrhagic shock encephalopathy. Certain diseases such as shigellosis and shiga-toxin producing *E. coli* will produce a severe encephalopathy. Other bacteria such as the campylobacter produce toxins that when absorbed will cause fits and a toxic encephalopathy. The fetor hepaticus of liver failure is due to the absorption of sulphur-containing thiols into the bloodstream (Chen *et al.*, 1970). These are produced by bacterial action on the sulphur-containing aminoacids cysteine and especially methionine, which also gives the smell to flatus. Inhalation of thiols can cause irreversible coma (Shults *et al.*, 1970). Mercaptans such as methanethiol (most potent), ethanethiol and dimethylsulphide are all produced in the colon. It is known that methionine given to patients with liver insufficiency will make the encephalopathy worse (Kinsell, 1949). When given intravenously to animals, thiols have an anaesthetic effect and produce coma that is enhanced by simultaneous administration of ammonia. It is thought that the mercaptans and ammonia from the bowel along with fatty acids could act synergistically in producing encephalopathy (Zieve et al., 1974; Zieve and Brunner, 1985).

The importance of toxicity of sulphur-containing substances has recently been boosted by the suggestion from the Birmingham group that Parkinson disease may be the result of hydrogen sulphide toxicity on the brain. Thiols produced from breakdown of methionine or cysteine are usually broken down by thiolmethyltransferase, which is in very high concentrations in gut mucosa and liver. Children who are deficient in thiolmethyltransferase enzymes may be normal unless exposed to hydrogen sulphide, when they may develop a severe encephalopathy very similar to mitochondrial encephalopathies (Sellars, personal communication). Inhalation of 0.1% by volume H_2S is fatal in people with normal thiolmethyltransferases. Sublethal doses causes damage to the most metabolically active parts of the brain, i.e. basal ganglia. It is thought that the thiols depress cerebral mitochondrial respiratory function (inhibit electron transfer) and have an effect on membrane transport (Waller, 1977; Vaklamp et al., 1979). Blood levels of thiols correlate with the degree of encephalopathy (MacClain et al., 1980).

Fatty acids: The liver metabolizes fatty acids by alteration in chain length or saturation. The concentration of free fatty acid in the blood rises at least threefold in hepatic encephalopathy and reaches high levels in children with Reye syndrome (Mamunes et al., 1975). Longer-chain fatty acids show definite neurotoxicity and may cause a reversible encephalopathy with coma (Zieve, 1985). They are thought to depress Na^+/K^+ ATPase and bind to the cell membranes. It might be expected that they would therefore affect depolarization. They also have a toxic effect on mitochondria in high concentration when they uncouple oxidative phosphorylation. This is the basis for the use of ketogenic diets in children with intractable epilepsy. This is believed to cause not only the development of ketosis as measured by plasma β-hydroxybutyrate concentrations but also the production of long-chain fatty acids. It has been suggested that octanoic acid in this situation acts as an anticonvulsant. When given to animals, octanoate causes a rise in intracranial pressure (Trauner and Adams, 1981) and alters the electrical activity of Purkinje cells (Borbola et al., 1974). They also inhibit Na^+/K^+ ATPase (Dahl, 1968). Short-chain fatty acids can cause coma but long-chain ones are more toxic and again affect mitochondrial permeability and energy coupling (Wojtczac, 1976). Medium-chain triglycerides given to patients with hepatic insufficiency do not cause an encephalopathy even though the CSF levels rise 500% (Linscheer et al., 1970; Weber, 1984). It is not known whether the direct effect of the fatty acids plays a part in encephalopathy, it seems more likely they work in conjunction with ammonia (as they inhibit glutamate dehydrogenase and mercaptans). Octanoate increases insulin secretion, decreases glucagon production and inhibits glycogenesis and thus may play a part in causing hypoglycaemia (Montague and Taylor, 1968; Edwards et al., 1969).

Amino acids: The liver is responsible for deamination of amino acids and it is not surprising that certain amino acid concentrations such as those of tyrosine, phenylalanine and methionine are raised in the plasma and CSF in liver disease (Baker, 1979). The concentration of free tryptophan is also raised but tryptophan is the only amino acid that is bound tightly to albumin and the low plasma albumin usually present in liver disease is probably responsible for the elevation of free tryptophan rather it being a reflection of failure of liver deamination. Tryptophan concentration is, however, also increased in CSF. The branched-chain amino acids leucine, isoleucine and valine are reduced in hepatic failure because it is thought they have been incorporated into muscle (Weber, 1984). Plasma alanine concentration is reduced in liver disease but, in most cases of hypoglycaemia with metabolic block, plasma alanine is raised. There is no evidence for a direct toxic effect or deficiency of essential amino acids playing a significant role in hepatic encephalopathy.

Bilirubin: The toxicity of bilirubin is seen in a pure setting in kernicterus in the newborn period. In haemolytic disease there is a vastly increased production of bilirubin. The enzyme glucuronyl transferase in the newborn liver is immature and not switched on since water-soluble bilirubin would not easily pass across the placenta. The rise in unconjugated serum bilirubin occurs without any change in ammonia, fatty acids, and mercaptans due to abnormal hepatocyte function but results from a high substrate concentration, which overloads the developmentally immature enzyme system.

In kernicterus (yellow staining of the brain.) it has been demonstrated that the yellow pigment is indeed bilirubin. The yellow pigment can be seen inside neurones and astrocytes on microscopy. It binds to membranes and can be seen in a granular form deposited on ganglioside in membranes.

Bilirubin is bound to serum albumin and it is only when the bilirubin-binding capacity is exceeded that free bilirubin in the plasma can pass freely into the central nervous system. Two moles of bilirubin bind to one mole of albumin. At normal plasma albumin concentrations this theoretically allows up to 80 mg% (1400 μmol) of bilirubin to be bound (Diamond, 1977). The premature infant has a lower plasma albumin. Fatty acids, salicylates, drugs, sodium benzoate, and hormones, such as thyroxine, may all bind to and compete for bilirubin binding sites on the albumin thus displacing bilirubin. Bilirubin in the unconjugated form is highly lipid-soluble while the conjugated form is water-soluble. It is therefore unconjugated free bilirubin which passes across the blood–brain barrier. It used to be believed that the blood–brain barrier matured with age and offered increasing resistance, but lipid-soluble substances such as bilirubin pass the blood–brain barrier without any hinderance at any age. In Crigler–Najjar syndrome kernicterus has been reported in the mature brain at 18 years (Blaschke *et al.*, 1974). Passage of substances across the blood–brain barrier depends upon: (1) binding to plasma proteins or other large molecules; (2) penetration of the endothelial cells, e.g. by pinocytosis; (3) lipid solubility; (4) degree of ionization — un-ionized compounds pass more easily than ionized ones and the degree of ionization depends upon the pK at plasma pH. (Phenobarbitone can change from 40 to 70% ionization at normal variations of plasma pH.); (5) the presence of active transport systems.

The blood–brain barrier is a very real entity and can break down allowing substances such as sucrose, trypan blue, fluorescein, ^{32}P, ^{131}I and labelled albumin into the brain extracellular space. This is the basis of vasogenic cerebral oedema and will be discussed later. Once through the blood–brain barrier the brain shows selective vulnerability and not all areas show equal uptake of bilirubin. In 35 cases reported by Claireaux in 1959 vulnerability was shown as follows:

Basal ganglia 32 cases
Cerebellum 25 cases
Hippocampus 24 cases
Medulla 24 cases
Subthalamic nucleus 19 cases
Thalamus 18 cases
Cerebral cortex 5 cases

The other paradox is that not all areas stained yellow undergo necrosis and actual damage. Clinically it appears to be an all-or-none phenomenan and there may be yellow staining of the basal ganglia at autopsy when the child died from some other cause without ever showing clinical evidence of kernicterus. The dentate nucleus and the olives, although often stained, very rarely show neuronal loss and gliosis. There is, therefore, selective vulnerability to the staining and even greater selective vulnerability to the gliosis. It is interesting that the basal ganglia, purkinje cells of the cerebellum and the hippocampus are also the most susceptible parts of the brain to hypoxia.

Microscopically the neurones are yellow. Nissl substance disappears, the nuclei become hyperchromatic, glycogen increases and the cell eventually dies to be replaced by gliosis. Because myelination is occurring at this stage, the fibrillary astrocytes formed as part of the scar or healing process may have their processes myelinated, resulting in a marbled appearance of certain nuclei such as the basal ganglia. By electron microscopy the mitochondria can be seen to enlarge, glycogen increases in the cells, and membraneous bodies appear in the purkinje cells.

In vitro bilirubin uncouples oxidative phosphorylation and has a definite toxic effect on isolated mitochondria. The simple explanation of kernicterus is that once bilirubin binding-capacities are exceeded, free lipid-soluble bilirubin enters the nervous system. There then appears to be selective vulnerability and a critical level at which interference with oxidative phosphorylation occurs. The most oxygen-dependent parts of the brain appeared to receive the maximum damage (consumption asphyxia). This does not appear, however, to be the only answer. One cannot simply take a plasma concentration and equate it with inevitable brain damage. There may be kernicterus at plasma bilirubin concentrations as low as 220 μmol/L in the premature infant and yet bilirubin concentrations of over 850 μmol/L may not cause clinical kernicterus in certain infants with rhesus isoimmunization. If one infuses albumin, the plasma-bound bilirubin rises as bilirubin is removed from tissues. The bilirubin concentration therefore rises but the risk of kernicterus lessens. There is no absolute value of bilirubin PO_2, phenylalanine, or ammonia at which brain damage occurs as neuronal toxicity is multifactorial. This is in part because measuring substances in plasma is doing it on the wrong side of the blood–brain barrier.

False neurotransmitters

In view of the variable and reversible nature of hepatic encephalopathy it has been thought that one likely mechanism was the production of substances that acted as false neurotransmitters (Fischer, 1974). It was felt, e.g. in proprionic acidaemia, that the hypotonia was due to the production of proprionyl choline, which showed competitive inhibition of acetylcholine receptors. There is, however, no evidence of a myasthenic component or excessive fatigue in these infants.

Serotonin was incriminated because of a rise in 5-hydroxyindoleacetic acid in the CSF. This was especially the case as there was a rise in free plasma tryptophan in hepatic encephalopathy, i.e. the precursor of 5-hydroxytryptamine. The rises in plasma tyrosine and phenylalanine were thought to indicate a possible block in production of thyroxine, adrenaline and dopamine.

Abnormal neurotransmitter substances, i.e. octopamine and tyramine (Faraj *et al.*, 1976), are produced in hepatic coma and the concentration in plasma are raised (Lam *et al.*, 1973). There appears to be a correlation between the level of octopamine and hepatic coma. This led to the use of bromocriptine in the treatment of hepatic coma. Intrathecal octopamine, however, has no effect when administered to animals (Zieve and Olsen, 1977). Dopamine levels have been found to be normal in brain and octopamine is not raised in the brains of patients dying from hepatic encephalopathy (Cuilleret, 1980).

The latest neurotransmitter in the field to be incriminated is GABA, which is produced by a bacterial action in the colon and is absorbed (Weber, 1984). This is the major inhibitory neurotransmitter and might be expected to cause an encephalopathy. GABA has been administered by mouth or intravenously for many years as theoretically an ideal anticonvulsant, but passage across the blood–brain barrier is minimal. Chemically related compounds, however, can be used as anaesthetic agents and will produce coma. GABA acts on the chloride ionophore and ammonia also has an effect, so that there could be a synergistic effect increasing the amount of brain inhibition. If the endothelial cells fail then enzymes such as GABA transaminase or dopamine transaminase that normally prevent entry into the brain may not stop the entry of increased concentrations of GABA and octopamine from plasma. Glutamine concentrations in brain are high and may cause an increase in endogenous GABA produced in the brain itself. This could explain how benzodiazepine antagonists rapidly reverse hepatic encephalopathy in some cases and also the low incidence of convulsions in true Reye syndrome.

In summary, therefore, there are a vast number of toxic compounds produced in hepatic coma that have an effect on brain mitochondrial function or act as neurotransmitters. No one substance appears to be unequivocally the main culprit. Synergism between different compounds such as ammonia, mercaptans, bilirubin and fatty acids may be responsible and add to the already compromised brain mitochondrial function.

Vascular damage

The endothelial cells of brain capillaries are unique in a number of ways. They are sealed together by tight endothelial junctions and there is an absence of fenestrations between cells seen in other capillary beds. This means that transfer of substances between plasma and brain interstitial fluid is transcellular across the endothelial cells and not intercellular.

The endothelial cells are surrounded by pericytes that have phagocytic properties and this, together with the foot processes of astrocytes, constitute the blood–brain barrier (Figure 1). The blood–brain barrier is metabolically very active, as reflected by the fact that these endothelial cells have up to five times more mitochondria than hepatocytes or muscle cells (Oldendorf and Brown, 1975). Hence, it is not surprising that metabolic diseases that affect mitochondrial function or the integrity of the endothelial cell can cause cerebral upsets, either by altering the surface characteristics of these cells, facilitating platelet adhesion and thrombus formation, or predisposing to vasogenic cerebral oedema.

Metabolic disorders known to cause cerebrovascular accidents (Natowicz and Kelley, 1987) are: sulphite oxidase deficiency; molybdenum cofactor deficiency; protein C deficiency; protein S deficiency; homocystinuria; OTC deficiency; Fabry disease; Leigh encephalopathy; Menke syndrome; MELAS syndrome; methylmalonic aciduria; and isovaleric aciduria. In the case of Leigh encephalopathy, for example, there are small-vessel thromboses with multiple small infarcts associated with vascular proliferation. Infarcted areas and abnormal vessels may calcify, and it is particularly likely to occur in the basal ganglia, which show necrosis, cavitation, oedema and

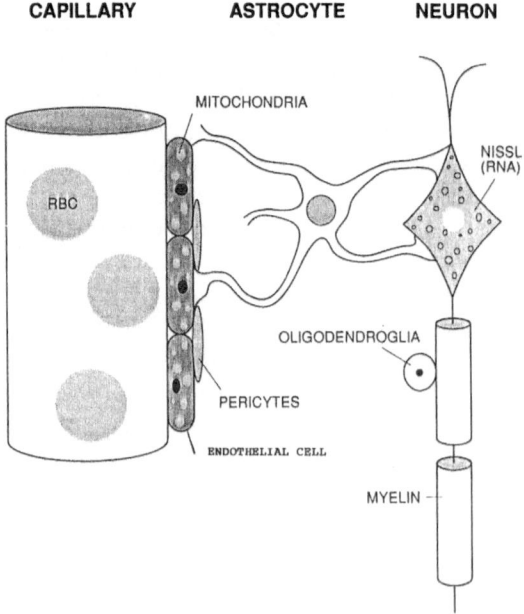

Figure 1 Schematic representation of the blood–brain barrier

calcification. This stresses the point that mitochondrial disorders can have a primary effect on the CNS, and not only act by deranging hepatocyte mitochondria.

Cerebral oedema

Swelling of the brain may be due to cerebral congestion or cerebral oedema, which is defined as an increase in volume of whole or part of the brain due to an increase in water content (Pappius and Feindel, 1976) (see Table 4). Cerebral oedema may be classified into extracellular, intracellular and myelinoclastic (Table 5) (Brown and Habel, 1976; Brown, 1991b).

Table 4 Brain swelling

Expanded intravascular volume
Increased intracellular water
Increased cell volume — metabolic storage
Myelin oedema (not same as white-matter oedema)

The brain swelling seen in hepatic encephalopathy and Reye syndrome is most likely due to a mixture of vasogenic cerebral oedema caused by an endothelial mitochondropathy and an increase in brain intravascular volume, that is to say, cerebral congestion.

Cerebral oedema causes a rise in intracranial pressure and this results in shifts and cones on the one hand and an impairment of cerebral circulation on the other. These effects are aggrevated by lumbar punctures (Brown, 1976). Cones through the tentorium and foramen magnum cause impaction syndromes leading to vascular impairment in the mid-brain and brain stem (Johnson and Yates, 1956). Clinically this manifests as hyperventilation followed by bradypnoea, loss of consciousness, pupillary dilatation, and loss of homeostasis leading to dopamine-dependent vasoparalytic shock. Monitoring of intracranial pressure (Table 6) is hence mandatory in the management of Reye syndrome and mitochondrial encephalopathies (Minns, 1977; Brown and Steer, 1986).

Table 5 Types of cerebral oedema

Extracellular oedema
Vasogenic
Hydrostatic
Hydrocephalic
Osmotic
Necrotic

Intracellular oedema
Osmotic
Failure of cell excretion of H_2O

Myelinoclastic oedema
Metabolic oedema
Toxic

Table 6   Methods of monitoring intracranial pressure

Lumbar puncture (transducer attached to needle)
Cysternal puncture
Subarachnoid puncture (neonatal via angle of fontanelle
Direct ventricular puncture via fontanelle
Burr hole and ventricular puncture
Burr hole and ventricular catheter
Perforation of skull with sternal marrow needle and catheter, into ventricle
Insertion of ventriculostomy reservoir
Surface catheter via burr hole
Surface transducer via burr hole
Insertion Leeds screw or Philadelphia bolt

Hypoxic ischaemic damage

We have already mentioned that metabolic disease can cause cerebrovascular accidents by major vessel occlusion leading to hypoxic ischaemic damage. Fits are common accompaniment of metabolic disease and these increase brain oxygen requirement by up to 400%. If this is allowed to persist, severe brain damage from consumptive asphyxia results. Cerebral oedema results in cerebral ischaemia.

Table 7   Possible reasons for failure to compensate for acute hypoxia

Glucose availability
Glucose-6-phosphatase deficiency
Partial glycogenoses
Adrenal hypoplasia, adrenal hyperplasia
Septo-optic dysplasia (abnormal glucoreceptors)
Pyruvate complex deficiency

Ketone availability
Medium-chain acyl-CoA deficiency
Multiple acyl-CoA deficiency
3-OH, 3-methylglutaryl-CoA lyase deficiency

Mitochondrial energy disorders
Carnitine deficiencies
Krebs cycle abnormalities
Cytochrome chain abnormalities

Cardiac output restriction
Myocardial disease
Drugs, e.g. β-blockers
Dysautonomia
Complicating hypovolaemia or septic shock

Respiratory failure
Airways obstruction — vomit, blood, saliva, tongue
Acute Mendelsohn syndrome aspiration, hydrochloric gastric acid
Central apnoae, muscle contraction
Controlled ventilation of respirator
Drugs, e.g. benzodiazepines and barbiturates

Table 8   Mechanisms of anoxic brain damage

Consumptive asphyxia (demand outstrips supply energy)
Excitotoxicity (glutamate stimulation of cell beyond energy supply)
Substrate failure (hypoglycaemia, failure of ketone production)
Intracellular acidosis (aggravated by excess substrate supply, e.g.
    glucose)
ATP depletion
Rupture of lysosomes (cell suicide)
Calcium invasion with cytotoxicity
Release of S–S/S–H groups
Free radicle toxicity (e.g. epoxides)
Failure of microcirculation from thromboplastin release
Osmotic disruption — release of idiogenic osmols and failure to
    excrete metabolic water

Many children with metabolic diseases are well until they are stressed by exercise (e.g. in carnitine palmitoyl transferase deficiency), starvation (medium-chain acyl dehydrogenase deficiency), receive a high protein load (arginosuccinic aciduria) or develop an infection. We see a small but steady number of neonates subjected to perinatal asphyxia who are devastated out of proportion with the degree of asphyxia. This may be due to a failure of compensatory mechanisms such as the mobilization of glucose from glycogen (Burchell *et al.*, 1989) (Table 7).

There are many possible ways that hypoxia may cause cell death (Table 8) and currently there is a lot of interest in excitotoxicity due to excessive glutamate production (Rothman and Alney, 1986). Hypoxic ischaemic damage leading to cell death is a major cause of chronic brain damage syndromes such as cerebral palsy, mental handicap and epilepsy and is the final common path by which permanent brain damage and handicap may arise in children with Reye syndrome or metabolic disease.

REFERENCES

Adams, R. D. and Foley, J. M. The neurological disorders associated with brain disease. In: Meritt, H. H. and Hare, C. C. (eds.) *Metabolic and Toxic Diseases of the Nervous System*, Vol. 32. Williams and Williams, Baltimore, 1953, pp. 198–237

Alberts, B., Bray, D., Lewis, J., Raff, M., Roberts, K. and Watson, J. D. The mitochondria. In: *The Cell.* Garland Press, New York, 1989, pp. 342–366

Ansevin, C. F. Reye syndrome: Serum induced alteration in brain mitochondrial function are blocked by fatty acids free albumin. *Neurology* 30 (1980) 160–166

Bakay, L., Crawford, J. D. and White, J. C. The effects of intravenous fluids on cerebrospinal fluid pressure. *Surg. Gynaecol. Obstet.* 99 (1954) 48–52

Baker, A. L. Amino acids in liver disease, a cause of hepatic encephalopathy. *J. Am. Med. Assoc.* 242 (1979) 355–356

Beks, J. W. F. and Kerckhoffs, H. P. M. Studies on the water content of cerebral tissues and intracranial pressure in vasogenic brain oedema. In: Brock, M. and Dietz, H. (eds.) *Intracranial Pressure 1*. Springer Verlag, Berlin, 1972, pp. 119–126

Benjamin, A. M. Control of glutaminase activity in rat brain cortex in vitro. Influence of glutamate, phosphate, ammonia, calcium and hydrogen ions. *Brain Res.* 208 (1981) 363–377

Bessman, S. P. and Bradley, J. E. Uptake of ammonia by muscle: its implications in ammoniogenic coma. *N. Engl. J. Med.* 253 (1955) 1143–1147

Bickford, R. G. and Butt, H. R. Hepatic coma and the electroencephalographic pattern. *J. Clin. Invest.* 34 (1955) 790–799

Blasberg, R. G. Clearance of serum albumin from brain extracellular fluid, a possible role in cerebral oedema. In: Pappius, H. M. and Feindel, W. (eds.) *Dynamics of Brain Oedema*. Springer Verlag, Berlin, 1972, pp. 98–102

Blaschke, T. F., Berk, P. D. and Scharschmidt, B. F. Crigler–Najjar syndrome an unusual course with development of neurologic damage at age 18. *Paediatr. Res.* 8 (1974) 573–590

Bonell, H. J. and Beckwith, J. B. Fatty liver in sudden childhood death, implications for Reye's syndrome? *Assoc. J. Dis. Child.* 140 (1986) 30–33

Borbola, J., Papp, J. G. and Szekeres, L. Effects of octanoate on the electrical activity of Purkinje cell. *Experientia* 30 (1974) 262–264

Bove, K. E., McAdams, A. J. and Partin, J. C. The hepatic lesion in Reye's syndrome. *Gastroenterology* 69 (1975) 685–697

Bougeneres, P. F., Rocchicciola, F. and Kolvra, S. Medium chain acyl CoA dehydrogenase deficiency in two siblings with a Reye like syndrome. *J. Paediatr.* 106 (1985) 918–921

Brain, W. R., Hunter, D. and Turnbull, H. M. Acute meningoencephalitis of childhood. Report of 6 cases. *Lancet* 1 (1929) 221–227

Brown, J. K. Lumbar puncture and its hazards. *Dev. Med. Child Neurol.* 18 (1976) 803–816

Brown, J. K. Valproate toxicity. *Dev. Med. Child. Neurol.* 30 (1988) 115–125

Brown, J. K. Mechanisms of production of raised intracranial pressure. In Minns, R. A. (ed.) *Problems of Intracranial Pressure in Childhood*. MacKeith Press, Oxford, 1991a, pp. 13–37

Brown, J. K. The pathological effects of raised intracranial pressure. In Minns, R. A. (ed.) *Problems of Intracranial Pressure in Childhood*. MacKeith Press, Oxford, 1991b, pp. 38–76

Brown, J. K. and Habel, A. H. Toxic encephalopathy and acute brain swelling in children. *Dev. Med. Child Neurol.* 17 (1976) 659–679

Brown, J. K., Ingram, T. T. S. and Seisha, S. S. Patterns of decerebration in infants and children. *J. Neurol. Neurosurg.* 36 (1973) 431–434

Brown, J. K. and Steer, C. R. S. Strategies in the management of acute encephalopathies. In: Gordon, N. and McKinlay, I. (eds.) *Neurologically Sick Children*. Blackwell Scientific, Oxford, 1986, pp. 219–294

Brown, R. E. and Madge, G. E. Fatty acid and mitochondrial injury in Reye's syndrome. *N. Engl. J. Med.* 286 (1972) 287–288

Bruton, C. J., Corsellis, J. A. N. and Russel, A. Hereditary hyperammoninaemia. *Brain* 93 (1970) 423–434

Burchell, A., Waddell, I. D., Stewart, L. and Hume, R. Perinatal diagnosis of type IC glycogen storage disease. *J. Inher. Metab. Dis.* 12 (1989), Suppl. 2, 315–317

Cavanagh, J. B. and Kyu, M. H. Type II Alzheimer changes experimentally produced in astrocytes in the rat. *J. Neurol. Sci.* 12 (1971) 63–75

Center for Disease Control. Follow up on Reye's syndrome. *United States Morbidity and Mortality weekly report.* 29 (1980) 321–322

Chen, S., Sieve, L. and Mahadevan, V. Mercaptans and dimethyl sulfide in the breath of patients with cirrhosis of the liver. *J. Lab. Clin. Med.* 75 (1970) 628–635

Claireaux, A. E. Hemolytic disease of the newborn. A clinical pathological study of 157 cases. *Arch. Dis. Child.* 25 (1950) 61–80

Coates, P. M., Hale, D. E. and Stanley, C. A. Systemic carnitine deficiency stimulating Reye's syndrome. *J. Paediatr.* 105 (1984) 679–682

Cuilleret, G., Pomier-Layarargues, G., Pons, F., Cadilhac, J. and Michel, H. Changes in brain catecholamine levels in human cirrhotic hepatic encephalopathy. *Gut* 21 (1980) 656–569

Dahl, D. R. Short chain fatty acid inhibition of rat brain Na/K. Adenosine triphosphatase. *J. Neurol. Chem.* 15 (1968) 815–820

Diamond, I., Bilirubin encephalopathy. In Goldensohn, E. S., Appel, S. H., (eds.) *Scientific Approaches to Clinical Neurology*. Lea and Febiger, Philadelphia, 1977, pp. 1212–1233

Editorial. Reye's syndrome and aspirin epidemiological association and inborn errors of metabolism. *Lancet* 2 (1987) 421–431

Edwards, J. C., Howell, S. C. and Taylor, K. W. Fatty acids as regulators of glucagon secretion. *Nature* 224 (1969) 808–809

Faraj, B. A., Bowers, P. A., Isaacs, J. W. and Rudman, D. Hypertyraminaemia in cirrhotic patients. *N. Engl. J. Med.* 294 (1976) 1360–1363

Filipe, J. I. and Lake, B. D. *Histochemistry in Pathology*. Churchill Livingstone, Edinburgh, 1983, pp. 53–69

Finberg, L., Luttrell, C. and Redd, H. Pathogenesis of lesions in the nervous system in hypernatraemic states. 2 experimental studies of gross anatomical changes and alterations of chemical composition of the tissues. *Paediatrics* 23 (1959) 46–53

Fischer, J. E. *False Neurotransmitters and Hepatic Coma*. Research Publications. Association Nervous and Mental Disorders, 53. Raven Press, New York, 1974, 53–73

Fishman, R. A. Effects of isotonic intravenous solutions on normal and increased intracranial pressure. *Arch. Neurol. Psychiatry* 70 (1953) 350–360

Gerschenfeld, H. M., Wald, F., Zadunaisky, J. A. and De Roberts, E. D. P. Functions of astroglia in the water ion metabolism of the central nervous system. An electron microscopic study. *Neurology* 9 (1959) 412–425

Glasgow, A. M., Eng, G. and Engel, A. G. Systemic carnitine deficiency simulating Reye's syndrome. *J. Paediatr.* 96 (1980) 889–891

Glasgow, J. F. T., Hicks, E. M., Jenkins, J. G., Keilty, S. R., Black, G. W. and Kannin, T. F. Reye's syndrome. *Br. J. Hosp. Med.* 34 (1985) 42–45

Glion, E., Szemberg, A. and Taubman, L. G. Glutamine estimation in cerebrospinal fluid in cases of liver cirrhosis and hepatic coma. *J. Lab. Clin. Med.* 53 (1959) 714–719

Grimm, G., Ferenci, P., Katzenschlager, R. and Madl, C. Improvement of hepatic encephalopathy treated with flumazenil. *Lancet* 2 (1988) 1392–1394

Habel, A. H. and Simpson, H. Osmolar relation between cerebrospinal fluid and serum in hyperosmolar hypernatraemic dehydration. *Arch. Dis. Child.* 51 (1976) 660–666

Hall, S. M. Reye's syndrome and aspirin. A review. *J. R. Soc. Med.* 79 (1986) 596–598

Hall, S. and Bellman, M. Reye's syndrome in the British Isles. First annual report of the joint British Paediatric Association and Communicable Disease Surveillance Center Surveillance Scheme. *Br. Med. J.* 288 (1984) 548–550

Hockwald, G. M., Marlin, A. E., Wald, A. and Malhan, C. Movement of water between blood brain and CSF as cerebral oedema. In: Pappius, J. H. M. and Feindel, W. (eds.) *Dynamics of Brain Edema*. Springer Verlag, Berlin, 1976, pp 129–137

Hourani, B. T., Harrlin, E. M. and Reynolds, T. B. Cerebrospinal fluid glutamine as a measure of hepatic encephalopathy. *Arch. Intern. Med.* 127 (1971) 1033–1036

Hurwitz, E. S. and Goodman, R. A. A cluster of cases of Reye's syndrome associated with chickenpox. *Paediatrics* 70 (1982) 901–906

Hurwitz, E. S., Nelson, D. B., Davis, C., Morens, D. and Schonberger, L. B. National surveillance for Reye's syndrome: a 5 year review. *Paediatrics* 70 (1982) 895–900

Huttenlocher, P. R., Schwartz, A. D. and Klatskin, G. Reye's syndrome: ammonia intoxication as a possible factor in encephalopathy. *Paediatrics* 43 (1969) 443–454

Johnson, R. T. and Yates, P. O. Brain stem haemorrhages in expanding supratentorial conditions. *Acta Radiol.* 46 (1956) 250–256

Kay, J. D. S., Hilton-Jones, D. and Hyman, N. Valproate toxicity and ornithine carbamyl transferase deficiency. *Lancet* 2 (1986) 1283–1284

Kinsell, L. W., Harper, H. A., Giese, G. K. and Margen, S. Studies in methionine metabolism. *J. Clin. Invest.* 28 (1949) 1439–1450

Laidlaw, J. and Read, A. E. The E.E.G. on hepatic encephalopathy. *Clin. Sci.* 24 (1963) 109–120

Lam, K. C., Tall, A. R., Goldstein, G. B. and Mistills, S. P. Role of a false neurochemical transmitter, octopamine in the pathogenesis of hepatic and renal encephalopathy. *Scand. J. Gastroenterol.* 8 (1973) 465–472

Levin, M., Kay, J. D. S. and Gould, J. D. Haemorrhagic shock and encephalopathy: a new syndrome with a high mortality in young children. *Lancet* 2 (1983) 64–67

Linscheer, W. G., Blum, A. L. and Platt, R. R. Transfer of medium chain fatty acids from blood to spinal fluid in patients with cirrhosis. *Gastroenterology* 58 (1970) 509–515

Lockwood, A. H. Ammonia induced encephalopathy. In: McCandless, S. W. (ed.) *Cerebral Energy Metabolism and Metabolic Encephalopathy.* Plenum Press, New York, 1985, pp. 203–207

Lockwood, A. H., Ginsberg, M. D., Butler, C. M. and Cuttierez, M. T. Selective effects of ammonia on regional brain glucose metabolism. *Ann. Neurol.* 12 (1982) 114–120

Lou, H. C., Lassen, N. A., Tweed, W. A., Johnson, G., Jones, M. and Palahniuk, R. K. Pressure passive cerebral blood flow and breakdown of the blood-brain barrier in experimental fetal asphyxia. *Acta Paediatr. Scand.* 68 (1979) 57–63

Lovejoy, F. H., Smith, A. L., Bressman, M. J., Wood, J. N., Victor, D. I. and Adams, P. E. Clinical staging in Reye's syndrome. *Am. J. Dis. Child.* 128 (1974) 36–41

Martinez-Hernandes, A., Bell, K. P. and Norenberg, M. D. Glutamine synthetase: glial localisation in brain. *Science* 195 (1977) 1356–1358

Mamunes, P., DeVries, G. H., Miller, C. D. and David, R. B. Fatty acid quantitation in Reye's syndrome. In: Pollack, J. D. (ed.) *Reye's Syndrome.* Grune and Stratton, New York, 1975, pp. 245–254

McClain, C. J., Zieve, L., Doizaki, W. M., Gilbertstadt, S. and Onstat, G. R. Blood methianethiol in alcoholic liver disease with and without hepatic encephalopathy. *Gut* 21 (1980) 318–323

Milhorat, T. H. *Cerebrospinal Fluid and the Brain Edemas.* Neuroscience Society, New York, 1987

Minns, R. A. Clinical application of ventricular pressure monitoring in children. *Zeitschrift fur Kinderchirurgie und Grenzgebiete* 224 (1977) 430–443

Montague, W. and Taylor, K. W. Regulation of insulin secretion by short chain fatty acids. *Nature* 217 (1968) 853

Natowicz, M. and Kelley, R. Mendelian etiologies of stroke. *Ann. Neurol.* 21 (1987) 175–189

Norenberg, M. D. A light and electron microscopic study of experimental portal–systemic (ammonia) encephalopathy. *Lab. Invest.* 36 (1977) 618–627

Norenberg, M. D. and Lapham, L. W. The astrocyte response in experimental portal–systemic encephalopathy: An electron microscopic study. *J. Neuropathol. Exp. Neurol.* 33 (1974) 422–435

Odell, G. B. and Schutta, M. S. Bilirubin encephalopathy. In: McCandless, D. (ed.) *Cerebral Energy Metabolism and Metabolic Encephalopathy.* Plenum Press, New York, 1985, pp. 229–261

Oldendorf, W. H. and Brown, J. W. Greater number of capiliary endothelial cell mitochondria in brain than muscle. *Proc. Soc. Exp. Biol. Med.* 149 (1975) 736–738

Pappius, H. M. and Feindel, W. (eds.) *Dynamics of Brain Edema.* Springer Verlag, Berlin, 1976

Partin, J. C., Partin, J. S., Schubert, W. K. and McLaurin, R. L. Brain ultrastructure in Reye's syndrome. *J. Neuropathol. Exp. Neurol.* 34 (1975) 425–444

Perry, L. T., Hansen, S. and MacLean, J. CSF and plasma glutamine elevation by anticonvulsant therapy, a potential diagnostic and therapeutic trap. *Clin. Res.* 33 (1975) 610A

Phelps, M. W., Hoffman, E. J. and Raybard, C. Factors which affect the uptake and retention of 13 NH3. *Stroke* 8 (1977) 694–702

Pollitt, R. J. Inherited disorders of straight chain fatty acid oxidation. *Arch. Dis. Child.* 62 (1987) 6–7

Raichle, M. E. and Grubb, R. L. Regulation of brain water permeability by centrally released vasopressin. *Brain Res.* 143 (1978) 191–194

Rennebohm, R. M., Heubi, J. E., Daugherty, C. C. and Daniels, S. R. Reye's syndrome in children receiving salicylate therapy for connective tissue disease. *J. Paediatr.* 107 (1985) 877–880

Reye, R. D. K., Morgan, G. and Baral, J. Encephalopathy and fatty degeneration of the viscera: A disease entity in childhood. *Lancet* 2 (1963) 749–752

Roe, C. R., Millington, D. S., Maltby, D. A. and Kinnebrew, P. Recognition of medium chain assay CoA dehydrogenase deficiency in asymptomatic siblings of children dying of sudden infant death or Reye like syndrome. *J. Paediatr.* 108 (1986) 13–18

Rothman, S. M. and Ulney, J. W. Glutamate and the pathophysiology of hypoxic–ischaemic brain damage. *Ann. Neurol.* 19 (1986) 105–111

Rothstein, J. D. and Herlong, H. F. Neurologic manifestation of hepatic disease. *Neurol. Clin.* 7 (1989) 563–578

Rudman, D., Glambos, J. T., Smith, R. B., Salam, A. and Warren, W. D. (1973). Comparison of the effects of various amino acids upon the blood ammonia concentration of patients with liver disease. *Am. J. Clin. Nutr.* 26 (1973) 916–925

Shults, W. T., Fountain, E. N. and Lynch, C. E. Methanethiol poisoning — irreversible coma and haemolytic anaemia following inhalation. *J. Am. Med. Assoc.* 211 (1970) 2153–2154

Sinniah, D. and Baskaran, G. Margosa oil poisoning in a case of Reye's syndrome. *Lancet* 1 (1981) 487–489

Stahl, J. Studies of the blood ammonia in liver disease. The diagnostic, prognostic and therapeutic significance. *Ann. Intern. Med.* 58 (1963) 1–24

Starko, K. M. and Mullick, F. G. Hepatic and cerebral pathology findings in children with fatal salicylate intoxication: further evidence of a causal relationship between salicylate and Reye's syndrome. *Lancet* 1 (1983) 326–329

Tanaka, K., Kean, E. A. and Johnson, B. Jamaican vomiting sickness: biochemical investigation of 2 cases. *N. Engl. J. Med.* 295 (1976) 461–467

Tanner, S. *Paediatric Hepatology.* Current Reviews in Paediatrics. Churchill Livingstone, Edinburgh, 1989, pp. 223–255

Trauner, D. A. and Adams, H. Intracranial pressure elevations during octanoate infusion in rabbits: an experimental model of Reye's syndrome. *Paediatr. Res.* 15 (1981) 1097–1099

Vaklamp, T., Meijer, A. J., Wilms, J. and Chamuleau, R. A. F. Inhibition of mitochondrial electron transfer in rats by ethanethiol and methane-thiol. *Clin. Sci.* 56 (1979) 147–156

Vergara, F., Plum, F. and Duffy, T. E. Alpha ketoglutaramate: increased concentration in CSF of patients in hepatic coma. *Science* 1983 (1974) 81–83

Waller, R. L. Methanethiol inhibition of mitochondrial respiration. *Toxicol. Appl. Pharmacol.* 42 (1977) 111–117

Warren, K. S. and Schenker, S. Effect of an inhibitor of glutamine synthesis (methionine sulfoximine) on ammonia toxicity and metabolism. *J. Lab. Clin. Med.* 64 (1964) 442–449

Wasterlain, C. E. and Posner, J. B. Cerebral edema in water intoxication. Clinical and chemical observations. *Arch. Neurol.* 19 (1968) 71–78

Weber, F. L. Hepatic encephalopathy. In: Williams, R. and Maddrey, W. C. (eds.) *Liver.* Butterworths, London, 1984, pp. 242–282

Weizman, Z., Mussafi, H. and Ishay, J. S. Multiple hornet stings with features of Reye's syndrome. *Gastroenterology* 89 (1985) 1407–1410

Wojtczac, L. Effects of long chain fatty acids and acetyl CoA on mitochondrial permeability and energy coupling processes. *J. Bioeng. Biomembranes* 8 (1976) 293–311

Zieve, L. Coma production with NH_4^+ synergistic factors. *Gastroenterology* 78 (1980) 1327

Zieve, L. Encephalopathy due to short and medium chain fatty acid. In: McCandless, D. W. (ed.) *Cerebral Energy Metabolism and Metabolic Encephalopathy.* Plenum Press, New York, 1985, pp. 163–177

Zieve, L. and Brunner, G. Encephalopathy due to mercaptans and phenols. In: McCandless, D. W. (ed.) *Cerebral Energy Metabolism and Metabolic Encephalopathy.* Plenum Press, New York, 1985, pp. 179–210

Zieve, L. and Olson, R. L. Can hepatic coma be caused by a reduction of brain noradrenaline or dopamine? *Gut* 18 (1977) 688–691

Zieve, L., Doizaki, W. M. and Zieve, F. J. Synergism between mercaptans and ammonia or fatty acids in the production of coma. *J. Lab. Clin. Med.* 83 (1974) 16–28

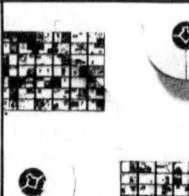

J. Inher. Metab. Dis. 14 (1991) 459–477
© SSIEM and Kluwer Academic Publishers.

Fetal and Neonatal Bile Acid Synthesis and Metabolism – Clinical Implications

W. F. BALISTRERI
*Children's Hospital Research Foundation, Elland and Bethesda Avenues,
Cincinnati, Ohio 45229, USA*

Summary: It has become apparent that with sophisticated technology we are now able to recognize defective bile acid metabolism in a wide variety of disease states. Recognition of specific aberrations, such as inborn errors in bile acid metabolism manifesting as neonatal cholestasis, offers new opportunities for therapeutic intervention. Future studies should determine the incidence of inborn errors in patients with enigmatic and unexplained liver diseases such as idiopathic neonatal hepatitis.

A sequence of metabolic and transport processes occurring in the liver (bile acid synthesis, conjugation and secretion) serves to maintain cholesterol balance, facilitate bile flow, and provide surface active detergent molecules which promote intestinal absorption of lipid. Proper functioning of this system involves an efficient ileal conservation mechanism, through which bile acid molecules are rescued from faecal loss and are recycled back to the liver – the enterohepatic circulation. Advances have been made in the characterization of bile acid metabolism and the enterohepatic circulation in healthy adults and children as well as in specific disease states (Dowling, 1972; Festi *et al.*, 1983; Hofmann *et al.*, 1983; LaRusso *et al.*, 1974). Marked differences in bile acid metabolic and transport processes have been noted in the developing infant (Balistreri *et al.*, 1981, 1983; Suchy, 1981b).

The key to our understanding of bile acid physiology and pharmacology has been the development of precise analytical methods. There are readily available assays for bile acids; availability of these kits has permitted bile acid measurements to be carried out by clinical chemistry laboratories throughout the world. In addition, sophisticated methodology such as mass spectrometry has allowed for the identification of specific abnormalities of bile acid metabolism.

In this review we will outline bile acid synthesis and metabolism in health, highlighting age-related differences, provide an overview of the enterohepatic circulation, and define where abnormalities in bile acid metabolism may occur.

BILE ACID CHEMISTRY

Bile acids (or salts), a group of compounds belonging to the steroid class, share a cyclopentanoperhydrophenanthrene nucleus (ABCD rings), and a side chain of variable length attached at the C-17 position, with a terminal carboxylic acid (Figure

1). The stereochemistry of the A/B rings, which influences the physicochemical properties of the bile acid in solution, is determined by the configuration of the hydrogen atom at position C-5 (Roda *et al.*, 1983; Hofmann, 1984). A wide variety of bile acids is found in the biological fluids of man and animal species (Haselwood, 1978); these differ from each other by the number and orientation of substituent groups in the nucleus. Bile acids are amphophilic, containing both a hydrophobic (non-polar) region, due to the hydrocarbon or steroid moiety, and a hydrophilic (polar) region, due to the hydroxyl and ionized carboxyl groups.

Bile acid synthesis in humans

Cholesterol is converted in the liver to highly polar primary bile acids; this serves as a major route of cholesterol elimination. The reactions catalysing the conversion of cholesterol to the primary bile acids involve several specific alterations to both the nucleus (hydroxylation) and the side chain (removal of a three carbon group); these are shown in Figure 2 and are detailed in Table 1. In humans the products are the two primary bile acids: cholic acid ($3\alpha,7\alpha,12\alpha$-trihydroxy-5β-cholanoic acid) and chenodeoxycholic acid ($3\alpha,7\alpha$-dihydroxy-5β-cholanoic acid). The newly synthesized bile acids are then conjugated at the carboxylic carbon (Figure 3). Following conjugation, bile acids are secreted into the bile, entering the gall bladder for temporary storage. With meal-stimulated gall bladder contraction, the primary bile acids enter the intestinal lumen where they participate in lipid digestion and absorption. The primary bile acids are then further metabolized in the lumen by the intestinal flora to form secondary bile acids; bacterial deconjugation (catalysed by bacterial hydrolase) and bacterial 7α-dehydroxylation occur (Figure 4). The products of these reactions are the secondary bile acids: deoxycholic acid ($3\alpha,12\alpha$-dihydroxy-5β-cholanoic acid), which arises from cholic acid, and lithocholic acid (3α-hydroxy-5β-cholanoic acid), derived from chenodeoxycholic acid. These secondary bile acids are then reabsorbed to some extent from the intestinal lumen and are recirculated to the liver where they are conjugated with glycine or taurine. Secondary bile acids participate in the enterohepatic circulation along with the primary bile acids; the approximate relative composition of adult biliary bile acids is therefore 36% cholic, 36% chenodeoxycholic, 24% deoxycholic and 1% lithocholic acid.

Lithocholic acid, the secondary monohydroxy bile acid formed from chenodeoxycholic acid by the intestinal flora, is insoluble in water and will precipitate out of solution in the colonic lumen. In contrast to cholic acid, which is a potent choleretic agent, lithocholic acid is capable of causing cholestasis. Lithocholic acid is toxic to cell membranes, including those of hepatocytes and red blood cells; cirrhosis, degeneration of hepatocytes, and bile duct and ductular cell reactions have been produced following lithocholic acid administration (Holsti, 1962; Palmer and Hruban, 1966; Palmer, 1972). These anatomical changes correlate with the inhibition of bile flow. Since lithocholic acid is a constituent of human bile and serum, protective mechanisms must exist in healthy subjects to prevent toxicity; these include sulphation and glucuronidation at the C-3 position to enhance water solubility and thus renal excretion (Matern *et al.*, 1984; Oelberg *et al.*, 1984).

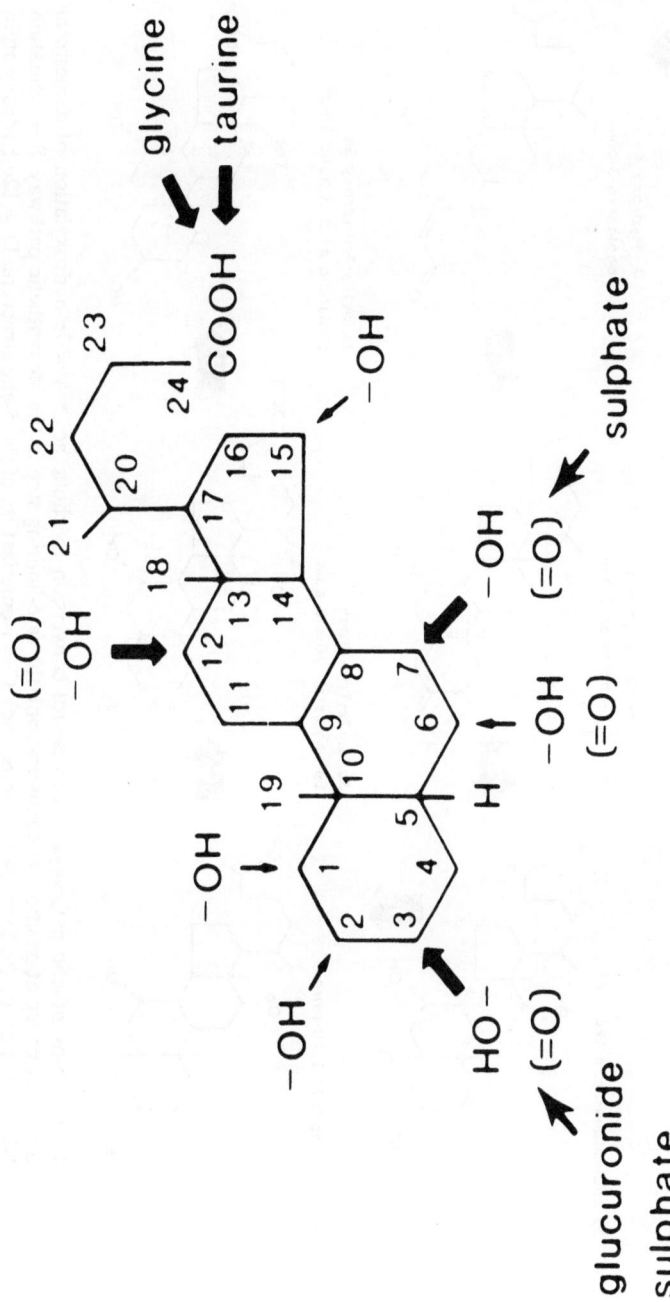

Figure 1 The structure of 5β-cholanoic acid, the bile acid nucleus; the numbering of the carbon atoms and the positions of substituent groups and conjugates are shown; the thickness of the arrow reflects the relative degree of quantitative importance. Reproduced with permission from Balistreri and Setchell (1988).

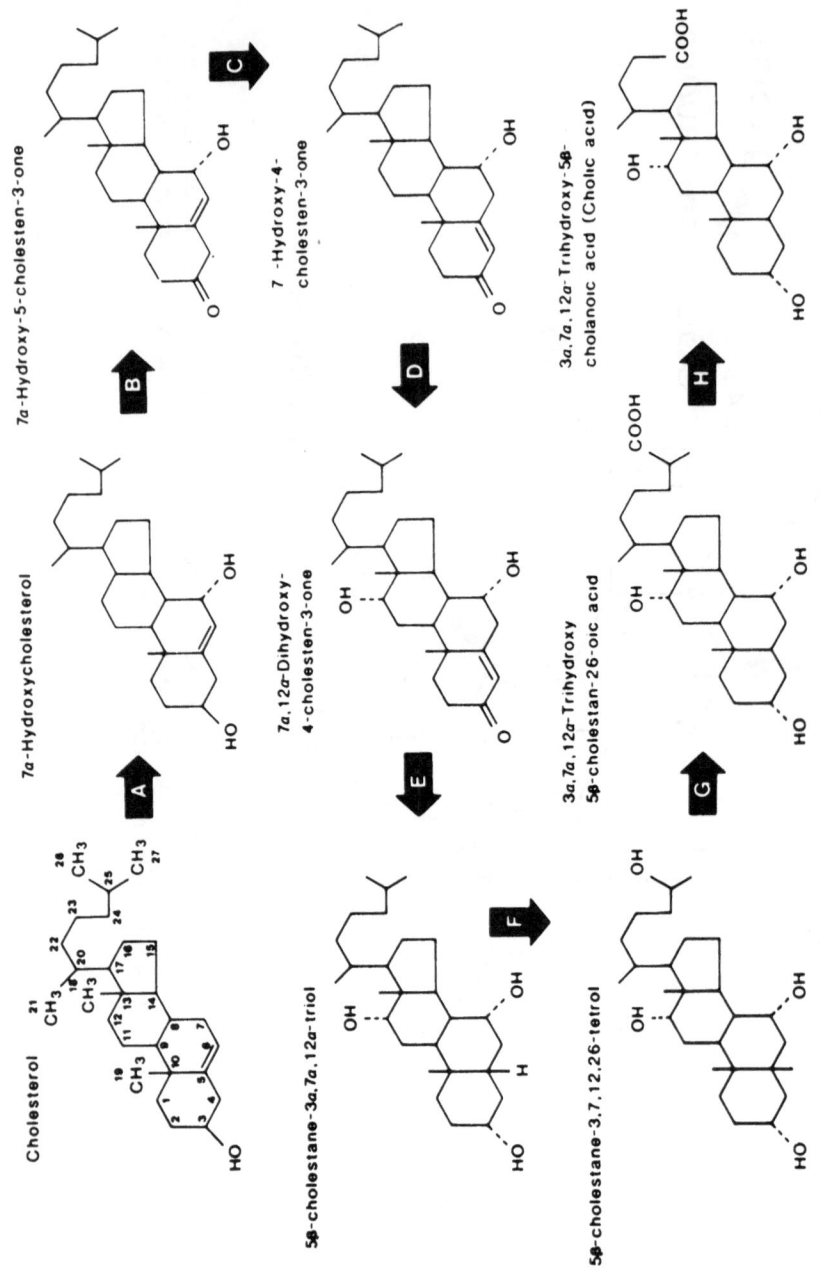

Figure 2 The biosynthetic pathways of cholesterol conversion to cholic acid: A = 7α-hydroxylation of cholesterol (addition of -OH group at position 7α configuration); the rate-limiting step in the biosynthetic pathway. B = oxidation of the 3β-hydroxyl group (to form 3-oxo compound). C = isomerization of the 5-ene structure. D = 12α-hydroxylation (for cholic acid only). E = saturation of the double bond and reduction of the 3-one group. F = hydroxylation of the side chain at C-26 position. G = side chain oxidation to cholestanoic acid. H = hydroxylation at C-24 and β-oxidation to reduce the length of side chain. Reproduced with permission from Balistreri and Setchell (1988).

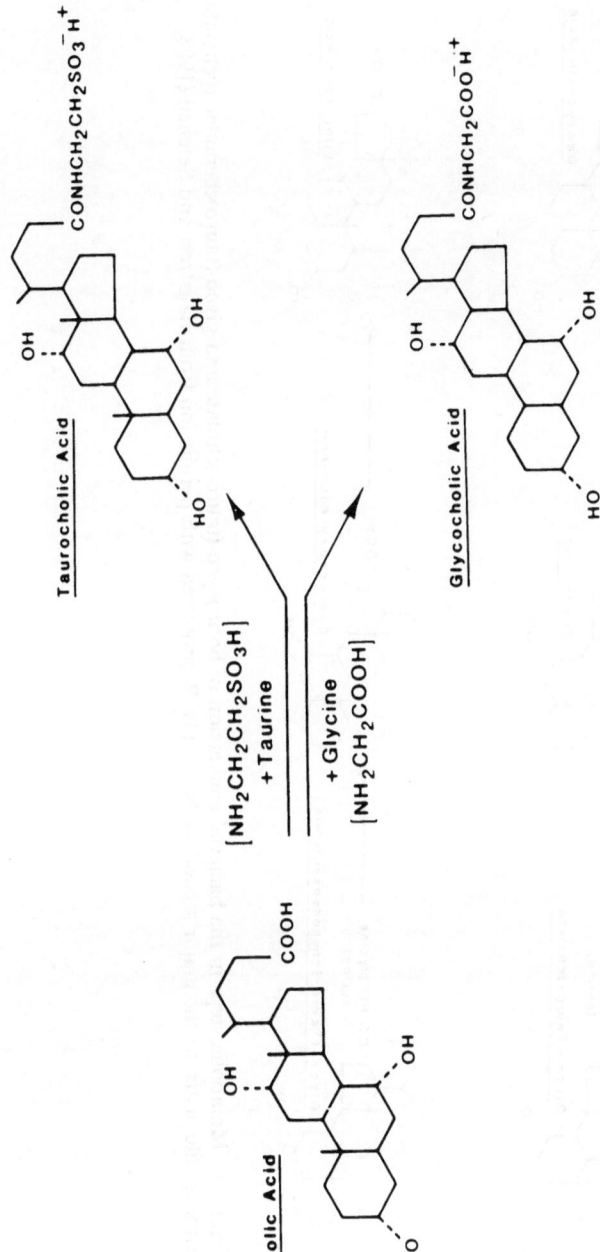

Figure 3 Conjugation of cholic acid at carboxylic acid carbon with either taurine or glycine. This reaction occurs via the formation of a coenzyme A derivative and is catalysed by a bile acid coenzyme A:amino acid *N*-acyltransferase and ligase. In healthy adults glycine conjugates predominate (3.5:1 ratio). Conjugation increases polarity and thus facilitates renal excretion. Reproduced with permission from Balistreri and Setchell (1988).

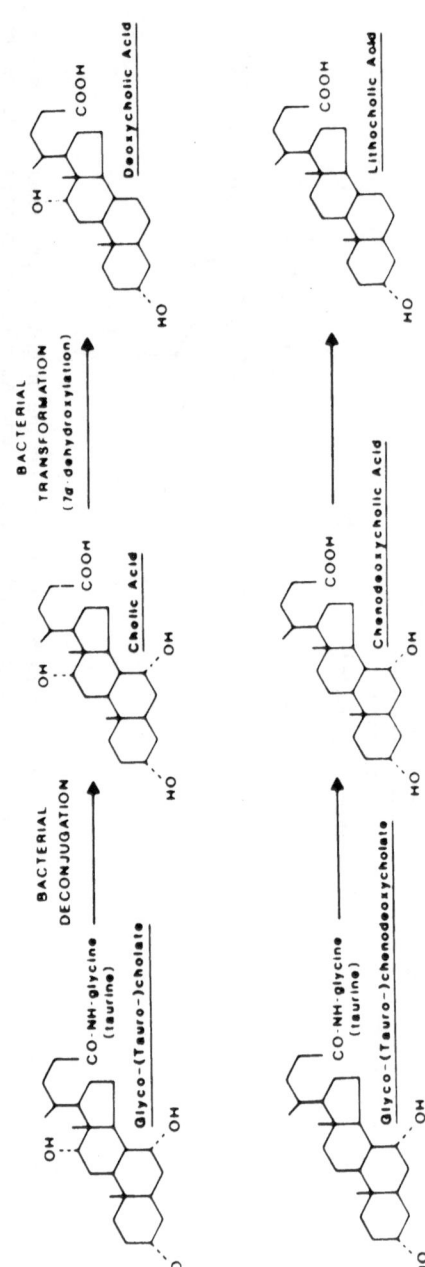

Figure 4 Metabolic steps in the bacterial conversion of both glyco-(tauro-)cholate and glyco-(tauro)chenodeoxycholate, primary bile acids, to the major secondary bile acids. Reproduced with permission from Balistreri and Setchell (1988).

Table 1 Reactions involved in the formation of bile acids from cholesterol (steps refer to arrows in Figure 2)

	Reaction	Enzyme involved	Subcellular location
Step A	C-7 hydroxylation	7α-Hydroxylase	Microsomal
Step B/C	Oxidation 3β-OH → 3-oxo and Δ^5 → Δ^4	3β-HSD/isomerase	Microsomal
Step D	C-12 hydroxylation (cholic acid)	12α-Hydroxylase	Microsomal
Step E	Reduction of Δ^4 → 5β(H)	Δ^4-3-Oxosteroid 5β-reductase	Cystolic
Step F	Reduction of 3-oxo → 3α-OH	3α-HSD	Cystolic
Step G	Side-chain hydroxylation at C-26	26-Hydroxylase	Mitochondrial
Step H	Side-chain oxidation → C-26 COOH	Alcohol/acetaldehyde dehydrogenae	Cystolic
Step I	(i) Formation of CoA derivative	Fatty acid β-oxidation system	Peroxisomal
	(ii) Hydroxylation at C-24	Fatty acid β-oxidation system	Peroxisomal
	(iii) β-Oxidation	Fatty acid β-oxidation system	Peroxisomal

Modified from Setchell (1990)

BILE ACID PHYSIOLOGY

There are multiple physiological functions mediated by bile acids (Table 2). They are of prime importance in processes such as micellular solubilization of lipid and nutrient absorption, therefore efficient conservation via recycling of these compounds is made possible by intestinal reabsorption and hepatic extraction – this recycling process is termed the enterohepatic circulation (Figure 5) (Dowling, 1972; Hofmann *et al.*, 1983; Hofmann and Roda, 1984). The sequence of events is as follows: Bile acids enter the duodenal lumen as mixed micelles following gall bladder contraction. In the lumen cholesterol and phospholipid are replaced in the micelle by the products of lipolysis (free fatty acids). Micelles facilitate fat absorption by: (1) accelerating hydrolysis by lipase; (2) solubilizing lipolytic products; and (3) delivering free fatty acids and monoglycerides to the intestinal mucosal surface for absorption. In order to carry out these functions a minimal bile acid concentration (approximately 2 mmol/L) must be present in the proximal small bowel lumen; this is termed the critical micellar concentration (Hofmann and Roda, 1984).

Bile acids then undergo reabsorption via two complementary mechanisms: (1) active transport in the terminal ileum (Dietschy *et al.*, 1966; Lack and Weiner, 1961, 1966; Dietschy, 1968; Schiff *et al.*, 1972; Wilson, 1981, 1990); the efficiency of ileal active transport is generally a function of polarity and conjugation state. Trihydroxy bile acids are transported more efficiently than dihydroxy bile acids, which in turn are transported more efficiently than monohydroxy bile acids; (2) passive (non-ionic) diffusion, which is dependent on the variable ability of each bile acid to remain undissociated at intestinal pH; the pKa of dihydroxy > trihydroxy bile acids and the pKa of glycine > taurine conjugates.

Subsequent to absorption, during passage in portal venous blood, a constant fraction will 'spill over' into peripheral serum. However, there is efficient hepatic extraction from portal venous blood therefore serum levels remain low ($< 4 \mu$mol/L)

Table 2   Physiological functions of bile acids (modified from Balistreri and Setchell (1988))

A. In the liver
   1. Generate bile flow (Boyer, 1980)
   2. Induce biliary lipid secretion (Gurantz and Hofmann, 1984; Hofmann and Roda, 1984)
   3. Modulate cholesterol biosynthesis
   4. ? Regulation of lipoprotein membrane receptors

B. In bile
   1. Desaturate bile (Gurantz and Hofmann, 1984; Hofmann and Roda, 1984)
   2. Transport cholesterol (Carey and Small, 1978)
   3. Buffer Ca^{2+} ion

C. In the intestine
   1. Form micelles (fat digestion) (Hofmann, 1963)
   2. Accelerate lipid (e.g. vitamin E absorption) transport (Hofmann and Borgstrom, 1964)
   3. Modulate motility (Flynn *et al.*, 1979)
   4. Modulate GI hormone output (Hanssen, 1980)
   5. Induce ion (and water) secretion (Mekhjian *et al.*, 1971; Chadwick *et al.*, 1979)

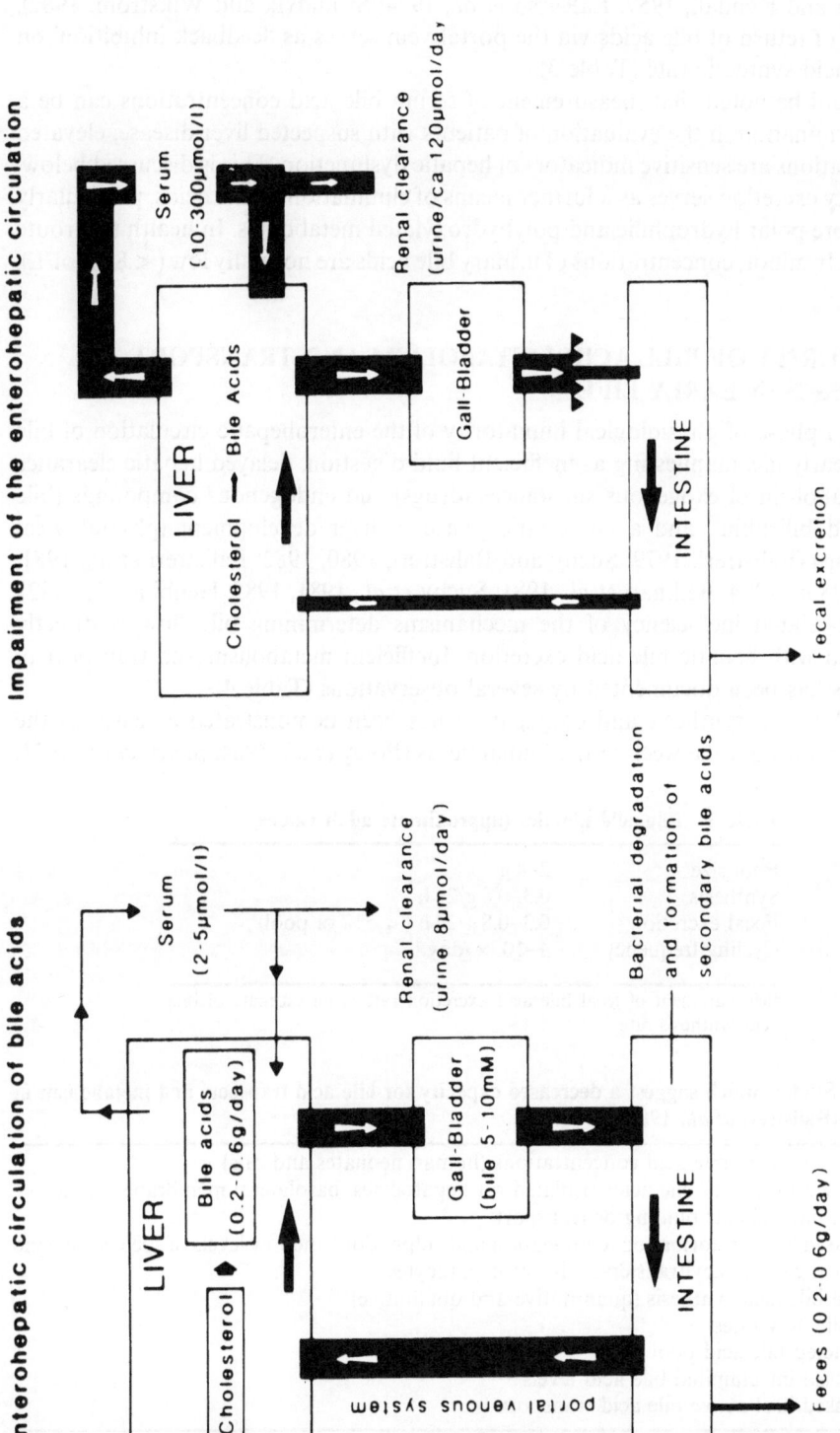

Figure 5 The main compartments and distribution of bile acids in the enterohepatic circulation; (left) schematic diagram of normal distribution and (right) impairment induced by cholestasis (note block in transfer to intestine). Reproduced with permission from Balistreri and Setchell (1988).

(Rudman and Kendall, 1957; LaRusso *et al.*, 1974; Strandvik and Wikstrom, 1982). The rate of return of bile acids via the portal vein serves as 'feedback inhibition' on the bile acid synthetic rate (Table 3).

It should be noted that measurement of serum bile acid concentrations can be a key determination in the evaluation of patients with suspected liver disease; elevated concentrations are sensitive indicators of hepatic dysfunction. This is discussed below.

Urinary excretion serves as a further means of elimination of bile acids, particularly of the more polar hydrophilic and polyhydroxylated metabolites. In health this route is relatively minor; concentrations of urinary bile acids are normally low ($< 8\,\mu\mathrm{mol/L}$).

IMMATURITY OF BILE ACID METABOLISM AND TRANSPORT PROCESSES IN EARLY LIFE

There is a phase of physiological immaturity of the enterohepatic circulation of bile acids in early life, manifesting as inefficient lipid digestion, delayed hepatic clearance and metabolism of exogenous substances (drugs) and endogenous compounds (bile acids and bilirubin), and a cholestatic phase of liver development (physiological cholestasis) (Balistreri, 1979; Suchy and Balistreri, 1980, 1982; Balistreri *et al.*, 1981, 1983a, 1983b, 1984; Belknap *et al.*, 1981; Suchy *et al.*, 1981, 1985; Heubi *et al.*, 1982). This age-related inefficiency of the mechanisms determining bile flow is directly correlated with hepatic bile acid excretion. Inefficient metabolism and transport of bile acids has been documented by several observations (Table 4).

Fetal bile salt synthesis and conjugation has been demonstrated as early as the 12th–16th intrauterine week in the human fetus (Poley *et al.*, 1964; Sharp *et al.*, 1971;

Table 3   Bile acid kinetics (approximate adult values)

Pool size	2–4 g
Synthesis	0.3–0.8 g/24 h
Fecal excretion	0.3–0.8 g/24 h ($< 5\%$ of pool)[a]
Cycling frequency	4–10 ×/day

[a]Measurement of fecal bile acid excretion rate is an estimate of bile acid synthesis rate

Table 4   Studies which suggest a decreased capacity for bile acid transport and metabolism in early life (Balistreri *et al.*, 1983b)

1. Decreased serum bile acid concentrations (human neonates and rats)
2. Decreased uptake of bile acids (isolated rat hepatocytes, basolateral membrane vesicles)
3. Altered intracellular binding or transport
4. Decreased biotransformation (conjugation and sulphation) and low levels of specific enzyme activity (ligase, *N*-acyltransferase) in rat hepatocytes
5. Altered bile acid synthesis (quantitative and qualitative)
6. Low bile flow rates
7. Contracted bile acid pool size
8. Decreased intraluminal bile acid levels
9. Decreased ileal active bile acid transport

Little *et al.*, 1975; Wahlen *et al.*, 1989). Taurine conjugates predominate in fetal life; this pattern is maintained to approximately six months of age. Secondary bile acids are also present in fetal bile and although the source is unknown, it has been suggested that they are derived either from maternal bile via transplacental transport or from primary synthesis through an alternative pathway.

The uptake, intracellular transport and metabolism (binding, translocation and synthesis) of bile acids is inefficient in the neonate. There is an elevation of serum bile acid concentrations in the newborn which is an indirect indicator of impaired hepatic clearance (Suchy *et al.*, 1981; Balistreri *et al.*, 1983). The specific activity of the enzymes involved in bile conjugation, sulphation and glucuronidation is low; the capacity of the suckling rat's liver to conjugate cholic acid is approximately 30% of that of the adult (Suchy and Balistreri, 1980; Suchy *et al.*, 1985). There is developmental immaturity of bile acid carriers in the brush border membrane of enterocytes in the terminal ileum (Moyer *et al.*, 1986). In the developing animal, ileal reabsorption of bile acids is decreased; active transport is absent in the postnatal period (Balistreri *et al.*, 1983b; Moyer *et al.*, 1986). As a direct reflection of underdeveloped intracellular events, there is a gradual age-related increase in bile acid pool size in humans and in various animal models (Balistreri *et al.*, 1983b). In addition to progressive quantitative changes in bile acid synthetic rate, there are qualitative differences. In the immature form of many species and in cholestatic liver disease, C-26 hydroxylation of cholesterol followed by oxidation of the side chain to yield 3β-hydroxy-5-cholenoic acid and lithocholate acid may occur, accounting for increased amounts of monohydroxy bile acids. Formation of these 'atypical' bile acids (DeWolf-Peeters *et al.*, 1971; Back and Walter, 1988) in the newborn results from the existence of a fetal biosynthetic pathway and a delay in the establishment of a mature synthetic sequence (Gustafsson, 1985). The pathophysiological effects of these atypical bile acids are unknown, but there may be a direct inhibitory effect on bile flow due to the absence of the choleretic and trophic primary bile acids. The resultant monohydroxy compounds such as lithocholate are intrinsically hepatotoxic and are capable of initiating or exacerbating cholestasis. Polyhydroxylated (tetrahydroxycholanoic) bile acids, found in the urine of normal infants (Strandvik and Wikstrom, 1982), are more soluble compounds and may present an efficient alternative route of elimination.

ABNORMALITIES OF BILE ACID METABOLISM

In view of the multiple processes involved in bile acid synthesis, conjugation and excretion, as well as hepatic and intestinal uptake, there are several potential sites for primary or secondary disturbances (Table 5). We will not discuss all of these potential disorders; however, we will summarize new information associated with hepatic disease related to inborn errors in bile acid metabolism. Inborn errors have led to further elucidation of bile acid metabolic pathways, for example, the study of patients with peroxisomal defects has contributed considerably to our understanding of peroxisomal as well as bile acid biochemistry.

Table 5 Abnormalities of bile acid metabolism

A. Defective bile acid synthesis

  1. Specific defects in bile acid synthesis

    (a) Cerebrotendinous xanthomatosis (CTX)

    (b) Intrahepatic cholestasis (familial neonatal hepatitis)

      (1) 3β-Hydroxysteroid dehydrogenase/isomerase deficiency (Clayton *et al.*, 1987)

      (2) Δ^4-3-oxosteroid 5β-reductase deficiency (Setchell *et al.*, 1988)

      (3) C_{24} steroid: 7α-hydroxylase (Javitt *et al.*, 1986)

    (c) Peroxisomal disorders (Setchell, 1987)

      (1) Genetic diseases with a general impairment of numerous peroxisomal functions and reduced or undetectable peroxisome numbers

        (a) Cerebro–hepato–renal (Zellweger's) syndrome

        (b) Infantile Refsum's disease

        (c) Neonatal adrenoleukodystrophy

        (d) Hyperpipecolic acidaemia[a]

        (e) Rhizomelic chondrodysplasia punctata[a]

      (2) Genetic diseases with generalized impairment of peroxisomal function but normal number of peroxisomes

        (a) Pseudo-Zellweger's syndrome

      (3) Genetic diseases with a single enzyme defect and a normal number of peroxisomes

        (a) X-linked adrenoleukodystrophy

        (b) Adult Refsum's disease

        (c) Acatalasaemia

  2. Acquired defects in bile acid synthesis (non-specific) secondary to parenchymal liver disease (cholestasis, cirrhosis)

B. Diminished bile acid uptake, intracellular metabolism or secretion

  1. Intrahepatic cholestasis (altered bile secretory apparatus)

  2. Parenchymal disease

    (a) regurgitation from cells

    (b) portosystemic shunting

C. Altered bile acid delivery to intestinal lumen

  1. Gall bladder disease

  2. Coeliac sprue

  3. Extrahepatic cholestasis (obstruction)

D. Interrupted enterohepatic circulation of bile acids (Hoffmann, 1967, 1972; Balistreri *et al.*, 1981)

  1. External bile fistula

  2. Contaminated small bowel syndrome (Schneider Viteri, 1974)

Continued

Table 5 *Continued*

---

3. Entrapment of bile acids in intestinal lumen by
   (a) cholestyramine
   (b) fibre
   (c) trivalent cations

E. Bile acid malabsorption

1. Primary bile acid malabsorption
   (a) Intractable diarrhoea (infants) (Balistreri *et al.*, 1977)
   (b) Irritable bowel (adults)

2. Secondary bile acid malabsorption
   (a) ileal disease
       (1) Crohn's disease
       (2) Ileal resection (Hofmann, 1967; Heubi and Balistreri, 1980)
       (3) Ileal bypass
       (4) Radiation enteritis
       (5) Postinfectious enteritis
   (b) Exogenous bile acid administration
   (c) Cystic fibrosis (Weber and Roy, 1985)

3. Tertiary bile acid malabsorption
   (a) Postcholecystectomy
   (b) Renal failure
   (c) Drugs

---

[a]The number of peroxisomes has not been documented in these disorders

Inborn errors in bile acid metabolism

Defective bile acid metabolism has been postulated to be an initiating or perpetuating factor in neonatal cholestatic disorders (Balistreri, 1987), the hypothesis being that inborn errors in bile acid metabolism, presumably due to an inherited enzymopathy, may be associated with either: (1) underproduction of the normal trophic and choleretic primary bile acids such as cholic acid; or (2) overproduction of primitive bile acid metabolites (monohydroxy bile acids) which might be hepatotoxic. With recent technological advances, specifically fast atom bombardment–mass spectrometry (FAB–MS), it has been possible to delineate specifically disorders of bile acid synthesis which are apparently associated with 'idiopathic' neonatal hepatitis. Non-volatile compounds can be analysed directly in biological samples or simple extracts via FAB–MS (Setchell, 1987). Mass spectra, generated from small microlitre volumes of urine, indicate the presence of steroid and bile acid conjugates. This technique, which is rapid and simple, has allowed specific defects to be identified (Clayton *et al.*, 1987; Setchell *et al.*, 1988).

A recently reported example of an inborn error of bile acid metabolism, manifesting as neonatal hepatitis, is Δ^4-3-oxosteroid 5β-reductase deficiency (Setchell *et al.*, 1988). We had the opportunity to evaluate monochorionic male twins born with marked cholestasis. A previous male sibling with neonatal hepatitis had died of liver failure at 4 months of age. When the twins were admitted, liver function tests revealed elevated serum aminotransferase levels, marked conjugated hyperbilirubinaemia, and a severe coagulopathy. Liver biopsies revealed marked lobular disarray, pseudoacinar transformation of hepatocytes, hepatocellular and canalicular bile stasis, and extramedullary haematopoiesis. Electron microscopy revealed bile canaliculi which were small and slit-like in appearance; there were few or absent microvilli containing a variable amount of electron-dense material. Initial screening of urine from both infants using FAB–MS indicated the presence of elevated amounts of taurine conjugates of hydroxy-oxo-cholenoic and dihydroxy-oxo-cholenoic acids. GC–MS confirmed the predominance of two major components identified as 3-oxo-7α-hydroxy-4-cholenoic and 3-oxo-7α,12α-dihydroxy-4-cholenoic acids. Gall bladder bile contained only trace amounts (less than $2\,\mu mol/L$) of bile acids. Δ^4-3-oxo bile acids represented the major urinary bile acids. Urinary excretion was therefore the major route for bile acid loss; estimates of bile acid synthesis rates from daily urinary output indicated markedly reduced total bile acid synthesis rates ($< 3\,mg$ per day). These biochemical findings indicated a defect in bile acid synthesis affecting the conversion of the 3-oxo-Δ^4 intermediates to the corresponding 3α-hydroxy-5β(H)-structures, a reaction catalysed by an NADPH-dependent Δ^4-3-oxosteroid-5β reductase enzyme (Figure 6) (Setchell *et al.*, 1988). The cholestasis and liver injury could have resulted from either: (1) the lack of synthesis of adequate amounts of primary bile acids, which provide a major driving force for bile secretion; or (2) the accumulation of Δ^4-3-oxo- and allo-bile acids which are potentially hepatotoxic. These physiological features may have been abetted by structural immaturity of the hepatocyte excretory pole. The morphological findings suggested that maturation of the canalicular membrane and the transport system for bile acid secretion may require exposure to primary bile acids in early development.

Oral bile acid therapy for patients with inborn errors

In the face of severe hepatic dysfunction we administered a combination of cholic acid and ursodeoxycholic acid (100 mg/day of each bile acid) orally in solution to our patients with Δ^4-3-oxosteroid 5β-reductase deficiency. Cholic acid was given in order to suppress endogenous bile acid synthesis and prevent the further accumulation of potentially hepatotoxic Δ^4-3-oxo- and allo-bile acids which arose in the presence of the enzyme deficiency. Ursodeoxycholic acid was given since it is a potent choleretic agent which has beneficial effects on the indices of liver function. Complete suppression of Δ^4-3-oxo and allo-bile acids occurred and normalization of liver function tests and bile canalicular morphology was also noted during bile acid therapy (Balistreri *et al.*, 1990; Setchell, 1990). These infants and a similarly affected younger sibling in whom treatment was indicated at 6 days of age continue to grow and thrive.

DETERMINATION OF SERUM BILE ACIDS – CLINICAL UTILITY

The physiological determinants of the serum levels of individual bile acids are well understood (DeBarros *et al.*, 1982). It has been shown that the fractional hepatic clearance remains constant during both fasting and digestion. This fraction is influenced by the bile acid structure – the fractional clearance of chenodeoxycholate

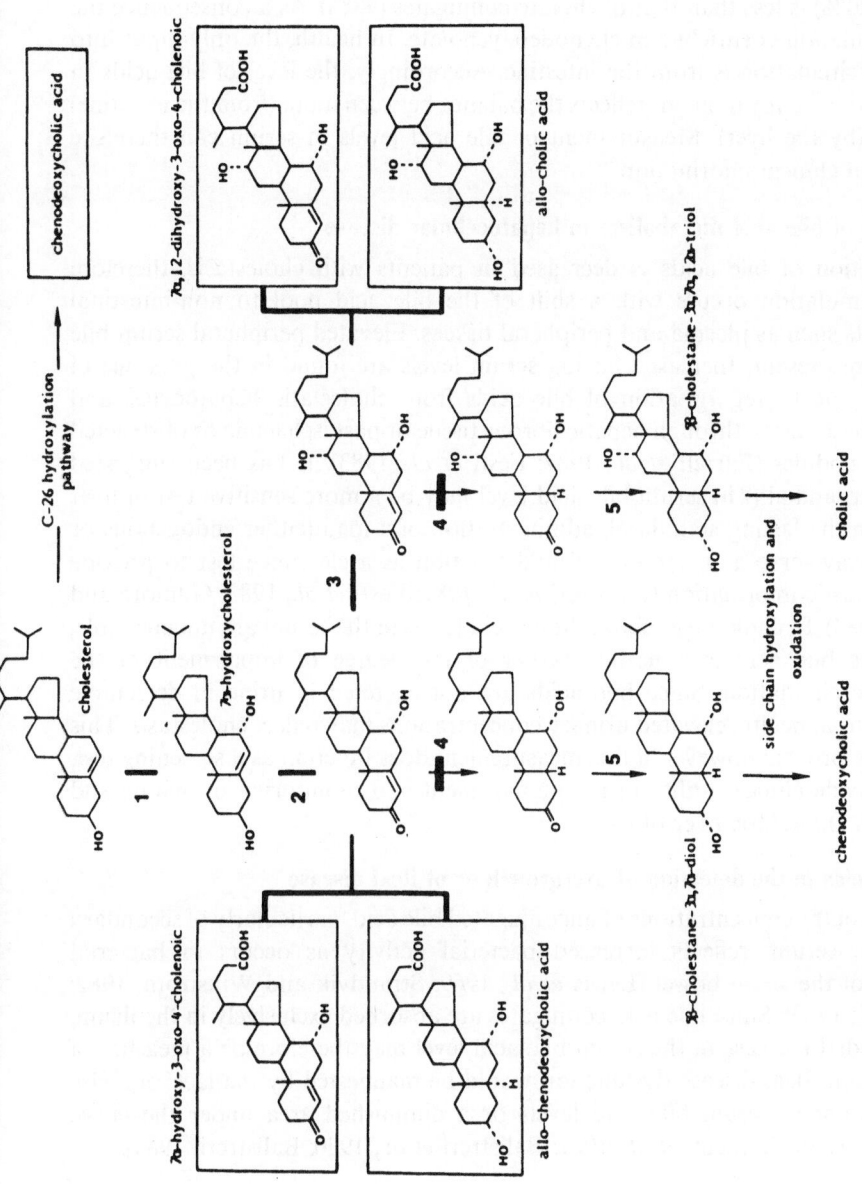

Figure 6 Δ^4-oxosteroid 5β-reductase deficiency. Biosynthetic pathways for synthesis of bile acids from cholesterol illustrating the point of the defect in synthesis (note block at step 4). This graph also depicts the resulting metabolism of the accumulated precursors. The key enzymes involved in the pathway are: (1) cholesterol 7α-hydroxylase; (2) 3β-hydroxysteroid dehydrogenase/isomerase; (3) 12α-hydroxylase; (4) Δ^4-3-oxosteroid-5β-reductase; (5) 3α-hydroxysteroid dehydrogenase. Defective Δ^4-3-oxosteroid 5β-reductase activity leads to accumulation of Δ^4-3-oxo bile acids and allo-bile acids (boxes). Reproduced with permission from Setchell et al. (1988).

J. Inher. Metab. Dis. 14 (1991)

conjugates (80%) is less than that of cholate conjugates (90%). As a consequence the systemic circulation is enriched in chenodeoxycholate. In health, the only input into the systemic circulation is from the intestine. Accordingly, the level of bile acids in peripheral blood at any moment reflects the balance between input (from the intestine) and uptake (by the liver). Measurement of bile acid levels in serum can therefore provide useful clinical information.

Disturbances of bile acid metabolism in hepatocellular disease

Biliary excretion of bile acids is decreased in patients with cholestasis, therefore hepatic accumulation occurs with a shift of the bile acid pool to non-intestinal compartments such as plasma and peripheral tissues. Elevated peripheral serum bile acid levels are present. Increased fasting serum levels are found in the presence of liver disease due to regurgitation of bile acids from cholestatic hepatocytes, and portosystemic shunting through hepatic fibrous tissue or past ischaemic or obstructed regenerative nodules (Farrell *et al.*, 1982; Festi *et al.*, 1983). It has been suggested that the postprandial (2 h) serum bile acid level may be a more sensitive test of liver function than the fasting state level; administration of a load (either endogenous or exogenous) may serve as a 'stress test' and function as a clearance test to provide further diagnostic information (Balistreri *et al.*, 1981; Festi *et al.*, 1983; Gilmore and Hofmann, 1983). In cholestasis, deoxycholic acid levels in the serum are undetectable, therefore this bile acid is a useful marker of the degree of impairment of the enterohepatic circulation. Since bile acids are not excreted in urine in detectable concentrations in health, elevated urinary concentrations may reflect cholestasis. This remains to be proven; however, if this measurement does function as a screening test, it would provide clinical utility in the management and monitoring of infants and children with cholestatic liver disease.

Serum bile acids in the detection of overgrowth or of ileal disease

An elevation of the concentrations of unconjugated bile acid, particularly of secondary bile acids in serum, reflects increased bacterial activity as occurs in bacterial overgrowth of the small bowel (Lewis *et al.*, 1969; Strandvik and Wikstrom, 1982; Setchell *et al.*, 1983). Since bile acid conjugates are absorbed exclusively in the ileum, the postprandial increase in the serum bile acid level may therefore be a measure of ileal absorption. Ileal disease/dysfunction would be manifested by the lack of a rise in the postprandial serum bile acid levels or a diminished area under the curve (LaRusso *et al.*, 1974; Suchy *et al.*, 1981; Balistreri *et al.*, 1980; Balistreri, 1984).

REFERENCES

Back, P. and Walter, K. Developmental pattern of bile acid metabolism as revealed by bile acid analysis of meconium. *Gastroenterology* 78 (1988) 671–676

Balistreri, W. F. Fat maldigestion – A reflection of immaturity of the enterohepatic circulation. In: Feeding the neonate < 1500 grams, nutrition and beyond. *Proceedings of the 79th Ross Conference on Pediatric Research*, Columbus, Ohio, Ross Laboratories (1979) pp. 1–6

Balistreri, W. F. Bile acid-induced intestinal dysfunction: implications to protracted infantile diarrhea and malnutrition. In E. Lebenthal (ed.) *Chronic Diarrhea in Children, Nestle*

Nutrition Workshop Series, Volume 6, Raven Press, New York (1984) pp. 347–364

Balistreri, W. F. (Foreword) Neonatal cholestasis: lessons from the past, issues for the future. In: W. F. Balistreri (ed.), *Seminars in Liver Disease. Neonatal Cholestasis, Volume* 7, *Number* 2, Thieme Medical Publishers, New York (1987) pp. 61–66

Balistreri, W. F. and Setchell, K. D. R. Clinical implications of bile acid metabolism. In: Silverberg, M. and Daum, F. (eds), *Textbook of Pediatric Gastroenterology, 2nd Edition*, Year Book Medical Publishers (1988) pp. 72–89

Balistreri, W. F., Partin, J. C. and Schubert, W. K. Bile acid malabsorption – a consequence of terminal ileal dysfunction in intractable diarrhea of infancy. *J. Pediatr.* 89 (1977) 21–28

Balistreri, W. F., Suchy, F. J. and Heubi, J. E. Serum bile acid response to a meal stimulus – A sensitive test of ileal function. *J. Pediatr.* 96 (1980) 582–589

Balistreri, W. F., Suchy, F. J., Farrell, M. K. and Heubi, J. E. Pathologic versus physiologic cholestasis: Elevated serum concentrations of a secondary bile acid in the presence of hepatobiliary disease. *J. Pediatr.* 98 (1981) 399–402

Balistreri, W. F., Heubi, J. E. and Suchy, F. J. Bile acid metabolism: Relationship of bile acid malabsorption and diarrhea. *J. Pediatr. Gastroenterol. Nutr.* 2 (1983a) 105–110

Balistreri, W. F., Heubi, J. E. and Suchy, F. J. Immaturity of the enterohepatic circulation in early life: factors predisposing to physiologic maldigestion and cholestasis. *J. Pediatr. Gastroenterol. Nutr.* 2 (1983b) 346–354

Balistreri, W. F., Zimmer, L., Suchy, F. J. and Bove, K. E. Bile salt sulfotransferase: Alterations during maturation and non-inducability during substrate ingestion. *J. Lipid Res.* 25 (1984) 228–235

Balistreri, W. F., A-Kader, H. H., Ryckman, F. C., Whitington, P. F., Heubi, J. E. and Setchell, K. D. Biochemical and clinical response to ursodeoxycholic acid administration in pediatric patients with chronic cholestasis. In Paumgartner, G., Stiehl, A. and Gerok, W. (eds.) *Bile Acids as Therapeutic Agents: from Basic Science to Clinical Practice* (Falk Symposium No. 58). Lancaster, Kluwer Academic Publishers, 1991, pp. 323–334

Belknap, W. M., Balistreri, W. F., Suchy, F. J. and Miller, P. C. Physiologic cholestasis II: Serum bile acid levels reflect the development of the enterohepatic circulation in rats. *Hepatology* 1 (1981) 613–616

Boyer, J. L. New concepts of mechanisms of hepatocyte bile formation. *Physiol. Rev.* 60 (1980) 303–315

Carey, M. C. and Small, D. M. The physical chemistry of cholesterol solubility in bile. *J. Clin. Invest.* 61 (1978) 998–1026

Chadwick, V. S., Gaginella, T. S., Carlson, G. L., DeBongnie, J. C., Phillips, S. F. and Hofmann, A. F. Effect of molecular structure on bile acid-induced alterations in absorptive function, permeability and morphology in perfused rabbit colon. *J. Lab. Clin. Med.* 94 (1979) 661–674

Clayton, P. T., Leonard, J. V., Lawson, A. M., Setchell, K. D. R., Andersson, S., Egestad, B. and Sjovall, J. Familial giant cell hepatitis associated with synthesis of 3β,7α-dihydroxy- and 3β,7α,12α-trihydroxy-5-cholenoic acids. *J. Clin. Invest.* 79 (1987) 1031–1038

DeBarros, S. G., Balistreri, W. F., Soloway, R. D., Weiss, S. G., Miller, P. C. and Soper, K. Response of serum bile acid concentrations to endogenous and exogenous input to the enterohepatic circulation. *Gastroenterology* 82 (1982) 647–652

DeWolf-Peeters, C., DeVos, R. and Desmit, V. Histochemical evidence of a cholestatic period in neonatal rats. *Pediatr. Res.* 5 (1971) 704–709

Dietschy, J. M. Mechanisms for the intestinal absorption of bile acids. *J. Lipid Res.* 9 (1968) 297–309

Dietschy, J. M., Salomon, H. S. and Siperstein, M. D. Bile acid metabolism: 1. Studies on the mechanisms of intestinal transport. *J. Clin. Invest.* 45 (1966) 832–846

Dowling, R. H. The enterohepatic circulation. *Gastroenterology* 62 (1972) 122–140

Farrell, M. K., Balistreri, W. F. and Suchy, F. J. Serum sulfated lithocholate as an indicator of cholestasis during parenteral and enteral nutrition in infants and children. *J. Parenteral Enteral Nutr.* 6 (1982) 30–33

Festi, D., Labate, A. M. M., Roda, A., Bazzoli, F., Frabboni, R., Rucci, P., Taroni, F., Aldini, R., Roda, E. and Barbara, L. Diagnostic effectiveness of serum bile acids in liver disease as evaluated by multivariate statistical methods. *Hepatology* **3** (1983) 707–713

Flynn, M., Darby, C., Hyland, J., Hammond, P. and Taylor, I. The effect of bile acids on colonic myoelectrical activity. *Br. J. Surg.* **66** (1979) 776–779

Gilmore, I. T. and Hofmann, A. F. Altered drug metabolism and elevated serum bile acids in liver disease: A unified pharmacokinetic explanation. *Gastroenterology* **78** (1980) 177–179

Gurantz, D. and Hofmann, A. F. Influence of bile acid structure on bile flow and biliary lipid secretion in the hamster. *Am. J. Physiol.* **247** (1984) 6736–6748

Gustafsson, J. Bile acid synthesis during development: Mitochondrial 12 hydroxylation in human fetal liver. *J. Clin. Invest.* **75** (1985) 604–607

Hanssen, L. E. Pure synthetic bile salts release immunoreactive secretin in man. *Scand. J. Gastroenterol.* **15** (1980) 461–463

Haselwood, G. A. D. *The Biological Importance of Bile Salts*, Elsevier North-Holland, New York, 1978

Heubi, J. E. and Balistreri, W. F. Bile salt metabolism in infants and children after protracted infantile diarrhea. *Pediatr. Res.* **14** (1980) 943–946

Heubi, J. E., Balistreri, W. F. and Suchy, F. J. Bile salt metabolism in the first year of life. *J. Lab. Clin. Med.* **100** (1982) 127–136

Hofmann, A. F. The function of bile salts in fat absorption: The solvent properties of dilute micellar solutions of conjugated bile salts. *Biochem. J.* **89** (1963) 57–68

Hofmann, A. F. The syndrome of ileal disease and the broken enterohepatic circulation: cholerehic enteropathy. *Gastroenterology* **51** (1967) 752–757

Hofmann, A. F. Bile acid malabsorption caused by ileal resection. *Arch. Int. Med.* **130** (1972) 597–605

Hofmann, A. F. The chemistry of bile in health and disease. *Hepatology* **4** (1984) 1S

Hofmann, A. F. and Borgstrom, B. The intraluminal phase of fat digestion in man: The lipid content of the micellar and oil phases of intestinal content obtained during fat digestion and absorption. *J. Clin. Invest.* **43** (1964) 247–257

Hofmann, A. F. and Roda, A. Physicochemical properties of bile acids and their relationship to biological properties: an overview of the problem. *J. Lipid Res.* **25** (1984) 1477–1482

Hofmann, A. F., Molino, G. and Belforte, G. Description and simulation of a physiological pharmacokinetic model for the metabolism and enterohepatic circulation of bile acids in man. Cholic acid in healthy man. *J. Clin. Invest.* **71** (1983) 1003–1022

Holsti, P. Bile acids as a cause of liver injury: Cirrhogenic effect of chenodeoxycholic acid in rabbits. *Acta Pathol. Microbiol. Scand.* **54** (1962) 479–481

Javitt, N. B., Kok, E., Gut, M., Rajagopalan, I. and Budai, K. Neonatal cholestasis: Identification of a metabolic error in bile acid synthesis (abstract). *Pediatr. Res.* (1986) 200

Lack, L. and Weiner, I. M. *In vitro* absorption of bile salts by small intestine of rats and guinea pigs. *Am. J. Physiol.* **200** (1961) 313–317

Lack, L. and Weiner, I. M. Intestinal bile salt transport structure activity relationships and other properties. *Am. J. Physiol.* **210** (1966) 1142–1147

LaRusso, N. F., Korman, M. G., Hoffman, N. E. and Hofmann, A. F. Dynamics of the enterohepatic circulation of bile acids. Postprandial serum concentrations of conjugates of cholic acid in health, cholecystectomy patients and patients with bile acid malabsorption. *N. Engl. J. Med.* **291** (1974) 689–692

Lewis, B., Panveliwalla, D., Tabaquali, S. and Wootten, I. D. P. Serum bile acids in stagnant-loop syndrome. *Lancet* **1** (1969) 219–220

Little, M., Smallwood, R. A., Lester, R., Piasecki, G. J. and Jackson, B. T. Bile salt metabolism in the primate fetus. *Gastroenterology* **69** (1975) 1315–1320

Matern, S., Matern, H., Farthmann, E. H. and Gerok, W. Hepatic and extrahepatic glucuronidation of bile acids in man. *J. Clin. Invest.* **74** (1984) 402–410

Mekhjian, H. S., Phillips, S. F. and Hofmann, A. F. Colonic secretion of water and electrolytes induced by bile acids: perfusion studies in man. *J. Clin. Invest.* **50** (1971) 1569–1577

Moyer, M. S., Heubi, J. E., Goodrich, A. L., Balistreri, W. F. and Suchy, F. J. Ontogeny of bile acid transport in brush border membrane from rat ileum. *Gastroenterology* 90 (1986) 1188–1196

Oelberg, D. G., Chari, M. V., Little, J. M., Adcock, E. W. and Lester, R. Lithocholate glucuronide is a cholestatic agent. *J. Clin. Invest.* 73 (1984) 1057–1063

Palmer, R. H. Bile acids, liver injury and liver disease. *Arch. Int. Med.* 130 (1972) 606–617

Palmer, R. H. and Hruban, Z. Production of bile duct hyperplasia and gallstones by lithocholic acid. *J. Clin. Invest.* 45 (1966) 1255–1261

Poley, J. R., Dower, J. C., Owen, C. A. and Stickler, G. B. Bile acids in infants and children. *J. Lab. Clin. Med.* 63 (1964) 838–846

Roda, A., Hofmann, A. F. and Mysels, K. J. The influence of bile salt structure on self association in aqueous solutions. *J. Biol. Chem.* 258 (1983) 6362–6370

Rudman, D. and Kendall, F. E. Bile acid content of human serum 1. Serum bile acids in patients with hepatic disease. *J. Clin. Invest.* 36 (1957) 530–535

Schiff, E. R., Small, N. C. and Dietschy, J. M. Characterization of the kinetics of the passive and active transport mechanisms for bile acid absorption in the small intestine and colon of the rat. *J. Clin. Invest.* 51 (1972) 1351–1362

Schneider, R. E. and Viteri, F. E. Luminal events of lipid absorption in protein-calorie malnourished children and relationship with nutritional recovery and diarrhea. I. Capacity of the duodenal content to achieve micellar solubilization of lipids. *Am. J. Clin. Nutr.* 27 (1974) 777–787

Setchell, K. D. R. Inborn errors of bile acid synthesis. *Semin. Liver Dis.* 7 (1987) 85–99

Setchell, K. D. R. Disorders of bile acid synthesis. In Walker, W. A., Durie, P. R., Hamilton, J. R., Walker-Smith, J. A. and Watkins, J. B. (eds.), *Pediatric Gastrointestinal Disease Volume 2*, New York, B. C. Decker, pp. 992–1013

Setchell, K. D. R. , Lawson, A. M., Blackstock, E. J. and Murphy, G. M. Diurnal changes in serum unconjugated bile acids in normal man. *Gut* 23 (1983) 637–642

Setchell, K. D. R., Harrison, D. L., Gilbert, J. M. and Murphy, G. M. Serum unconjugated bile acids – qualitative and quantitative profiles in ileal resection and bacterial overgrowth. *Clin. Chim. Acta* 152 (1985) 297–306

Setchell, K. D. R., Suchy, F. J., Welsh, M. B., Zimmer-Nechemias, L., Heubi, J. and Balistreri, W. F. Δ^4-3-oxosteroid 5β-reductase deficiency described in identical twins with neonatal hepatitis – a new inborn error in bile acid synthesis. *J. Clin. Invest.* 82 (1988) 2148–2157

Sharp, H. L., Peller, J., Carey, J. B. and Krivit, W. Primary and secondary bile acids in meconium. *Pediatr. Res.* 5 (1971) 274–279

Strandvik, B. and Wikstrom, S. A. L. Tetrahydroxylated bile acids in healthy human newborns. *Eur. J. Clin. Invest.* 12 (1982) 301–305

Suchy, F. J. and Balistreri, W. F. Maturation of bile acid conjugation in heptocytes from fetal and suckling rats. *Gastroenterology* 78 (1980) 1324

Suchy, F. J. and Balistreri, W. F. Ileal dysfunction in Crohn's disease assessed by postprandial serum bile acid response. *Gut* 22 (1981) 948–952

Suchy, F. J. and Balistreri, W. F. Taurocholate uptake in hepatocytes from developing rats. *Pediatr. Res.* 16 (1982) 282–285

Suchy, F. J., Balistreri, W. F., Heubi, J. E., Searcy, J. E. and Levin, R. S. Physiologic cholestasis: elevation of the primary serum bile acid concentrations in normal infants. *Gastroenterology* 80 (1981) 1037–1041

Suchy, F. J., Courchene, S. M. and Balistreri, W. F. Ontogeny of hepatic bile acid conjugation in the rat. *Pediatr. Res.* 19 (1985) 97–107

Wahlen, E., Egestad, B., Strandvik, B. and Sjovall, J. Ketonic bile acids in urine of infants during the neonatal period. *J. Lipid Res.* 12 (1989) 1847–1857

Weber, A. M. and Roy, C. C. Bile acid metabolism in children with cystic fibrosis. *Acta Paediatr. Scand.* 317 (1985) 9–15

Wilson, F. A. Intestinal transport of bile acids. *Am. J. Physiol.* 4 (1981) G83

Wilson, F. A. Modern approaches to bile acid transport proteins. *Hospital Practice* (April 1990) 79–94

J. Inher. Metab. Dis. 14 (1991) 478–496

Inborn Errors of Bile Acid Metabolism

P. T. CLAYTON

Department of Child Health, Institute of Child Health, 30 Guilford Street, London WC1N 1EH, UK and Hospital for Sick Children, Great Ormond St, London, UK

Summary: Cholesterol is converted to cholic acid and chenodeoxycholic acid by a series of reactions involving modifications to the steroid nucleus and oxidation of the side chain. These reactions can be affected by a number of inborn errors of metabolism. When this happens unusual bile acids or bile alcohols are synthesized; these can be identified using gas chromatography–mass spectrometry and fast atom bombardment mass spectrometry techniques. Two defects affecting the modifications to the steroid nucleus have been described; both present with cholestatic liver disease of neonatal onset. The better characterized of the two – 3β-hydroxy-$\Delta 5$-C27-steroid dehydrogenase deficiency – leads to excretion of 3β-7α-dihydroxy-5-cholenoic acid and $3\beta,7\alpha,12\alpha$-trihydroxy-5-cholenoic acid in the urine. The liver disease improves dramatically on treatment with chenodeoxycholic acid. Deficient activity of 3-oxo-$\Delta 4$-steroid 5β-reductase is thought to be the cause of familial liver disease in some infants who excrete 7α-hydroxy-3-oxo-4-cholenoic acid and $7\alpha,12\alpha$-dihydroxy-3-oxo-4-cholenoic acid in the urine. However, diagnosis of this disorder is problematical; a similar pattern of metabolite excretion can occur as a result of liver damage caused by viruses or inborn errors of pathways unrelated to bile acid synthesis. Defective side chain oxidation in patients with cerebrotendinous xanthomatosis (CTX) leads to synthesis of bile alcohols such as 5β-cholestane-$3\alpha,7\alpha,12\alpha,25$-tetrol and 5β-cholestane-$3\alpha,7\alpha,12\alpha,23,25$-pentol. Patients with CTX do not have cholestatic liver disease. Their major problems (neurological disease, atherosclerosis and xanthomata) are caused by accumulation of cholestanol and cholesterol in the tissues. Bile acid precursors are probably diverted into synthesis of cholestanol. Chenodeoxycholic acid suppresses the production of abnormal metabolites from cholesterol (by inhibition of cholesterol 7α-hydroxylase) and leads to improvement in the neurological disease. Defective side chain oxidation also occurs in peroxisomal disorders but this time it leads to accumulation of C27 bile acids such as $3\alpha,7\alpha,12\alpha$-trihydroxy-5β-cholestanoic acid (trihydroxycoprostanic acid, THCA). This compound is readily detected in the bile and plasma of patients with defects of peroxisome biogenesis. In patients with defects of a single peroxisomal β-oxidation enzyme (the 3-hydroxyacyl-CoA component of the bifunctional protein or the thiolase), the major C27 bile acid in bile may be $3\alpha,7\alpha,12\alpha,24$-tetrahydroxy-$5\beta$-cholestanoic acid (varanic acid). In addition to the above inborn errors, others which are less well characterized undoubtedly exist, as do defects of bile acid transport across membranes.

The primary bile acids (the taurine and glycine conjugates of chenodeoxycholic acid and cholic acid) are synthesized from cholesterol in the liver. The synthetic pathway is regulated by feedback inhibition; bile acids passing through the liver in the enterohepatic circulation inhibit the first step in the synthetic pathway, cholesterol 7α-hydroxylase. An inborn error affecting bile acid synthesis may have effects attributable to bile acid deficiency or to accumulation of intermediates and the metabolites of these intermediates.

Two of the effects of bile acid deficiency are readily predictable. The major component of bile secretion is bile-acid dependent – it is driven by the active transport of bile acids from the hepatocytes into the canaliculi. Thus inborn errors affecting the synthesis of bile acids may produce cholestasis, reduced bile flow. The rôle of bile acids in the intestinal lumen is to facilitate the digestion and absorption of fats and fat-soluble vitamins. Thus reduced luminal bile acid concentrations are associated with steatorrhoea and symptoms of fat-soluble vitamin malabsorption. Where cholestasis and malabsorption are due to bile acid deficiency these problems should be correctable by therapeutic administration of cholic and/or chenodeoxycholic acid.

The fact that intermediates in bile acid synthesis accumulate is also not surprising – not only is their usual route of metabolism blocked but their production is accelerated by loss of the bile acid feedback on cholesterol 7α-hydroxylase. In cerebrotendinous xanthomatosis the metabolites which accumulate can be converted to cholestanol, and cholestanol accumulation plays an important rôle in the pathogenesis of neurological damage and xanthomata (Björkhem, 1985). Treatment is directed at suppressing the activity of cholesterol 7α-hydroxylase, using a bile acid known to inhibit the enzyme, chenodeoxycholic acid.

Some of the disorders which affect bile acid synthesis also affect other pathways (e.g. disorders of peroxisome biogenesis where many peroxisomal pathways are interrupted). In such cases the neurological and hepatic disease may be attributable to something other than interruption of the bile acid synthesis pathway. None the less, bile acid analyses can be a useful means of diagnosis.

DIAGNOSIS OF INBORN ERRORS OF BILE ACID METABOLISM

There are three groups of patients in whom we have diagnosed inborn errors affecting bile acid synthesis:

(i) infants and children with unexplained cholestatic liver disease (especially if familial, present from the neonatal period and associated with steatorrhoea and fat-soluble vitamin malabsorption);

(ii) infants and children with (predominantly) neurological problems suggestive of a peroxisomal disorder – motor delay and hypotonia, ocular abnormalities (particularly a reduced electroretinogram and pigmentary retinopathy), seizures, dysmorphic features, failure to thrive, sensorineural deafness, hepatomegaly;

(iii) patients suspected of having cerebrotendinous xanthomatosis. In adults the combination of tendon xanthomata, low intelligence, progressive spasticity and ataxia and cataracts may make the diagnosis obvious. In children the only symptoms may be mental retardation and minimal spasticity and/or ataxia.

To achieve early diagnosis of the treatable disorders it would probably be necessary to screen all patients with neonatal cholestasis and all patients with developmental delay. Analytical methods are therefore required which can be used on large numbers of samples, which can detect any abnormal species of bile acid or bile alcohol (be it present as the free compound, conjugated with glycine or taurine or as the sulphate or glucuronide) and which can also provide some quantitative information. For the majority of patients, we use a combination of a quantitative gas chromatography–mass spectrometry (GC–MS) method on the plasma (Clayton and Muller, 1980; Clayton et al., 1987a) and fast atom bombardment mass spectrometry (FAB–MS) on the urine (Lawson et al., 1986). For some patients we also analyse bile by FAB–MS (Clayton et al., 1990). If the urine or the bile contain unusual bile acids or bile alcohols then an appropriate method is chosen for further analysis of the sample by GC–MS. The choice of relatively simple methods has enabled us to obtain experience of metabolite patterns in over 600 plasma and urine samples from children (and a few adults) with a variety of hepatobiliary, neurological and other disorders.

PATHWAYS FOR SYNTHESIS OF BILE ACIDS FROM CHOLESTEROL

In the major pathway for bile acid synthesis, modifications to the cholesterol nucleus (Figure 1) occur prior to oxidation of the side chain (Figure 2) (Björkhem, 1985). Thus, intermediates are produced with a bile acid nucleus and the cholesterol side chain, 5β-cholestane-$3\alpha,7\alpha$-diol and 5β-cholestane-$3\alpha,7\alpha,12\alpha$-triol. Side chain oxidation can occur by two routes. The major pathway starts with hydroxylation at C-26 (Figure 2, left side) and further oxidation produces the 27-carbon bile acids, $3\alpha,7\alpha$-dihydroxy-5β-cholestanoic acid (dihydroxycoprostanic acid, DHCA) and $3\alpha,7\alpha,12\alpha$-trihydroxy-5β-cholestanoic acid (trihydroxycoprostanic acid (THCA). THCA and DHCA then undergo β-oxidation in the peroxisomes to produce chenodeoxycholic and cholic acids respectively. Where the 26-hydroxylation pathway is blocked, some synthesis of cholic acid can occur by the 25-hydroxylation pathway (Figure 2, right side).

DISORDERS AFFECTING MODIFICATIONS TO THE CHOLESTEROL NUCLEUS

The pathway by which cholesterol is converted to 5β-cholestane-$3\alpha,7\alpha$-diol and 5β-cholestane-$3\alpha,7\alpha,12\alpha$-triol is shown in Figure 1. Because the names of some of the enzymes involved in this pathway are rather long, it is proposed that the steps are numbered as indicated in the figure and the inborn errors are referred to as bile acid synthesis defect 1 (BSD 1) if the first step in the pathway (cholesterol 7α-hydroxylase) is affected, BSD 2 if the second step (3β-hydroxy-$\Delta5$-C27-steroid dehydrogenase) is affected, and so on. BSD 2 is now well documented; there are problems in defining the true characteristics of BSD 3 (3-oxo-$\Delta4$-steroid 5β-reductase deficiency) and no

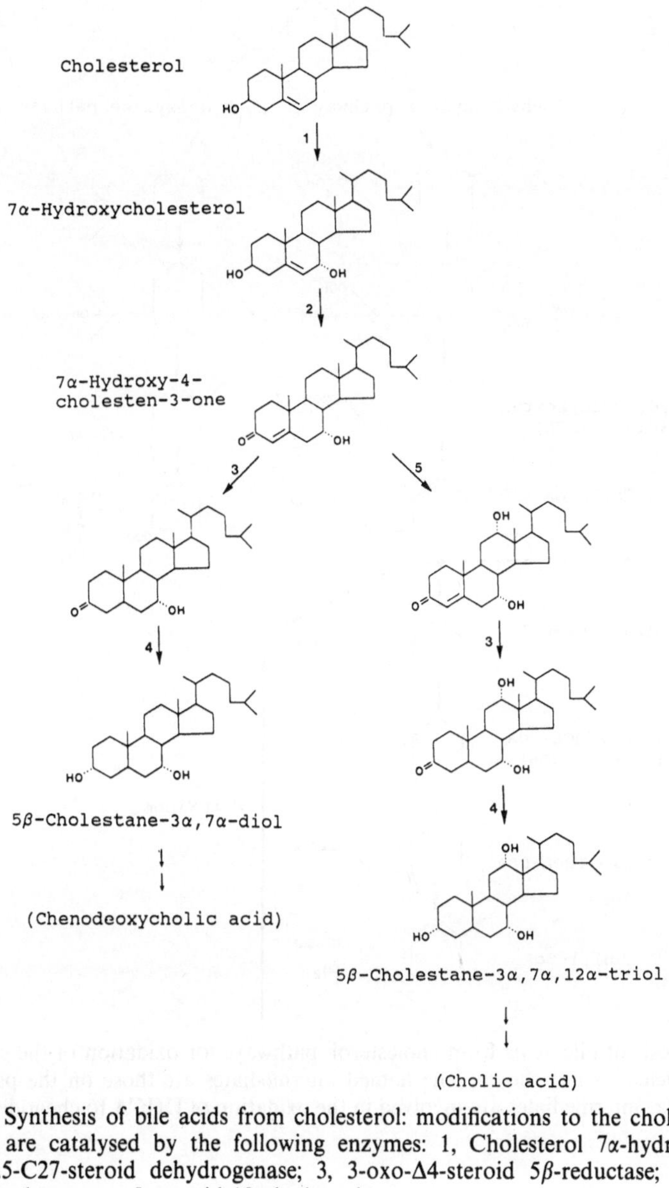

Figure 1 Synthesis of bile acids from cholesterol: modifications to the cholesterol nucleus. Reactions are catalysed by the following enzymes: 1, Cholesterol 7α-hydroxylase; 2, 3β-hydroxy-Δ5-C27-steroid dehydrogenase; 3, 3-oxo-Δ4-steroid 5β-reductase; 4, 3α-hydroxy-steroid dehydrogenase; 5, steroid 12α-hydroxylase

other defects in this pathway have yet been described. Studies of BSD 2 have made it clear that side chain oxidation of intermediates can occur efficiently when the nuclear modifications cannot be completed. Thus the major abnormal metabolites are C24 bile acids with an unsaturated nucleus.

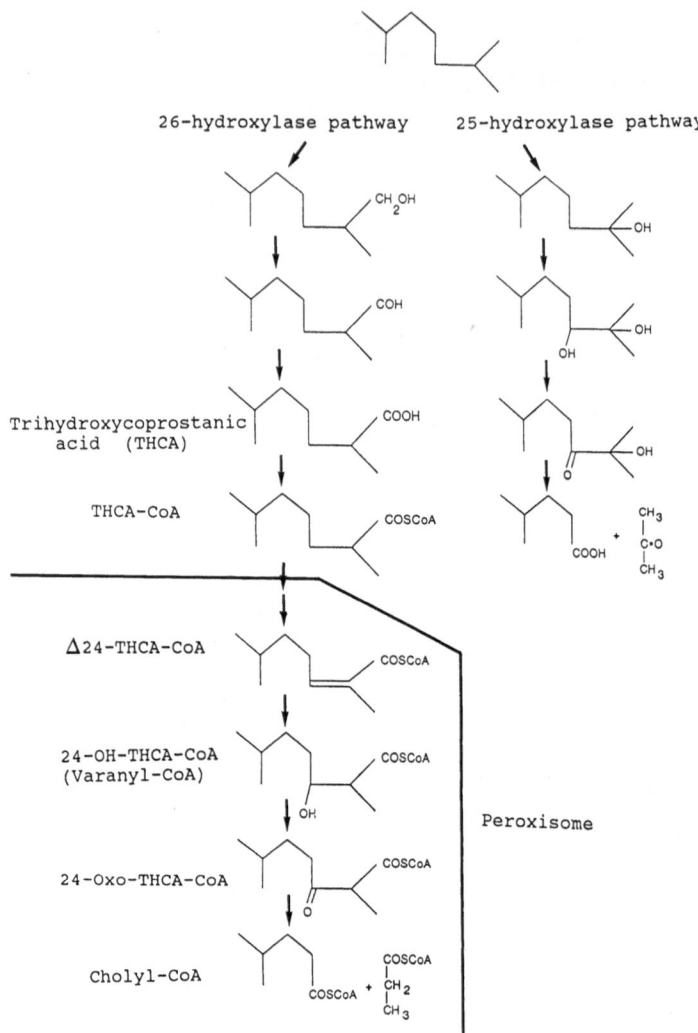

Figure 2 Synthesis of bile acids from cholesterol: pathways for oxidation of the side chain. The bile acid nucleus is not shown. The named intermediates are those on the pathway to cholic acid. Similar intermediates are involved in the oxidation of DHCA to chenodeoxycholic acid in the peroxisomes

BSD 2: 3β-hydroxy-Δ5-C27-steroid dehydrogenase deficiency

The effect of this enzyme deficiency is shown in Figure 3. 7α-Hydroxycholesterol cannot be converted to 7α-hydroxy-4-cholesten-3-one and undergoes side chain oxidation with or without 12α-hydroxylation to produce 3β,7α-dihydroxy-5-cholenoic acid and 3β,7α,12α-trihydroxy-5-cholenoic acid. These bile acids undergo sulphation at C-3 as well as partial conjugation with glycine and they appear in large amounts in the urine.

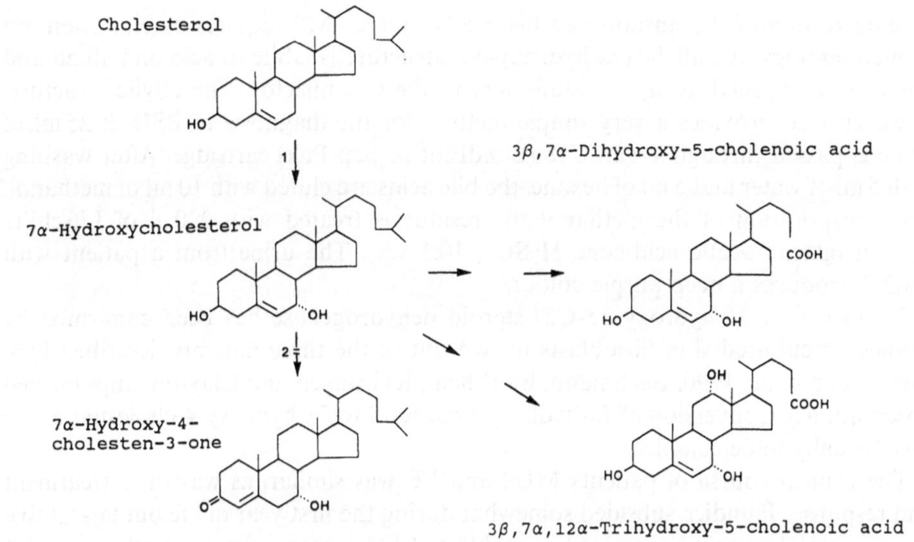

Figure 3 Site of the defect in BSD (3β-hydroxy-$\Delta5$-C27-steroid dehydrogenase). 7α-Hydroxycholesterol cannot be converted to 7α-hydroxy-4-cholesten-3-one and undergoes side chain oxidation ($\pm$ 12α-hydroxylation) to produce 3β-7α-dihydroxy-5-cholenoic acid and $3\beta,7\alpha,1\alpha$-trihydroxy-5-cholenoic acid

Three children with this condition have been seen at the Hospital for Sick Children, Great Ormond Street. The first (MU2) was Arabic, the offspring of a first cousin marriage, and he had a family history of two affected siblings who had died (Clayton *et al.*, 1987b; Buchmann *et al.*, 1990; Ichimiya *et al.*, 1990). The second (AB) was Caucasian. The third (FF) was Arabic and again the product of a first cousin marriage. Thus if we include the siblings of the first patient we have data on five children. All five affected children had cholestatic jaundice commencing in the neonatal period and still present at 3 months. The three children who were fully documented all developed clinical rickets early in infancy. One had a bleeding diathesis at 9 months which responded to parenteral vitamin K, and all had steatorrhoea. Two developed pruritus at around 7 months. Routine biochemical investigations revealed a plasma bilirubin of 16–250 μmol/L, aspartate aminotransferase (AST) 55–980 iu/L (normal 20–50 iu/L), alkaline phosphatase (at 3–4 months) of 1230–2014 iu/L (normal 250–1000 iu/L), calcium 1.68–2.30 mmol/L (normal 2.13–2.62), vitamin E < 4 μmol/L (normal 11.5–35 μmol/L), and prothrombin ratio 1–3 (corrected by parenteral vitamin K). Liver biopsies have shown a non-specific hepatitis progressing to a micronodular cirrhosis. Giant cells were prominent in early biopsies. Bile pigment was visible in hepatocytes, canaliculi and bile ducts in patients with a high plasma bilirubin.

Analysis of the plasma bile acids by GC–MS shows very low or undetectable concentrations of chenodeoxycholic and cholic acids. Analysis of the urine by FAB–MS shows ions m/z 469, 485, 526 and 542 attributable to sulphated $3\beta,7\alpha$-dihydroxy-5-cholenoic acid and $3\beta,7\alpha,12\alpha$-trihydroxy-5-cholenoic acid and their glycine conjugates.

Demonstration of the unsaturated bile acids by GC–MS requires careful attention to methodology; the allylic (7α-hydroxy-Δ5) structure is labile to acid and alkali and the 7α-trimethylsilyl group is readily lost in the GC injector. The allylic structure, however, also provides a very simple method for the diagnosis of BSD 2: 25 ml of urine is passed through a 6 ml C18 (BondElut or Sep-Pak) cartridge. After washing with 5 ml of water and 5 ml of hexane, the bile acids are eluted with 10 ml of methanol. After evaporation of the methanol the residue is treated with 200 μl of Lifschütz reagent (glacial acetic acid/conc H_2SO_4, 10:1 v/v). The urine from a patient with BSD 2 produces a deep purple colour.

Deficiency of 3β-hydroxy-Δ5-C27-steroid dehydrogenase has been confirmed by studies on cultured skin fibroblasts in two out of the three patients described here (Buchmann *et al.*, 1990; Buchmann, Björkhem, Kvittingen and Clayton, unpublished observations). Conversion of 7α-hydroxycholesterol to 7α-hydroxy-4-cholesten-3-one was virtually undetectable.

The clinical course of patients MU2 and FF was similar, as was their treatment and response. Jaundice subsided somewhat during the first year of life but fat-soluble vitamin malabsorption remained a problem. FF became anicteric at the age of 1 year, but plasma transaminases were still elevated (AST 68 iu/L) and a liver biopsy showed a non-specific hepatitis with some individual hepatocyte necrosis and bridging fibrosis. Treatment with chenodeoxycholic acid was commenced at a dose of 125 mg (the contents of one capsule) daily ($12 \, \text{mg kg}^{-1} \text{day}^{-1}$). There was symptomatic improvement (better appetite, less steatorrhoea), he remained anicteric and the AST fell within 4 weeks to inside the normal range, where it has remained. A liver biopsy performed after 4 months of treatment showed a definite improvement. An inflammatory infiltrate was still present in portal tracts but it was less marked and there was less hepatocyte necrosis and bridging fibrosis. In the case of MU2, treatment did not start until the age of 4.3 years (Ichimiya *et al.*, 1990), but there was still a dramatic improvement in symptoms (including pruritus) and in plasma bilirubin and transaminases. On treatment with chenodeoxycholic acid both FF and MU2 have required no significant fat-soluble vitamin supplementation.

The third patient we have treated with bile acids, AB, had more severe liver disease in infancy than either of the other two. Her plasma bilirubin at 7 months was 188 μmol/L, the AST was 760 iu/L and a biopsy showed an aggressive hepatitis with hepatocyte necrosis and bridging fibrosis. She was treated initially with chenodeoxycholic acid ($15 \, \text{mg}^{-1} \text{kg}^{-1} \text{day}$) and later with $7 \, \text{mg}^{-1} \text{kg}^{-1} \text{day}$ of chenodeoxycholic acid and $7 \, \text{mg}^{-1} \text{kg}^{-1} \text{day}$ of cholic acid. Over the course of a year her bilirubin returned to normal and the transaminases fell progressively. A repeat liver biopsy showed a more normal parenchyma and less inflammation.

Untreated, BSD 2 led to cirrhosis and death prior to the age of 5 years in the siblings of MU2. However, Watkins and colleagues have diagnosed BSD 2 in a child who was still alive at the age of 12 years, albeit with signs of chronic liver disease (J. B. Watkins, K. D. R. Setchell and colleagues, 1990, personal communication). It is clear that the outcome of the liver disease varies in different patients. None the less the beneficial effect of bile acid therapy in individual patients has been unequivocally demonstrated.

The effect of chenodeoxycholic acid therapy on the concentrations of bile acids and bile alcohols in bile, plasma, urine and faeces has been studied by Ichimiya and colleagues (H. Ichimiya, B. Egestad, H. Nazer, E. S. Baginski, P. T. Clayton and J. Sjövall, unpublished observations). Treatment was associated with a dramatic reduction in the plasma concentrations and urinary excretions of 3β-hydroxy-$\Delta 5$ bile acids and bile alcohols but the amounts of these compounds present in the faeces actually increased. This suggests that chenodeoxycholic acid works at least in part by promoting bile acid-dependent bile flow and this allows 3β-hydroxy-$\Delta 5$ compounds to enter the bile rather than passing into the blood and being excreted in the urine. There may be some inhibition of cholesterol 7α-hydroxylase but this is certainly incomplete.

The family histories of patients with BSD 2 suggest autosomal recessive inheritance. Prenatal diagnosis should theoretically be possible; it has not yet been attempted.

BSD 3: 3-oxo-$\Delta 4$-steroid 5β-reductase deficiency

Screening children with familial cholestatic liver disease by FAB–MS of urine reveals some patients whose urine spectrum is dominated by ions m/z 444, 460, 494 and 510, which can be shown by GC–MS analysis to originate from the glycine and taurine conjugates of 7α-hydroxy-3-oxo-4-cholenoic acid and $7\alpha,12\alpha$-dihydroxy-3-oxo-4-cholenoic acid (Clayton *et al.*, 1988b; Setchell *et al.*, 1988). The most likely explanation for this finding is that these patients have reduced activity of hepatic 3-oxo-$\Delta 4$-steroid 5β-reductase (reaction 3 in Figure 1) and that 3-oxo-$\Delta 4$ bile acid precursors undergo side chain oxidation and conjugation. Preserved activity of hepatic 3-oxo-$\Delta 4$-steroid 5α-reductase would explain the presence of allo (5α[H]) bile acids in the body fluids of these patients. The major question is whether any of these patients have an inborn error of metabolism directly affecting 3-oxo-$\Delta 4$-steroid 5β-reductase. Systematic analysis of urine samples from patients with cholestatic liver disease of known cause revealed that 3-oxo-$\Delta 4$ bile acids could be the dominant urinary bile acids in patients with inborn errors in pathways other than those of bile acid synthesis, e.g. fumarylacetoacetase deficiency (tyrosinaemia), α_1-antitrypsin deficiency. They were the dominant urinary bile acids in an infant with fulminant hepatitis B but disappeared from the urine when the hepatitis resolved. Thus, a secondary reduction in the activity of hepatic 3-oxo-$\Delta 4$-steroid 5β-reductase can be a consequence of liver damage – perhaps when there is extensive damage to the endoplasmic reticulum (microsomes) which certainly occurs with both hepatitis B and α_1-antitrypsin deficiency. Unfortunately, 3-oxo-$\Delta 4$-steroid 5β-reductase cannot be measured in cultured fibroblasts so that fibroblast studies cannot be used to distinguish between a primary enzyme deficiency and secondary inhibition.

Patients excreting 3-oxo-$\Delta 4$ bile acids have been given bile acids with varying results. In one patient chenodeoxycholic acid produced an exacerbation of cholestasis and a rise in transaminases (Nazer, Gunasekaran and Sjövall, personal communication). This is perhaps not surprising as pretreatment concentrations of chenodeoxycholic acid in plasma (and probably also in hepatocytes) are elevated and chenodeoxycholic acid is known to be hepatotoxic. However, the work of Setchell and colleagues (1988) has shown clearly that 3-oxo-$\Delta 4$ bile acids are poorly secreted into bile and therefore synthesis of these bile acids instead of chenodeoxycholic and cholic acid probably does contribute to the pathogenesis of cholestasis. They have tried treating one patient with ursodeoxycholic acid, then cholic acid with chenodeoxycholic acid and finally ursodeoxycholic acid with cholic acid. The latter seemed the most satisfactory treatment and they reported improvements in bilirubin and transaminases and in the liver biopsy (Balistreri, 1991).

DISORDERS AFFECTING CONVERSION OF 5β-CHOLESTANE-3α,7α-DIOL TO DHCA AND 5β-CHOLESTANE-3α,7α,12α-TRIOL TO THCA

Side chain oxidation commences with hydroxylation in the C-26 position; subsequent oxidation of C26-hydroxylated bile alcohols is catalysed by liver alcohol dehydrogenase and aldehyde dehydrogenase.

Cerebrotendinous xanthomatosis; 26-hydroxylase deficiency

Cerebrotendinous xanthomatosis (CTS) has been comprehensively reviewed recently (Björkhem and Skrede, 1989). It is an autosomal recessive disorder which leads to the accumulation of cholestanol and cholesterol in most tissues, but particularly in brain, in xanthomata and in bile. Characteristically, mental retardation or regression in childhood is followed, in adolescence or early adult life, by spastic paresis, cerebellar ataxia, cataracts, and tendon xanthomata. Premature atherosclerosis may occur and there is usually progressive neurological deterioration. In 1974, Setoguchi and colleagues demonstrated that patients with CTX had a defect in bile acid biosynthesis involving incomplete oxidation of the side chain. Björkhem and colleagues have now shown convincingly that the defect is in the mitochondrial 26-hydroxylase which is active on bile acid intermediates such as 5β-cholestane-3α,7α,12α-triol (see Björkhem and Skrede, 1989 for references). The accumulating metabolites are metabolized by hydroxylation in the side chain at positions other than C-26. Thus the major metabolite in bile is (the glucuronide of) 5β-cholestane-3α,7α,12α,25-tetrol, and in urine cholestane pentol glucuronides predominate, the major one being (23S)-5β-cholestane-3α,7α,12α,23,25-pentol. The cholestane pentol glucuronides produce a large peak at m/z 627 on FAB–MS analysis of urine (Egestad et al., 1985; Clayton, P. T. and Lawson, A. M. ,1986, unpublished observations). Plasma chenodeoxycholic acid, cholic acid and deoxycholic acid concentrations are low (Beppu et al., 1982). Using our usual method for plasma bile acid analysis, we have identified the following compounds on the GC–MS trace of a patient with CTX: 5β-cholestane-3α,7α,12α-triol, 5β-cholestane-3α,7α,12α,25-tetrol and 7α,12α-dihydroxy-4-cholesten-3-one; other workers have shown raised plasma concentrations of 7α-hydroxy-4-cholesten-3-one and 7α-hydroxycholesterol in untreated CTX (Björkhem et al., 1987; Koopman et al., 1987). Thus there is evidence for the accumulation of most of the intermediates in Figure 1, as one might expect with the combination of a block in the metabolism of 5β-cholestane-3α,7α-diol and 5β-cholestane-3α,7α,12α-triol and loss of feedback inhibition of cholesterol 7α-hydroxylase.

In patients with CTX, some synthesis of cholic acid can occur because 5β-cholestane-3α,7α,12α,25-tetrol can be converted to (24S)-3α,7α,12α,24,25-pentol and thence to cholic acid plus acetone (Figure 2, right hand side) (Shefer *et al.*, 1976).

Patients with CTX do not suffer from cholestatic liver disease or lipid malabsorption; synthesis of cholic acid by the 25-hydroxylase pathway may go some way towards explaining this. However, it is also possible that the bile alcohols produced by these patients can be actively secreted into bile, driving bile acid-dependent bile flow and participating in micellar solubilization of lipids. It should be remembered that bile alcohols (and C27 bile acids) perform this function efficiently in other species (Hoshita, 1985).

The major problems in CTX stem from cholestanol (and cholesterol) accumulation in tissues, particularly the central nervous system. The possible causes of increased synthesis of cholestanol have been critically reviewed by Björkhem and Skrede (1989). The most likely explanation is that accumulating bile acid intermediates are converted into cholestanol. Increased synthesis of cholesterol may be due to loss of bile acid inhibition of HMG-CoA reductase or it may be secondary to the accumulation of cholestanol.

CTX was the first inborn error of bile acid synthesis to be treated with bile acids. As already noted, the main aim of therapy is to inhibit cholesterol 7α-hydroxylase and prevent the accumulation of bile acid intermediates. Chenodeoxycholic acid has been shown to lower plasma cholestanol concentrations, and depress synthesis of cholesterol and cholestanol (Salen *et al.*, 1975). It also leads to the disappearance of bile alcohols from the urine of treated patients (Wolthers *et al.*, 1983; Batta *et al.*, 1985); ursodeoxycholic acid is not effective as would be expected since it is not an inhibitor of cholesterol 7α-hydroxylase (Kooopman *et al.*, 1984; Heuman *et al.*, 1988). Most importantly, a number of patients treated with chenodeoxycholic acid have shown reversal of neurological disability with a rise in IQ and improved strength and independence (Salen *et al.*, 1983; Berginer *et al.*, 1984). Obviously it would be desirable to start treatment before developmental delay or neurological signs become apparent. Koopman and colleagues (1987) have suggested that large populations of infants/children could be screened for CTX by using a simple commercial kit assay for 7α-hydroxylated steroids in urine. FAB–MS with automatic sample introduction could also be used to look for cholestane pentol glucuronides (m/z 627) in large numbers of samples. However, normal infant urine contains enough cholestane pentol glucuronide to produce a peak on the FAB–MS trace, so some method of quantitation would be required.

Heterozygotes for CTX can be detected by the increase in urinary 5β-cholestane-$3\alpha,7\alpha,12\alpha,23,25$-pentol which occurs following cholestyramine (Koopman *et al.*, 1986). Mitochondrial 26-hydroxylase can be determined in cultured skin fibroblasts (Skrede *et al.*, 1986); if the enzyme can also be measured in amniocytes or chorionic villus cells then prenatal diagnosis will be possible. However, unless the current mean age of diagnosis is reduced, pregnancies at risk will rarely be identified.

DISORDERS AFFECTING β-OXIDATION OF DHCA AND THCA

Prior to peroxisomal β-oxidation, THCA (or DHCA) must be converted to the CoA derivative; this occurs in the endoplasmic reticulum (Prydz *et al.*, 1988; Schepers *et al.*, 1989). The THCA-CoA must then be transported into the peroxisome; a carrier protein may be involved. The peroxisomal pathway for β-oxidation of THCA-CoA (Figure 2) commences with a THCA-CoA oxidase which is distinct from the acyl-CoA oxidase involved in fatty acid oxidation (Casteels *et al.*, 1988). The CoA ester of Δ24-THCA is then acted on firstly by the enoyl-CoA hydratase component of the bifunctional protein (producing the CoA ester of 24-hydroxy-THCA (varanic acid)) and secondly by the 3-hydroxyacyl-CoA dehydrogenase component of the bifunctional protein. Finally, the CoA ester of 24-oxo-THCA undergoes thiolytic cleavage to produce cholyl-CoA. The bifunctional protein and the thiolase involved in this pathway are the same as those involved in peroxisomal β-oxidation of fatty acids, including very long chain fatty acids (VLCFA).

Defects of peroxisome biogenesis

The disorders of peroxisome biogenesis (Zellweger syndrome and its milder variants, infantile Refsum disease, neonatal adrenoleukodystrophy and hyperpipecolic acid-aemia) have been extensively reviewed elsewhere (Schutgens *et al.*, 1986; Wanders *et al.*, 1988; Lazarow and Moser, 1989). Analysis of plasma bile acids from infants with these disorders invariably shows the presence of C27 bile acids and a C29-dicarboxylic acid ($3\alpha,7\alpha,12\alpha$-trihydroxy-27-carboxymethyl-5β-cholestan-26-oic acid) first identified by Janssen and colleagues (1982) (Clayton *et al.*, 1987a). In infants THCA is the major C27 bile acid; in older children DHCA may be present at much higher concentrations than THCA. FAB–MS analysis of the urine of infants with defects of peroxisome biogenesis may show peaks attributable to THCA (m/z 449) and its taurine conjugate (m/z 556); however, the constant feature is a peak at m/z 572 attributable to nuclear-hydroxylated derivatives of THCA such as 1β-hydroxy-THCA and 6α-hydroxy-THCA (Lawson *et al.*, 1986). In children over the age of 18 months, there is insufficient taurotetrahydroxycholestanoic acid in the urine to produce a clear peak at m/z 572 on the FAB–MS trace so this is an unreliable method for diagnosis in this age group.

The reason for the relatively low concentration of DHCA in the plasma of infants with defects of peroxisome biogenesis and the origin of some of the other metabolites have been elucidated by tracer studies. Kase and colleagues (1990) have shown that in infants with defects of peroxisome biogenesis, much of the DHCA is converted to THCA by 12α-hydroxylation. THCA can be converted to nuclear-hydroxylated derivatives and to the C29-dicarboxylic acid (Kase *et al.*, 1985).

Hanson and colleagues (1979) suggested that patients with Zellweger syndrome may produce quite large amounts of varanic acid. However, there were technical limitations to this study; without the use of capillary gas chromatography it is difficult to separate varanic acid from isomeric compounds with similar mass spectra, including nuclear hydroxylated derivatives of THCA and C25- and C26-hydroxylated derivatives of THCA. More recent studies suggest that in patients with defects of peroxisome biogenesis, varanic acid is produced in small amounts, probably by microsomal hydroxylation of THCA (Clayton *et al.*, 1987a, 1990).

The detection of a plasma or urine bile acid profile suggestive of a defect of peroxisome biogenesis should always be followed up by other tests of peroxisome function (platelet/fibroblast dihydroxyacetone phosphate acyltransferase as a minimum) to show that the patient really does have impairment of peroxisomal pathways other than the β-oxidation pathway.

Some patients with disorders of peroxisome biogenesis have clinically apparent cholestasis; most have quite marked hepatic fibrosis or cirrhosis. It has been suggested that THCA may contribute to liver damage but there is no proof of this, and there are many other biochemical abnormalities which could be contributing.

Measurement of THCA in amniotic fluid has been used for the prenatal diagnosis of pregnancies at risk from Zellweger syndrome (Stellaard *et al.*, 1988).

Defects affecting all peroxisomal β-oxidation proteins

There have been two reports of patients with clinical features similar to Zellweger syndrome in whom peroxisomes were identifiable in biopsy material but in whom immunoblotting techniques showed an absence of the three peroxisomal β-oxidation proteins (Paturneau-Jouas *et al.*, 1988; Suzuki *et al.*, 1988a,b). THCA and DHCA were present in the plasma and there was evidence of accumulation of other substrates normally metabolized by β-oxidation in the peroxisomes – increased plasma very long chain fatty acids and increased excretion of dicarboxylic acids in the urine. Further investigation revealed a deficiency of dihydroxyacetone phosphate acyltransferase; thus the peroxisomes appear normal but lack the β-oxidation enzymes and the dihydroxyacetone phosphate acyltransferase. The reason for this remains to be elucidated.

Defects of individual peroxisomal β-oxidation proteins

Defects of peroxisomal β-oxidation proteins have recently been reviewed by Wanders and colleagues (1990). Affected patients have severe hypotonia, developmental delay, seizures and a large fontanelle. Liver function tests are not severely deranged and liver histology shows only mild periportal fibrosis.

Two types of disorder affecting the peroxisomal bifunctional protein have been described. Watkins and colleagues (1989) described a patient who lacked immunoreactive bifunctional protein and had an elevated plasma concentration of THCA. From the nature of the defect, one might predict that the patient would also accumulate Δ24-THCA: however, this bile acid was not specifically sought. In a sibship with a defect in the 3-hydroxyacyl-CoA dehydrogenase component of the bifunctional protein, varanic acid was the major bile acid in duodenal juice (Clayton *et al.*, 1988a, 1990; Wanders *et al.*, 1990). GC–MS analysis suggested that it was almost entirely the 24R,25S isomer of varanic acid which was accumulating and this was confirmed by HPLC linked to FAB–MS (Rosankiewicz, J. R., Lawson, A. M. and Clayton, P. T., unpublished observation). This suggests that in man, as in the rat (Une *et al.*, 1984), peroxisomal β-oxidation proceeds via the 24R,25S isomer of varanic acid. The plasma of these infants contained varanic acid and THCA in similar amounts and no C29 dicarboxylic acid. The urine contained taurine-conjugated tetrahydroxycholestanoic and tetrahydroxycholestenoic acids, producing ions m/z 572 and 570 respectively on FAB–MS.

The first defect of peroxisomal β-oxidation to be described was peroxisomal 3-

oxoacyl-CoA thiolase deficiency (Goldfischer *et al.*, 1986; Schram *et al.*, 1987). Analysis of plasma from this patient revealed the presence of THCA and varanic acid at low concentration (Clayton *et al.*, 1990). Concentrations of C27 bile acids in urine were also low – below the threshold of detection of the FAB–MS technique. Thus plasma very long chain fatty acid analysis is superior to plasma and urine bile acid analyses for the detection of thiolase deficiency. Analysis of bile, however, showed an interesting profile – one which was clearly distinguishable from the profiles of patients with other peroxisomal defects. The major C27 bile acid was varanic acid (as was observed in deficiency of the 3-hydroxyacyl-CoA component of the bifunctional protein). However, capillary GC–MS separated two isomers of this compound and careful scrutiny of the trace suggested that the second peak may have been a doublet; HPLC linked to FAB–MS confirmed that there were three isomers of varanic acid present in the bile (Rosankiewicz, J. R., Lawson, A. M. and Clayton, P. T., unpublished observation). The likely explanation is that when metabolism of 24-oxo-THCA to cholic acid is blocked it can be converted to isomers of varanic acid other than the 24R,25S isomer.

Unknown defects leading to the accumulation of THCA

The early descriptions of patients with trihydroxycoprostanic acidaemia include some patients who could not be clinically defined as having Zellweger syndrome and, at the time of these descriptions, back-up tests for peroxisomal dysfunction were not available (Eyssen *et al.*, 1972; Hanson *et al.*, 1975; Parmentier *et al.*, 1979). In retrospect it is probable that most of these patients had defects of peroxisome biogenesis. However, the only abnormalities recorded in the siblings reported by Hanson and colleagues were liver disease, deafness and rickets. The liver disease and deafness are compatible with a disorder of peroxisome biogenesis but no dysmorphic features or developmental delay were recorded; thus the precise defect remains undefined.

Recently a number of patients have been described in whom accumulation of THCA has been demonstrated but in whom very long chain fatty acids are normal (excluding a defect of peroxisome biogenesis, a defect of bifunctional protein and a defect of peroxisomal thiolase). Possible mechanisms for the THCA accumulation would include defects of THCA-CoA synthetase, the transport mechanism which allows THCA-CoA to enter the peroxisome and THCA-CoA oxidase. None of these mechanisms has yet been proved although it has been suggested that the accumulation of the C29 dicarboxylic acid (noted in all but one of the patients) excludes a defect of THCA-CoA synthetase on the basis that the C29 acid is probably produced by chain elongation of THCA-CoA (rather than of THCA itself). The patients are a rather diverse group. Christensen and colleagues (1990) described a girl who was normal until 18 months and then developed ataxia, hypotonia and hyporeflexia which improved on a low phytanic acid diet. Pryzembel and colleagues (1990) described a small-for-dates infant who continued to fail to thrive postnatally, showed no psycho-motor development and developed hepatic dysfunction leading to death from hepatic failure at $6\frac{1}{2}$ months. He had some dysmorphic features, hypertonia and unco-ordinated eye movements. Wanders and colleagues (1990) described twins with severe hypotonia plus psychomotor delay, dysmorphic features and ocular abnormalities. Mild hepatomegaly was noted but not severe hepatic dysfunction. Poll-The and colleagues (1988) described siblings who had episodes of hypoketotic hypoglycaemia with hydroxydicarboxylic aciduria and who also had peripheral neuropathy and pigmentary retinopathy but normal mental development. Hepatic peroxisomes looked structurally abnormal. The authors proposed that these children had a defect affecting both mitochondrial and peroxisomal β-oxidation.

Barth and colleagues (1990) have described two siblings with elevated levels of very long chain fatty acids, C27 bile acids and phytanic acid but otherwise normal peroxisomal function tests. These infants clearly had some defect of peroxisomal β-oxidation but the precise nature of the defect could not be defined. The clinical picture was rather different from that of patients with proven defects of the bifunctional protein or thiolase, and involved progressive psychomotor deterioration (with loss of myelin apparent on magnetic resonance imaging), retinopathy and peripheral neuropathy as well as hypotonia, feeding difficulties and seizures. Fontanelle size was normal.

ANOTHER POSSIBLE DEFECT OF SIDE CHAIN OXIDATION

We are currently studying a child with severe familial cholestasis starting in the neonatal period who has low concentrations of chenodeoxycholic acid and cholic acid in plasma and whose urine contains, as the major metabolite, 5β-cholestane-$3\alpha,7\alpha,12\alpha,24,25$-pentol. One possible explanation would be a defect in the 25-hydroxylase pathway (Figure 2, right hand side, one of the last three reactions). However, this would be at variance with the commonly held view that the 25-hydroxylase pathway plays a minor role in bile acid synthesis.

DISORDERS AFFECTING ENTEROHEPATIC CIRCULATION (TRANSPORT DEFECTS)

Maintenance of the bile acid pool within the enterohepatic circulation requires two active uptake mechanisms – one in the ileum transporting bile acids from the intestinal lumen to the portal circulation and one in the liver clearing bile acids from portal blood into the hepatocytes.

Heubi and colleagues (1979, 1982) have described two unrelated boys with congenital diarrhoea, steatorrhoea and growth failure. Investigations revealed evidence of bile acid malabsorption and further studies using ileal biopsies showed a significant reduction in the active uptake of taurocholate. There was no microscopic evidence of mucosal disease in the ileum and other aspects of ileal function were normal. It was concluded that the two boys had an inborn error affecting the ileal transport mechanism. The diarrhoea was attributed to exposure of the colonic mucosa to high bile acid concentrations.

A defect in the transport of bile acids from the hepatocytes into the canaliculi would be expected to produce familial cholestasis with steatorrhoea and fat-soluble vitamin malabsorption, but with high plasma and urinary chenodeoxycholic acid and cholic acid concentrations (unlike the synthesis defects). There are many patients who fulfil these criteria. Some have hypoplastic intrahepatic bile ducts while others have normal hepatic histology; none of them has yet been shown to have a primary defect of bile acid transport.

POSSIBLE DISORDERS AFFECTING PROCESSING OF BACTERIAL METABOLITES

While the bile acid pool is within the intestinal lumen, bacterial metabolism of bile acids occurs. Taurine and glycine conjugates are split, 7α-dehydroxylation produces deoxycholic acid from cholic acid and lithocholic acid from chenodeoxycholic acid, and bacterial dehydrogenases convert 3α-, 7α- and 12α-hydroxy groups to the 3-oxo, 7-oxo and 12-oxo groups respectively. In the liver deconjugated bile acids are converted to the CoA derivatives and then reconjugated with glycine or taurine. Hepatic hydroxysteroid dehydrogenases convert 3-oxo, 7-oxo and 12-oxo bile acids back to the 3α-, 7α- or 12α-hydroxy parent compound.

Hofmann and Standvik (1988) have speculated on the likely consequences of a disorder of bile acid conjugation – steatorrhoea and diarrhoea, fat-soluble vitamin malabsorption and a high ratio of cholic acid to chenodeoxycholic acid in the plasma. No such patient has yet been described.

Similarly, no-one has yet unequivocally demonstrated the existence of an inborn error affecting one of the hepatic hydroxysteroid dehydrogenases, but work in Japan has raised the possibility of a deficiency of the 12α-hydroxysteroid dehydrogenase in some adults with cirrhosis. In 1968, Hoshita and colleagues demonstrated the presence of $3\alpha,7\alpha$-dihydroxy-12-oxo-5β-cholanic acid (12-oxo-chenodeoxycholic acid) in the fistula bile of 6 out of 17 patients suffering from hepatobiliary disease. Kikuchi (1972) postulated that 12-oxochenodeoxycholic acid was produced from cholic acid in the gut and that, in some patients, passage through the liver resulted in conjugation of the oxo bile acid with taurine and glycine without reduction of the 12-oxo group. Amuro and colleagues (1980) showed that in some Japanese patients with cirrhosis, 12-oxochenodeoxycholic acid is the major bile acid in the urine. They also suggested that this may be attributable to an impaired ability of the patient's liver to reduce oxo bile acids.

We have only come across one infant with hepatobiliary disease in whom 12-oxo bile acids were the major urinary bile acids (Clayton, P. T., Mowat, A. P. and Lawson, A. M., unpublished observation). Further investigation revealed that the child was being given dehydrocholic acid (Decholin, 3,7,12-trioxo-5β-cholanic acid) as a choleretic. It would appear that 12-oxochenodeoxycholic acid is a major metabolite of dehydrocholic acid, presumably because the hepatic 12α-hydroxysteroid dehydrogenase is less efficient than the 3α- and 7α-hydroxysteroid dehydrogenases. Dehydrocholic acid is used quite extensively in Japan; it is important that this explanation for the results of Amuro and colleagues be excluded.

OTHER DISORDERS

Kibe and colleagues (1980) found a series of unusual bile alcohols in the bile of a 65-year-old Japanese man with cholestasis due to gallstones in the common bile duct.

The bile alcohols were identified as 26,27-dinor-5β-cholestane-3α,7α,12α,24,25-pentol, 24-methyl-26,27-dinor-5β-cholestane-3α,7α,12α,24-tetrol and 3α,7α,12α-trihydroxy-26,27-dinor-5β-cholestan-24-one. Synthesis of cholic and chenodeoxycholic acid appeared to be normal and the cause of the production of unusual bile alcohols was not elucidated.

Physicians studying hepatobiliary disease are very aware of the fact that there are many inherited disorders whose biochemical basis is not understood. There are probably more inborn errors of bile acid metabolism waiting to be discovered.

ACKNOWLEDGEMENTS

I am grateful to the Child Health Research Appeal Trust for financial support and to Aspreys plc for their generous donation of GC–MS equipment. Cholic acid for therapeutic use was generously donated by Dr Herbert Falk. I am indebted to Dr Alex Lawson for help with mass spectrometry and to all the clinicians who have sent me patients and/or samples. Most of all I owe my thanks to the parents who were prepared to put their faith in theoretically sound but clinically unproven forms of treatment.

REFERENCES

Amuro, Y., Endo, T., Higashino, K., Uchida, K. and Yamamura, Y. Urinary and fecal keto bile acids in liver cirrhosis. *Clin. Chim. Acta* 114 (1981) 137–147

Balistreri, W. F. Fetal and neonatal bile acid synthesis and metabolism – clinical implications. *J. Inher. Metab. Dis.* 14 (1991) 459–477

Barth, P. G., Wanders, R. J. A., Schutgens, R. B. H., Bleeker-Wagemakers, E. M. and van Heemstra, D. Peroxisomal β-oxidation defect with detectable peroxisomes: a case with neonatal onset and progressive course. *Eur. J. Pediatr.* 149 (1990) 722–726

Batta, A. K., Shefer, S., Batta, M. and Salen, G. Effect of chenodeoxycholic acid on biliary and urinary bile acids and bile alcohols in cerebrotendinous xanthomatosis; monitoring by high performance liquid chromotography. *J. Lipid Res.* 26 (1985) 690–698

Beppu, T., Seyama, Y., Kasama, T., Serizawa, S. and Yamakawa, T. Serum bile acid profiles in CTX. *Clin. Chim. Acta* 118 (1982) 167–175

Berginer, V. M., Salen, G. and Shefer, S. Long term treatment of CTX with chenodeoxycholic acid therapy. *N. Engl. J. Med.* 311 (1984) 1649–1652

Björkhem, I. Mechanism of bile acid biosynthesis in mammalian liver. In Danielsson, H. and Sjövall, J. (eds.), *Sterols and Bile Acids. New Comprehensive Biochemistry, Vol. 12*, Elsevier, Amsterdam, New York and Oxford, 1985, pp. 231–278

Björkhem, I. and Skrede, S. Familial diseases with storage of sterols other than cholesterol: cerebrotendinous xanthomatosis and phytosterolaemia. In Scriver, C. R., Beaudet, A. L., Sly, W. S. and Valle, D. (eds.) *The Metabolic Basis of Inherited Disease*, 6th edn, McGraw-Hill, New York, 1989, pp. 1283–1302

Björkhem, I., Skrede, S., Buchmann, M. S., East, C. and Grundy, S. Accumulation of 7α-hydroxy-4-cholesten-3-one and cholesta-4,6-dien-3-one in patients with CTX. Effect of treatment with chenodeoxycholic acid. *Hepatology* 7 (1987) 226–271

Buchmann, M. S., Kvittingen, E. A., Nazer, H., Gunasekaran, T., Clayton, P. T. and Sjövall, J. Lack of 3β-hydroxy-Δ5-C$_{27}$-steroid dehydrogenase/isomerase in fibroblasts from a child with urinary excretion of 3β-hydroxy-Δ5-bile acids – a new inborn error of metabolism. *J. Clin. Invest.* 86 (1990) 2034–2037

Casteels, M., Schepers, L., Van Eldere, J., Eyssen, H. and Mannaerts, G. P. Inhibition of 3α,7α,12α-trihydroxy-5β-cholestanoic acid oxidation and of bile acid secretion in rat liver by fatty acids. *J. Biol. Chem.* 263 (1988) 4654–4661

Christensen, E., Van Eldere, J., Brandt, N. J., Schutgens, R. B. H., Wanders, R. J. A. and Eyssen, H. J. A new peroxisomal disorder: Di- and trihydroxycholestanaemia due to a presumed trihydroxycholestanoyl-CoA oxidase deficiency. *J. Inher. Metab. Dis.* 13 (1990) 363–366

Clayton, P. T. and Muller, D. P. R. A simplified gas-liquid chromatographic method for the estimation of non-sulphated plasma bile acids. *Clin. Chim. Acta* 105 (1980) 401–405

Clayton, P. T., Lake, B. D., Hall, N. A., Shortland, D. B., Carruthers, R. A. and Lawson, A. M. Plasma bile acids in peroxisomal dysfunction syndromes: analysis by capillary gas chromatography–mass spectrometry. *Eur. J. Pediatr.* 146 (1987a) 166–173

Clayton, P. T., Leonard, J. V., Lawson, A. M., Setchell, K. D. R., Andersson, S., Egestad, B. and Sjövall, J. Familial giant cell hepatitis associated with synthesis of 3β,7α-dihydroxy- and 3β,7α,12α-trihydroxy-5-cholenoic acids. *J. Clin. Invest.* 79 (1987b) 1031–1038

Clayton, P. T., Lake, B. D., Hjelm, M., Stephenson, J. B. P., Besley, G. T. N., Wanders, R. J. A., Schram, A. M. and Tager, J. M. Bile acid analyses in 'pseudo-Zellweger' syndrome; clues to the defect in peroxisomal β-oxidation. *J. Inher. Metab. Dis.* 11 (1988a) (Suppl. 2) 165–168

Clayton, P. T., Patel, E., Lawson, A. M., Carruthers, R. A., Tanner, M. S., Strandvik, B., Egestad, B. and Sjövall, J. 3-Oxo-Δ4 bile acids in liver disease. *Lancet* 1 (1988b) 1283–1284

Clayton, P. T., Patel, E., Lawson, A. M., Carruthers, R. A. and Collins, J. Bile acid profiles in peroxisomal 3-oxoacyl-CoA thiolase deficiency. *J. Clin. Invest.* 85 (1990) 1267–1273

Egestad, B., Pettersson, P., Skrede, S. and Sjövall, J. Fast atom bombardment mass spectrometry in the diagnosis of cerebrotendinous xanthomatosis. *Scand. J. Clin. Lab. Invest.* 45 (1985) 443–446

Eyssen, H., Parmentier, G., Compernolle, F., Boon, J., Eggermont, E. Trihydroxycoprostanic acid in the duodenal fluid of two children with intrahepatic bile duct anomalies. *Biochim. Biophys. Acta* 273 (1972) 212–221

Goldfischer, S., Collins, J., Rapin, I., Neumann, P., Neglia, W., Spiro, T., Ishii, T., Roels, F., Vamecq, J. and Van Hoof, F. Pseudo-Zellweger syndrome: deficiencies in several peroxisomal oxidative activities. *J. Pediatr.* 108 (1986) 25–32

Hanson, R. F., Isenberg, J. N., Williams, G. C., Hachey, D., Szczepanik, P., Klein, P. D. and Sharp, H. L. The metabolism of 3α,7α,12α-trihydroxy-5β-cholestan-26-oic acid in two siblings with cholestasis due to intrahepatic bile duct anomalies. *J. Clin. Invest.* 56 (1975) 577–587

Hanson, R. F., Szczepanik-Van Leeuwen, P., Williams, G. C., Grabowski, G. and Sharp, H. L. Defects of bile acid synthesis in Zellweger's syndrome. *Science (Washington DC)* 203 (1979) 1107–1108

Heubi, J. E., Balistreri, W. F., Partin, J. C., Schubert, W. K. and McGraw, C. A. Refractory infantile diarrhoea due to primary bile acid malabsorption. *J. Pediatr.* 94 (1979) 546–551

Heubi, J. E., Balistreri, W. F., Fondacaro, J. D., Partin, J. C. and Schubert, W. K. Primary bile acid malabsorption: Defective *in vitro* ileal active bile acid transport. *Gastroenterology* 83 (1982) 804–811

Heumann, D. M., Hernandez, C. R., Hylemon, P. B., Kubaska, W. M., Hartman, C. and Vlahcevic, Z. R. Regulation of bile acid synthesis. I. Effects of unconjugated ursodeoxycholate and cholate on bile acid synthesis on chronic bile fistula rat. *Hepatology* 8 (1988) 358–365

Hofmann, A. F. and Strandvik, B. Defective bile acid amidation: predicted features of a new inborn error of metabolism. *Lancet* 2 (1988) 311–313

Hoshita, T. Bile alcohols and primitive bile acids. In Danielsson, H. and Sjövall, J. (eds.) *Sterols and Bile Acids. New Comprehensive Biochemistry*, Vol. 12, Elsevier, Amsterdam, New York and Oxford, 1985, pp. 231–278

Hoshita, T., Yashima, H., Okada, S. and Yamada, T. Isolation of 3α,7α-dihydroxy-12-oxo-5β-cholanoic acid from the bile of patients with hepatobiliary diseases. *Hiroshima J. Med. Sci.* 17 (1968) 105–113

Ichimiya, H., Nazer, H., Gunasekaran, T., Clayton, P. and Sjövall, J. Treatment of chronic liver disease caused by 3β-hydroxy-$\Delta5$-C27-steroid dehydrogenase deficiency with chenodeoxycholic acid. *Arch. Dis. Child.* 65 (1990) 1121–1124

Kase, B. F., Björkhem, I., Haga, P. and Pedersen, J. I. Defective peroxisomal cleavage of the C_{27}-steroid side chain in the cerebro–hepato–renal syndrome of Zellweger. *J. Clin. Invest.* 75 (1985) 427–435

Kase, B. F., Pedersen, J. I., Wathne K.-O., Gustafsson, J. and Björkhem, I. On the importance of peroxisomes in the formation of chenodeoxycholic acid in human liver. Metabolism of $3\alpha,7\alpha$-dihydroxy-5β-cholestanoic acid in an infant with Zellweger syndrome. *Pediatr. Res.* 29 (1990) 64–69

Kibe, A., Nakai, S., Kuramoto, T. and Hoshita, T. Occurrence of bile alcohols in the bile of a patient with cholestasis. *J. Lipid Res.* 21 (1980) 594–599

Kikuchi, H. The metabolic sequence for the occurrence of an anomalous bile acid, 12-ketochenodeoxycholic acid, found in the bile of hepatobiliary diseased patients. *J. Biochem. (Tokyo)* 72 (1972) 165–172

Koopman, B. J., Wolthers, B. G., van der Molen, J. V., Nagel, G. T., Waterreus, R. J. and Oosterhuis, H. J. G. H. Capillary gas chromatographic determination of urinary bile acids and bile alcohols in CTX patients proving the ineffectivity of ursodeoxycholic acid treatment. *Clin. Chim. Acta* 142 (1984) 103–111

Koopman, B. J., Waterreus, R. J., Brekel, H. W. C. and Wolthers, B. G. Detection of carriers of CTX. *Clin. Chim. Acta* 158 (1986) 179–186

Koopman, B. J., van der Molen, J. C., Wolthers, B. G. and Vanderpas, J. B. Determination of some hydroxycholesterols in human serum samples. *J. Chromatog.*, 416 (1987) 1–13

Lawson, A. M., Madigan, M. J., Shortland, D. B. and Clayton, P. T. Rapid diagnosis of Zellweger syndrome and infantile Refsum's disease by fast atom bombardment–mass spectrometry of urine bile salts. *Clin. Chim. Acta* 161 (1986) 221–231

Lazarow, P. B. and Moser, H. W. Disorders of peroxisome biogenesis. In Scriver, C. R., Beaudet, A. L., Sly, W. S. and Valle, D. (eds.) *The Metabolic Basis of Inherited Disease*, 6th edn., McGraw-Hill, New York, 1989, pp. 1479–1509

Parmentier, G. G., Janssen, G. A., Eggermont, E. A. and Eyssen, H. J. C_{27} bile acids in infants with coprostanic acidaemia and occurrence of a $3\alpha,7\alpha,12\alpha$-trihydroxy-5β-C_{29} dicarboxylic bile acid as a major component in their serum. *Eur. J. Biochem.* 102 (1979) 173–183

Paturneau-Jouas, M., Taillard, F., Gansmuller, A., Schutgens, R., Mikol, J., Aigrot, M. S. and Sereni, C. Clinical, biochemical, pathological 'Zellweger-like' disorder with morphological normal peroxisomes. In Salvayre, R., Douste-Blazy, L. and Gatt, S. (eds.) *Lipid Storage Disorders: Biological and Medical Aspects, NATO ASI series, Life Sciences*, vol. 150, 1988, pp. 805–809

Poll-Thé, B. T., Bonnefont, J. P., Ogier, H., Charpentier, C., Pelet, A., Le Fur, J. M., Jakobs, C., Kok, R. M., Duran, M., Divry, P., Scotto, J. and Saudubray, J. M. Familial hypoketotic hypoglycaemia associated with peripheral neuropathy, pigmentary retinopathy and C_6–C_{14} hydroxydicarboxylic aciduria. A new defect in fatty acid oxidation? *J. Inher. Metab. Dis.* 11 Suppl. 2 (1988) 183–185

Prydz, K., Kase, B. F., Björkhem, I. and Pedersen, J. I. Subcellular localisation of $3\alpha,7\alpha$-dihydroxy- and $3\alpha,7\alpha,12\alpha$-trihydroxy-5β-cholestanoyl-coenzyme A ligase(s) in rat liver. *J. Lipid Res.* 29 (1988) 997–1004

Pryzembel, H., Wanders, R. J. A., van Roermund, C. W. T., Schutgens, R. B. H., Mannaerts, G. P. and Casteels, M. Di- and trihydroxycholestanoic acidaemia with hepatic failure. *J. Inher. Metab. Dis.* 13 (1990) 371–374

Salen, G., Meriwether, T. W. and Nicolau, G. Chenodeoxycholic acid inhibits increased cholesterol and cholestanol synthesis in patients with cerebrotendinous xanthomatosis. *Biochem. Med.* 14 (1975) 57–74

Salen, G., Shefer, S. and Berginer, V. M. Familial diseases with storage of sterols other than cholesterol: Cerebrotendinous xanthomatosis and sitosterolaemia with xanthomatosis. In Stanbury, J. B., Wyngarden, J. B., Frederickson, D. S., Brown, M. S. and Goldstein, J. L.

(eds.) *The Metabolic Basis of Inherited Disease*, 5th edn., McGraw-Hill, New York, 1983, pp. 713–730

Schepers, L., Casteels, M., Verheyden, K., Parmentier, G., Asselberghs, S., Eyssen, H. J. and Mannaerts, G. P. Subcellular distribution and characteristics of trihydroxycoprostanoyl-CoA synthetase. *Biochem. J.* 257 (1989) 221–229

Schram, A. W., Goldfischer, S., van Roermund, C. W. T., Brouwer-Kelder, E. M., Collins, J., Hashimoto, T., Heymans, H. S. A., Van den Bosch, H., Schutgens, R. B. H., Tager, J. M. and Wanders, R. J. A. Human peroxisomal 3-oxoacyl-CoA thiolase deficiency. *Proc. Natl. Acad. Sci. USA* 84 (1987) 2494–2496

Schutgens, R. B. H., Heymans, H. S. A., Wanders, R. J. A., van den Bosch, H. and Tager, J. M. Peroxisomal disorders: a newly recognised group of genetic diseases. *Eur. J. Pediatr.* 144 (1986) 430–440

Setchell, K. D. R., Suchy, F. J., Welsh, M. B., Zimmer-Nechemias, L., Heubi, J. and Balistreri, W. F. Δ^4-3-Oxosteroid 5β-reductase deficiency described in identical twins with neonatal hepatitis. A new inborn error in bile acid synthesis. *J. Clin. Invest.* 82 (1988) 2148–2157

Setoguchi, T., Salen, G., Tint, G. S. and Mosbach, E. H. A biochemical abnormality in cerebrotendinous xanthomatosis: Impairment of bile acid biosynthesis associated with incomplete degradation of the cholesterol side chain. *J. Clin. Invest.* 531 (1974) 1393–1401

Shefer, S., Cheng, F. W., Dayal, B., Hauser, S., Tint, G. S., Salen, G. and Mosbach, E. H. A 25-hydroxylation pathway of cholic acid biosynthesis in man and rat. *J. Clin. Invest.* 57 (1976) 897–903

Skrede, S., Björkhem, I., Kvittingen, E. A., Buchmann, M. S., East, C. and Grundy, S. Demonstration of 26-hydroxylation of C_{27}-steroids in human skin fibroblasts, and a deficiency of this activity in CTX. *J. Clin. Invest.* 78 (1986) 729–735

Stellaard, F., Langelaar, S. A., Kok, R. M., Kleijer, W. J., Schutgens, R. B. H. and Jakobs, C. Prenatal diagnosis of Zellweger syndrome by determination of trihydroxycoprostanic acid in amniotic fluid. *Eur. J. Pediatr.* 148 (1988) 175–176

Suzuki, Y., Shimozawa, N., Orii, T., Igarashi, N., Kono, N., Matsui, A., Inoue, Y., Yokota, S. and Hashimoto, T. Zellweger-like syndrome with detectable hepatic peroxisomes: a variant form of peroxisomal disorder. *J. Pediatr.* 113 (1988a) 841–845

Suzuki, Y., Shimozawa, N., Orii, T., Igarashi, N., Kono, N., Hashimoto, T. Molecular analysis of peroxisomal β-oxidation enzymes in infants with Zellweger syndrome and Zellweger-like syndrome: further heterogeneity of the peroxisomal disorders. *Clin. Chim. Acta.* 172 (1988b) 65–76

Une, M., Morigami, I., Kihira, K. and Hoshita, T. Stereospecific formation of (24E)-$3\alpha,7\alpha,12\alpha$-trihydroxy-5β-cholest-24-en-26-oic acid and (24R,25S)-$3\alpha,7\alpha,12\alpha,24$-tetrahydroxy-$5\beta$-cholestan-26-oic acid from either (25R)- or (25S)-$3\alpha,7\alpha,12\alpha$-trihydroxy-5β-cholestan-26-oic acid by rat liver homogenate. *J. Biochem. (Tokyo)* 96 (1984) 1103–1007

Wanders, R. J. A., Heymans, H. S. A., Schutgens, R. B. H., Barth, P. G., van den Bosch, H. and Tager, J. M. Peroxisomal disorders in neurology. *J. Neurol. Sci.* 88 (1988) 1–39

Wanders, R. J. A., van Roermund, C. W. T., Schelen, A., Schutgens, R. B. H., Tager, J. M., Stephenson, J. B. P. and Clayton, P. T. A bifunctional protein with deficient enzymic activity: Identification of a new peroxisomal disorder using novel methods to measure the peroxisomal β-oxidation enzyme activities. *J. Inher. Metab. Dis.* 13 (1990a) 375–379

Wanders, R. J. A., van Roermund, C. W. T., Schelen, A., Schutgens, R. B. H., Zeman, J., Kozich, V., Hyanek, J., Casteels, M. and Mannaerts, G. P. Di- and trihydroxycoprostanaemia in twin sisters. *J. Inher. Metab. Dis.* 14 (1991) 357–360

Watkins, P. A., Chen, W. W., Harris, C. J., Hoefler, G., Hoefler, S., Blake, D. C., Balfe, A., Kelley, R. I., Moser, A. B., Beard, M. E. and Moser, H. W. Peroxisomal bifunctional enzyme deficiency. *J. Clin. Invest.* 82 (1989) 771–777

Wolthers, B. G., Volmer, M., van der Molen, J., Koopman, B. J., De Jager, A. E. J. and Waterreus, R. J. Diagnosis of cerebrotendinous xanthomatosis (CTX) and effect of chenodeoxycholic acid therapy by analysis of urine using capillary gas chromatography. *Clin. Chim. Acta* 131 (1983) 53–65

J. Inher. Metab. Dis. 14 (1991) 497–511

α_1-Antitrypsin Deficiency and Liver Disease: Clinical Presentation, Diagnosis and Treatment

M. Hussain, G. Mieli-Vergani and A. P. Mowat*
*Department of Child Health, King's College Hospital, Denmark Hill,
London SE5 8RX, UK*

Summary: The α_1-antitrypsin deficient subject (protease inhibitor (PI) phenotype ZZ) has an increased susceptibility to liver disease. The condition is most commonly identified in early infancy as a conjugated hyperbilirubinaemia with hepatitis (11%) or a bleeding state due to vitamin K malabsorption (2%). 50% of cases have cirrhosis and 25% die in the first decade of life. A further 2% present with cirrhosis in later childhood. Adult males are at risk of hepatoma development with or without cirrhosis. Diagnosis is by isoelectric focussing or allele-specific oligonucleotide hybridization. The treatment is that of cholestasis and cirrhosis including transplantation. The pathobiology of the deficiency state, the mechanism of liver damage and the vulnerability of the newborn liver are discussed in this review. A plea is made for a trial of infusions of α_1-antitrypsin in early infancy, as is used safely but without proven efficacy in the emphysematous PIZZ subject. Prospects of therapy by gene modification are also reviewed.

INTRODUCTION

α_1-antitrypsin was isolated by Schultz and colleagues in 1955. An association with liver disease and α_1-antitrypsin deficiency was first identified in two brothers with cirrhosis by Freier and colleagues in 1968. Since then genetic deficiency of α_1-antitrypsin has had a major impact on clinical practice in paediatric hepatology (Sharp et al., 1969). The deficiency state PIZZ (PI = protease inhibitor, genotype ZZ) is the second most common single diagnosis after biliary atresia in infants with hepatitis syndrome in populations of European descent. The clinical, laboratory and pathological features are frequently indistinguishable from those of biliary atresia. The prognosis is much worse than that of idiopathic hepatitis of infancy. Although presenting less frequently in later life, it must be excluded in any child or adult presenting with chronic liver disease (Mowat, 1987). It is the most common metabolic disease for which liver transplantation is performed (Cohen et al., 1989; Starzl et al., 1989).

*Correspondence

α_1-antitrypsin is a small monomeric glycoprotein (molecular weight 52 kDa). It has a single polypeptide core of 394 residues with carbohydrates forming three complex side chains (Cox, 1989; Crystal, 1990). The plasma glycoprotein is made in the liver as shown by the change in phenotype following liver transplantation (Cohen et al., 1989). It readily diffuses into tissue fluids. It is also synthesized in other tissues, particularly in the gastrointestinal tract and in macrophages (Perlmutter et al., 1989).

α_1-antitrypsin inhibits a wide range of serine proteases; its principal target is thought to be neutrophil elastase. This enzyme functions as an extracellular protease. Its prime substrate is elastin but it also attacks many other proteins, including a variety of proteins in the coagulation and complement cascades, E. coli cell wall components and all major components of extracellular matrix (Carrell, 1986; Travis, 1988). Within the liver the latter effect could have profound functional and structural sequelae. α_1-antitrypsin is thus thought to inhibit tissue-damaging protease.

The rise in serum α_1-antitrypsin concentration in common with other acute phase reactants during tissue injury is assumed to preserve the balance between released proteases and protease inhibitors. The active centre of antitrypsin (methionine 358–serine 359) is easily inactivated by oxidants, for example by myeloperoxidase from activated neutrophils. Inactivation can also occur if the exposed molecular loop between amino acids 342 and 358 is cleaved by enzymes from such common organisms as Pseudomonas aeruginosa. If proteases are uninhibited then tissue damage may be severe. Free neutrophil elastase causes inactivation of antithrombin and C1-inhibitor. A catastrophic increase in intravascular coagulation, complement activation and kallikrein-catalysed kinin release can then occur (Wewers, 1989).

α_1-antitrypsin is encoded by a single structural gene, the PI locus 10.2 kb in length, on chromosome 14q31-32.3. The inheritance of α_1-antitrypsin is codominant, with each allele functioning separately. More than 75 genetic variants of the glycoprotein have been identified (Crystal, 1990); many have normal serum concentrations. The common phenotype is PIMM of which there are four subtypes. Two common phenotypes, PI S and Z, produce low serum concentrations: Pi S homozygotes have about 60% and Pi Z homozygotes about 15% of the α_1-antitrypsin concentrations of Pi M homozygotes. Other rare alleles such as PIM_{maltom} and PIZ_{tun} (Whitehouse et al., 1989) also have low concentrations. Pi null produces no detectable serum α_1-antitrypsin.

Clinical implications

The clinically important variant is PIZ, with a homozygote frequency of between 1 in 1660 to 1 in 7000 newborns of European descent (Brantly et al., 1988b). It arises from a point mutation at codon 342 which results in the replacement of glutamic acid by lysine. The Z polypeptide is synthesized at normal rates but there is deficient secretion of the glycoprotein from the endoplasmic reticulum, the rate being approximately 15% of that of the M variant. It is a much slower inhibitor of neutrophil elastase (Brantly et al., 1988a). The PIZZ individual is at risk of gradually developing emphysema evident in early adult life, particularly if a heavy cigarette smoker; up to 60% may be affected (Carrell, 1986). The risk is also great in the rare null homozygote. There are isolated reports of emphysema in PISZ subjects (Cox, 1989).

The process of gradual destruction of the alveolar wall occurs over the course of many years which makes direct study of the pathogenesis very difficult. There is much indirect evidence implicating protease–antiprotease imbalance in pathogenesis, in particular ineffective inhibition of neutrophil elastase by α_1-antitrypsin. The pathological change appears to develop in the centri-acinar area where macrophages which produce elastase accumulate (Wewers, 1989).

LIVER DISEASE

Sveger (1988) has been responsible for a remarkable epidemiological study of 120 PIZZ infants identified initially in a cohort of 200 000 Swedish newborn infants screened for low serum concentrations of α_1-antitrypsin. At 6 months of age up to 70% of the infants had biochemical evidence of hepatitis (i.e. inflammation of the liver) with at least 2–3% progressing to cirrhosis (Sveger, 1988). In this cohort 11% had an icteric hepatitis (equivalent to 1/15 384 live births).

In an epidemiological study in south-east England of infants identified as having a conjugated hyperbilirubinaemia lasting at least two weeks, the incidence of PIZZ associated disease was remarkably similar at 1/19 200 live births. The PIZZ frequency in England is estimated at 1 in 3400 live births (Psacharopoulos and Mowat, 1979).

Adult males have an increased incidence of cirrhosis and hepatocellular carcinoma (Eriksson et al., 1986). Cholangiocarcinoma has also been reported in two PIZZ siblings (Parham et al., 1989).

Diagnosis

α_1-antitrypsin phenotyping, preferably by isoelectric focussing, is required for diagnosis. It is an essential investigation in infants with hepatitis syndrome or suspected biliary atresia and in older children with chronic liver disease. The deficiency state may be suspected by visual scanning of serum protein electrophoretic strips if α_1 globulin is not seen, or by the typical appearance on liver biopsy after 12 weeks of age (see below). Since serum levels, measured by immunological techniques, may be increased or decreased by associated diseases or drugs, these are unreliable for making a diagnosis (Cox, 1989).

Presenting features of liver disease

Hepatitis syndrome in infancy: The most common presentation is as an acute icteric hepatitis which follows directly from neonatal physiological jaundice (Table 1). It is suspected when conjugated hyperbilirubinaemia develops. The first sign is a change in the urine colour; it becomes distinctly yellow or even slightly brown. The clinical significance of this observation is frequently missed since the colour is not unlike that of adult urine in health. After one week of age infants have urine which is colourless or only faintly yellow even if they have an unconjugated hyperbilirubinaemia. The onset of jaundice may be at any time in the first four months of life, the mean age at recognition being between two and three weeks. Jaundice lasts on average for

Table 1 Presenting features of liver disease: experience at King's College Hospital, 1971–89

Neonatal ascites	0
Hepatitis of infancy	
Conjugated jaundice	178
Spontaneous bleeding	7
Complications of cirrhosis	
Ascites	1
Bleeding varices	2
Hepatosplenomegaly	3
Jaundice	1
Total	192

three months but may persist for as long as a year. It is most severe in the first two weeks of life when maximum serum bilirubin concentrations ranging from 60 to 360 μmol/L may occur. The stools may contain no yellow or green pigment, mimicking biliary atresia. The infants commonly have slow weight gain and some may show irritability or lethargy. They are at risk of septicaemia which can cause a devastating deterioration in liver function with marked prolongation of the prothrombin time. In the UK referral to a paediatric service is as likely to be for these reasons as for jaundice which in this age group is often discounted as physiological, although in all instances the jaundice is conjugated and is accompanied by persistently yellow urine. All have hepatomegaly and approximately 50% have splenomegaly (Psacharopoulos and Mowat, 1977; Mowat, 1984; Cox, 1989). Rarely the presentation is with ascites in the newborn period (Ghishan et al., 1983).

Bleeding diathesis in the first two months of life: In approximately 5% the presenting feature is a severe bleeding episode at 2–6 weeks of age, the onset being later in infants who had received parenteral vitamin K at delivery. Bleeding may take the form of exsanguinating bleeding from the umbilicus or superficial injury, or may be intracranial. The latter may be followed by long term neurological abnormality with mental retardation and spasticity. Frequently such children require ventricular peritoneal shunts for the relief of hydrocephalus (Hope et al., 1982; Psacharopoulos et al., 1983). Invariably in these infants there is clinical evidence of liver disease, including jaundice, which has been ignored. In such children the prothrombin time (prothrombin ratio) is greatly prolonged. It reverts to normal within six hours with intravenous vitamin K. Such bleeding may be prevented by early recognition of the presence of liver disease and the administration of vitamin K.

In infants presenting with or without bleeding the jaundice gradually clears but a proportion will have persisting hepatomegaly or splenomegaly. Biochemical tests of liver function remain abnormal.

Cirrhosis in later childhood: Less commonly children present with asymptomatic hepatosplenomegaly or with complications of cirrhosis such as ascites or haematemesis, with no prior history of jaundice in infancy. We have recently seen a 9-month-old child present with an apparent liver tumour which was eventually shown to be a massive cirrhotic nodule.

Cirrhosis and hepatoma in later life: There appears to be a statistically significant increased risk of cirrhosis and primary hepatoma in males over the age of 50 (Eriksson *et al.*, 1986). Hepatoma can occur in the absence of cirrhosis (Cox, 1989). α-fetoprotein levels, usually elevated in hepatoma, are infrequently elevated in the PIZZ subject with this tumour. Interestingly, PIMM infants with hepatitis frequently have very high α-fetoprotein concentrations, but in the PIZZ infant with hepatitis of similar severity elevations are minor (Johnston *et al.*, 1976).

Pathological features

Liver biopsy in the acute stages shows features indistinguishable from idiopathic neonatal hepatitis except that giant cell transformation is rarely prominent. There may be conspicuous fatty infiltration around the portal tracts. The histological features may be very similar to those of extrahepatic biliary atresia. Fibrous tissue in the portal tract and intralobular fibrosis may be prominent. Cirrhosis may be evident as early as 8 weeks of age and it may be macronodular, micronodular or take a so-called biliary form. If there is marked bile duct proliferation and portal tract fibrosis in early infancy, cirrhosis is likely to supervene in the first decade. In contrast, where there is little portal tract fibrosis in initial biopsy cirrhosis is less likely. Hepatocellular carcinoma may develop in adults, both with and without cirrhosis. The extrahepatic ducts are small if cholestasis is severe, but are not atretic.

A distinctive pathological feature is the presence of diastase-resistant, PAS positive, magenta coloured globules 2–20 nm in diameter seen most prominently in the periportal hepatocytes, but only after the age of 12 weeks (Talbot and Mowat, 1975). These globules appear to correspond to the amorphous material which on electron microscopy is seen to distend the endoplasmic reticulum of some hepatocytes. Other intracellular organelles are normal. The material reacts with the specific fluorescein-tagged antibody to α_1-antitrypsin, giving a bright fluorescence not seen in the hepatocytes of non-PIZ subjects. The accumulation of this material, which is antigenically similar to normal (PIM) serum α_1-antitrypsin, occurs in PIZ subjects whether liver disease is present or not. It can be detected as early as 19 weeks gestation (Malone *et al.*, 1990).

Subsequent course of liver disease

Of the patients in Sveger's study, two have died from cirrhosis and one dying of aplastic anaemia and another dying in an accident were found to have cirrhosis at *post mortem*, although there had been no biochemical or clinical evidence of liver disease during life. All four had cholestasis in infancy. The percentage with raised transaminases fell gradually throughout childhood from 70% at six months of age. At 12 years of age 3 out of 15 with hepatitis in infancy and 14 out of 102 with anicteric disease still had raised transaminases. None have developed clinical evidence of liver disease (Sveger 1988).

Three of the seven infants in the SE England study died of cirrhosis by the age of 3 years and one of the survivors now aged 18 years is clinically well but has cirrhosis. Two have no evidence of liver disease (Dick and Mowat, 1985). Further information on the progression of liver disease is limited to the reported experience of centres such as our own which see a large number of referred cases (Nebbia *et al.*, 1983; Psacharopoulos *et al.*, 1983; Ghishan and Green, 1988; Cox, 1989). Together these comprise approximately 200 patients. It is impossible to assess the size of the referral population or to know which factors determined referral.

The course of the liver disease is similar irrespective of the mode of presentation in infancy. About 5% remain jaundiced, progress to decompensated cirrhosis and die in the first year of life. The majority of cases appear to recover from the acute hepatitis; the jaundice clears and growth and rate of weight gain improve. A period of well-being ensues. Clinical examination in the majority, however, will show persistent hepatomegaly with or without splenomegaly. Standard biochemical tests of liver function such as aspartate and alanine aminotransferase, γ-glutamyl transpeptidase and alkaline phosphatase remain elevated.

The subsequent evolution of the liver disease in our cases has followed four main patterns. In approximately 25% of these patients the clinical and biochemical abnormalities gradually improve and results come within the normal range at ages ranging from 3–10 years. In these the liver is not hard and there is no splenomegaly. Liver changes as seen on biopsy are limited to slight widening of the portal tracts and a minimal increase in hepatic fibrosis. Survival into the third decade without features of cirrhosis has been recorded in such patients.

Approximately 25% have died from complications of cirrhosis at ages ranging from six months to 17 years (Table 2). These patients will have had clinical and biopsy evidence of cirrhosis with a hard liver and splenomegaly. After a period ranging from a few months to 13 years hepatic decompensation occurred, as evidenced by ascites, hyponatraemia, recurrence of jaundice, haematemesis or severe failure to thrive. Haematuria and/or albuminuria due to glomerular lesions is an infrequently reported complication (Strife *et al.*, 1983; Levy *et al.*, 1986) which may be followed by severe systemic hypertension after transplantation (Noble-Jamieson *et al.*, 1990).

Table 2   Age at death from cirrhosis: experience at King's College Hospital, 1971–89

Age	No. of deaths[a]
Less than 1 year	7
1–3 years	5
3–12 years	14
17 years	1

Mean: 6.1 years (27 deaths)

[a]Excludes patients receiving liver grafts

Death from liver disease occurred within two months to four years of the onset of such developments.

Approximately 25% survive through the first decade although they have histologically confirmed cirrhosis. Will all subsequently decompensate? A further 25% without liver biopsy evidence of cirrhosis have persistently abnormal liver function tests with or without clinical features of portal hypertension. In some of these cases without clinical abnormality, liver function tests may eventually become normal.

In general the prognosis of liver disease in childhood is related to the severity and duration of the acute hepatic dysfunction in early infancy, but in the individual patient liver biopsy is the more reliable guide to prognosis (Nebbia et al., 1983; Psacharopoulos et al., 1989). In those who will die or develop cirrhosis, liver biopsies in the first six months of life show marked portal tract changes with increased fibrosis and oedema or established cirrhosis. Intrahepatic bile duct hypoplasia has been associated with a good prognosis. Although such patients have increased lung volumes (Greenough et al., 1988), early progression to emphysema is unusual (Buist et al., 1990). In adults the coexistence of emphysema and cirrhosis is rarely recognized (Cox, 1989).

Liver disease with other PI phenotypes

Although liver disease has been reported in both infants and adults with phenotypes SZ, SS and FZ (Kelly et al., 1989) and an increased prevalence of MZ has been found in adult patients with cirrhosis and chronic active hepatitis, these may be chance observations (Cox, 1989). A further problem is that the PIZZ phenotype may give an SZ-like appearance, particularly in the presence of liver disease (Whitehouse et al., unpublished observations). In our experience of almost 2000 infants and children with chronic liver disease, PIZZ is the only phenotype represented more commonly than in the healthy population.

The pathogenesis of liver damage and progressive liver disease

The physiological rôle of α_1-antitrypsin and the suspected pathogenesis of emphysema have been considered above. The cause of liver damage and progressive liver disease is unknown. The similarity in severity of liver disease in up to 80% of siblings suggests that a second genetic factor may contribute to liver disease (Psacharopoulos et al., 1983). Amongst possible genetically influenced mechanisms which may be implicated in pathogenesis are defects in chemotaxis (Cox, 1989) and liver specific autoimmune reactions and thus increased lymphocyte-induced hepatocyte cytotoxicity. Such cytotoxicity can be inhibited by the addition of a purified liver membrane lipoprotein preparation, suggesting that an immune reaction to liver membrane antigens may be involved in the pathogenesis of liver injury (Modelli et al., 1984). In a study of HLA phenotypes and class II (HLA-DR) gene polymorphism in 140 PIZZ subjects, 92 with liver disease, the class II DR3B gene was associated with liver disease while DR4 was apparently protective (Doherty et al., 1990). The associations are weak, however, and other factors must be implicated.

We have observed one identical twin who died of cirrhosis at 10 years of age, while his brother, now aged 19, has no clinical or biochemical evidence of liver disease and had only slightly increased hepatic fibrosis on liver biopsy at 8 years of age. Clearly environmental factors must play a rôle, but what these might be remains a matter for speculation. The relatively high incidence of low birth weight suggests that some factor may be operating *in utero*. Postnatally, the absorption of macromolecules which are trapped in the Kupffer cells may initiate liver damage by stimulating protease release. Breastfeeding has been associated with a lower incidence of severe liver disease in some studies but this is not universal; the concentration of α_1-antitrypsin in breast milk is 30–40% that of serum. A poorer prognosis in males has also been suggested but again this is not consistent in all series (Cox, 1989; Labrune et al., 1989).

Two hypotheses are currently being considered in pathogenesis. The first considers that accumulation of α_1-antitrypsin in the hepatocyte causes the process(es) that lead to severe liver damage. Against this is the observation that only 70% of PIZZ infants have abnormal liver function tests and at most 20–40% develop in the course of a lifetime clinically significant liver disease despite accumulation. It is conceivable that in certain circumstances these intracellular accumulations could produce cell surface changes which would initiate an immune attack on the hepatocyte or cause hepatocellular necrosis. With the marked heterogeneity of liver function across the hepatic lobule even early in life (Sokal et al., 1989), it is possible that these effects could be enhanced at particular parts of the lobule. Since abnormally folded proteins within cells can increase the synthesis of proteins induced by thermal or chemical stress (so called stress proteins), a possible mechanism underlying liver damage might be the accumulation of such proteins. It has recently been shown that peripheral blood monocytes from PIZZ individuals with liver disease have enhanced synthesis of proteins in the heat shock/stress gene family (SP90, SP70, ubiquitin). Synthesis is further increased by heat (42°C) and endotoxin. This change did not occur in PIZZ subjects with emphysema and no liver disease, or in PIMM individuals with advanced liver disease. Ubiquitin mRNA in liver was also significantly increased in PIZZ livers removed at grafting compared with MZ or MM livers (Perlmutter et al., 1989). Further studies will be required to determine whether these changes are due to a separate genetic defect related to the metabolism of stress proteins or α_1-antitrypsin transport from the cell. Equally, extrinsic factors may influence the metabolism of either or both.

The evidence stated in favour of the accumulation hypothesis is that no liver disease occurs in PIQ0 homozygotes who have no PAS positive globules in the liver and that liver disease does occur in the other rare phenotypes with accumulation of α_1-antitrypsin, i.e. PIM$_{malton}$. In fact, studies of the liver histology in either the exceedingly rare and genetically pleomorphic PIQ0 or in PIM$_{malton}$ are limited to only one or two cases (Cox, 1989; Curiel et al., 1989). Further supportive evidence is the effect of the transfer of the Z gene to transgenic mice which does cause accumulation and hepatitis, i.e. hepatic inflammation, but no increase in hepatic fibrosis occurs.

The second hypothesis, protease–antiprotease imbalance generally considered to be the cause of emphysema, has also been extended to the liver damage although it

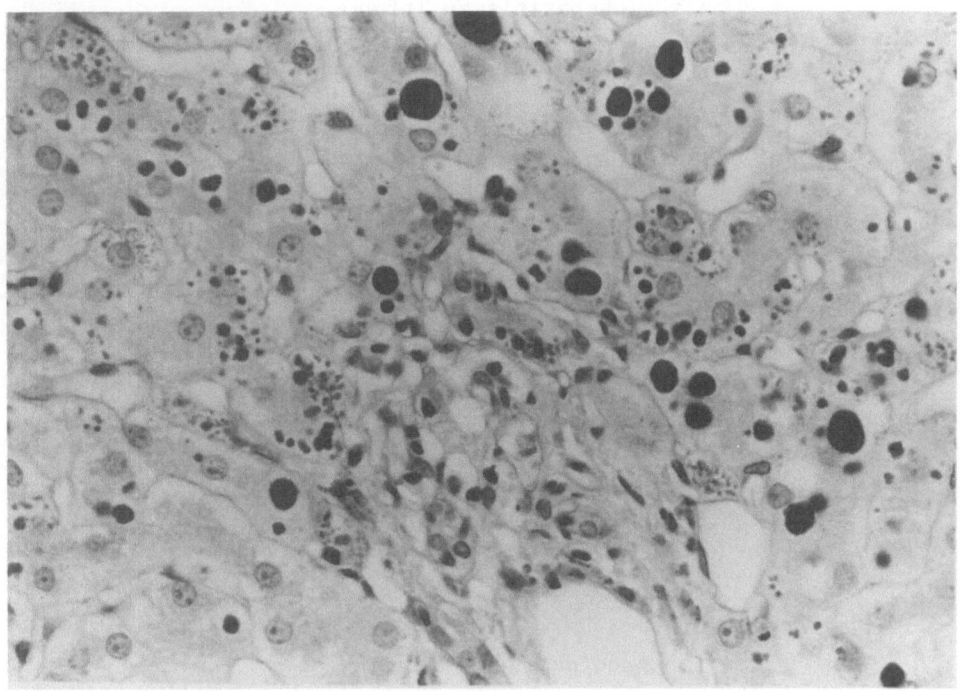

Figure 1 Photomicrograph of the liver biopsy section stained with PAS after diastase digestion showing a normal portal tract surrounded by hepatocytes containing within their cytoplasm dense dark globules of varying size of α_1-antitrypsin. These are magenta coloured

is difficult to obtain direct evidence of what may be happening in the hepatic microenvironment. With 1 g of elastase and 1 g of collagenase being produced daily, uninhibited action of such enzymes could cause disastrous tissue destruction and inflammation. Leukocyte or macrophage proteases released during inflammation could directly damage hepatocytes or extracellular matrix components. These are now known to be much more than structural macromolecules. They interact with parenchymal cells through specific receptors and thus influence cell function. They also interact with inflammatory cells (Ruoslahti and Pierschbacher, 1988). An increased degree of complement activation (C3d/C3 ratio) has been found in children with liver disease, particularly if severe, presumably associated with diminished protease inhibition. It has yet to be shown that complement activation causes liver damage in this disorder. The evidence quoted against this is the absence of liver disease in the PIQ0 variant (see above), while in favour is the observation that 23% of PISZ infants have increased serum transaminases. These subjects do not have significant accumulation but do have low serum levels. By 12 years of age only 2% had elevated levels. This pattern of abnormality in serum transaminase mirrors that seen in the PIZZ subject (Sveger, 1988) and emphasises the susceptibility of the newborn to liver dysfunction.

Any hypothesis should account for the fact that most liver disease starts in the

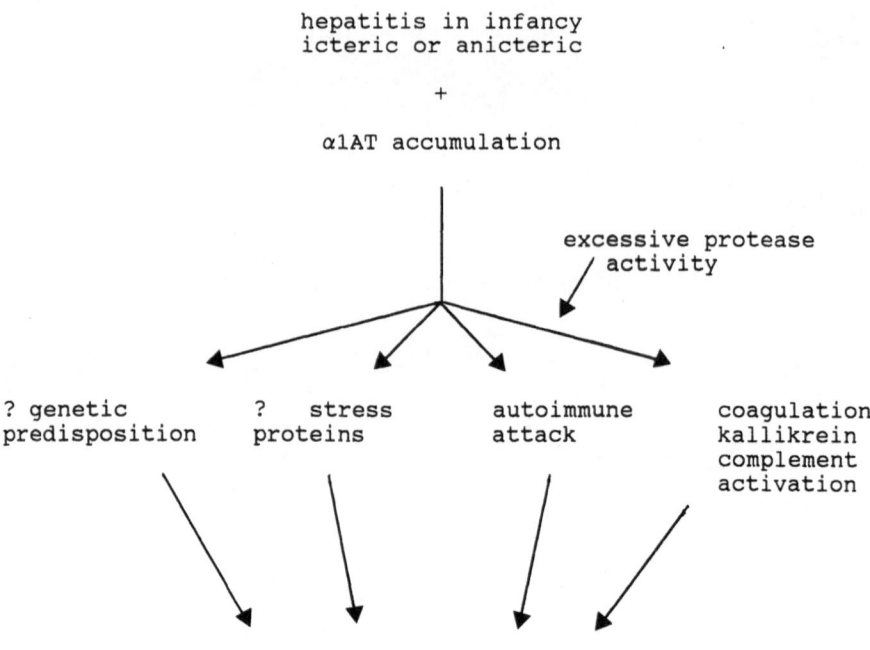

Figure 2 An illustration of factors which may be involved in perpetuating inflammation and stimulating the accumulation of components of the extracellular matrix, leading to increased intrahepatic fibrosis, cirrhosis and possible malignancy

first weeks of life. Many aspects of liver function and structure (e.g. liver cell plates two cells thick) are relatively immature or inefficient in the first months of life which may account for the high frequency of liver disease presenting at this time (Peters, 1983). The hepatic extracellular matrix may be particularly susceptible in early infancy when many metabolites of matrix components are present in high concentration in serum (Udall, 1985; Trivedi, 1989), suggesting that the developmental leakiness of the newborn gut could allow foreign proteins into the portal circulation. When trapped in the liver they might stimulate protease release and induce hepatitis which could become progressive if there were insufficient protease inhibitors present to inactivate the proteases. Bacterial colonization of the gut at this time could also increase the protease load coming to the liver. Viral infection in the liver as evidenced by the demonstration of alpha interferon in Kupffer cells and inflammatory cells is particularly common at this age (Davies *et al.*, unpublished observations), and could also cause monocyte elastase production.

From the above it seems that α_1-antitrypsin accumulation may initiate changes which when associated with an unexplained increased synthesis of stress proteins may cause liver damage. Not all hepatocytes may be equally affected. What effect the increased rate of stress protein synthesis has on monocyte function is unknown. Does it increase protease release? Does it increase the production of oxidants which

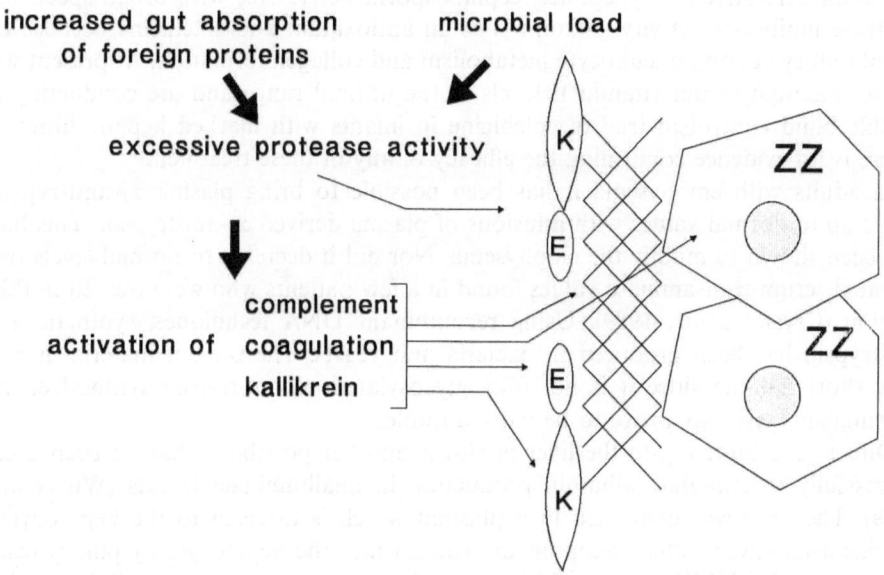

Figure 3 Diagrammatic representation of possible sites of liver injury and of mechanisms which may aggravate liver damage in early infancy in the PIZZ child. Proteases carried from the gut in the portal blood or liberated within the liver substance may, in the absence of the enzyme inhibitor, cause damage to the Kupffer cells (K), the specialized endothelial lining cells (E), components of the extracellular matrix (XX) or the PIZZ hepatocyte arranged in plates two cells thick. The accumulation of α_1-antitrypsin in the endoplasmic reticulum may have caused the cell membrane to be particularly susceptible to protease attack. Excessive protease activity also activates the complement, coagulation and Kallikrein cascades, initiating an intense inflammatory response with all its possible sequelae

further inactivate α_1-antitrypsin? These changes occur in a microenvironment very susceptible to attack by neutrophil elastase but very depleted in its main defence, i.e. α_1-antitrypsin. In early infancy the liver is clearly at its most vulnerable.

Management

The management is that of chronic cholestasis and of cirrhosis (Mowat, 1987). There is no specific treatment for liver disease associated with α_1-antitrypsin deficiency short of liver transplantation. Liver transplantation should be planned as soon as cirrhosis decompensates or if it is complicated by recurrent variceal bleeding not readily prevented by injection therapy, or by renal complications. The results are similar to those in other forms of cirrhosis except that hypertension may be more frequent. Liver transplantation corrects the serum phenotype to that of the donor (Cohen et al., 1989). The longest follow-up is only 16 years, therefore it is too early to determine whether this treatment will prevent emphysema (Starzl et al., 1989).

There is no evidence that the course of the disease is influenced by phenobarbitone given as an enzyme inducer, or corticosteroids or penicillamine given as anti-inflammatory agents. Other agents which theoretically might limit the disease include aprotinin derivatives, polypeptides, cephalosporin derivatives with broad spectrum protease inhibitory activity, vitamin E as an antioxidant and colchicine because of its inhibitory action on leukocyte metabolism and collagen formation. At present we try to maintain serum vitamin E levels in the normal range and are conducting a double blind controlled trial of colchicine in infants with marked hepatic fibrosis. There is no evidence confirming the efficacy of any of these treatments.

In adults with emphysema it has been possible to bring plasma α_1-antitrypsin levels up to normal values with infusions of plasma derived α_1-antitrypsin. This has not been shown to modify the emphysema. Nor did it decrease to normal levels the elevated serum transaminase values found in a few patients who were treated in this fashion (Crystal et al., 1989). Using recombinant DNA techniques, synthetic α_1-antitrypsin has been produced in bacteria and yeasts. The present material has a very short half-life since it is not fully glycosylated. α_1-antitrypsin synthesized in mammalian cells may prove to be more durable.

Direct gene targeting to the liver in vivo is another possibility, having been used successfully to stimulate albumin production in analbuminaemic rats (Wu et al., 1989). The gene was contained in a plasmid which is targeted to the hepatocyte-specific asialoglycoprotein receptor and carried into the hepatocyte by pinocytosis. In this way the PIMZ state would be created. Another theoretical possibility is the correction of the hepatic secretory problem by insertion of another gene which makes a complementary change in the polypeptide, allowing it to assume the normal tertiary configuration which may facilitate secretion (Brantly et al., 1988a; Schwarzenberg and Sharp, 1990). Modifications to α_1-antitrypsin can be produced which make it more resistant to oxidative inactivation (George et al., 1984). Perhaps more immediately practicable and attractive, to paediatric hepatologists if not to pulmonary physicians, would be a trial of exogenous serum-derived α_1-antitrypsin, given intravenously at 1–4 weekly intervals, as is being used in emphysema but commencing as soon as significant liver damage is identified, perhaps in conjunction with a neonatal screening programme. It should be possible to construct a trial of therapy lasting 6–12 months which in the course of at most a decade, and perhaps much sooner, would indicate whether such therapy was efficacious.

GENETIC COUNSELLING

For parents who are Z heterozygotes each fetus has a 25% chance of being a PIZ homozygote; if one parent is a homozygote each fetus has a 50% chance of being a homozygote. This state could formerly only be detected by fetal blood sampling from the umbilical vessels at 16 weeks gestation (Corney et al., 1987). In families in whom a previously affected child has had severe liver disease the chances are 75% that a second PIZZ child will follow a similar course. In these circumstances families will frequently opt for termination of pregnancy. Earlier antenatal diagnosis is now possible by examining the DNA of chorionic villus samples using synthetic oligonucleotide probes specific for the M and Z gene, or by restriction fragment length polymorphism. With the polymerase chain reaction results can be made available within a few days of sampling at 11 weeks gestation. Preliminary studies confirm the validity of such techniques (Povey, 1990).

REFERENCES

Brantly, M., Courtney, M. and Crystal, R. G. Repair of the secretion defect in the Z form of α_1-antitrypsin by the addition of a second mutation. *Science* 242 (1988a) 1700–1702

Brantly, M., Nukiwa, T. and Crystal, R. G. Molecular basis of α_1-antitrypsin deficiency. *Am. J. Med.* 84 (1988b) 13–31

Carrell, R. W. α_1-antitrypsin: molecular pathology, leukocytes and tissue damage. *J. Clin. Invest.* 78 (1986) 1427–1431

Cohen, A., O'Grady, J., Mowat, A. P. and Williams, R. Liver transplantation for metabolic disorders. In: *Baillière's Clinical Gastroenterology* 3 (1989) 767–786

Corney, G., Whitehouse, D. B., Hopkinson, D. A., Rodeck, C. H., Nicolaides, K., Norman, M. and Mowat, A. P. Prenatal diagnosis of α_1-antitrypsin deficiency by fetal blood sampling. *Prenatal Diagnosis* 7 (1987) 101–108

Cox, D. W. α_1-antitrypsin deficiency. In: Scriver, C. R., Beaudet, A. L., Sly, W. S. and Valle, D. (eds.), *The Metabolic Basis of Inherited Disease*, 6th edn., McGraw-Hill, New York, 1989, pp. 2409–2437

Crystal, R. G. α_1-antitrypsin deficiency, emphysema and liver disease. Genetic basis and strategies for therapy. *J. Clin. Invest.* 85 (1990) 1343–1351

Crystal, R. G., Brantly, M. L., Hubbard, R. C., Curiel, D. T., States, D. J. and Holmes, M. D. The α_1-antitrypsin gene and its mutations. Clinical consequences and strategies for therapy. *Chest* 95 (1989) 196–208

Curiel, D. T., Holmes, M. D., Okayama, H. *et al.* Molecular basis of the liver and lung disease associated with α_1-antitrypsin deficiency allele M_{malton}. *J. Biol. Chem.* 264 (1989) 13938–13945

Dick, M. C. and Mowat, A. P. Hepatitis syndrome in infancy. An epidemiological survey with 10-year follow-up. *Arch. Dis. Child.* 60 (1985) 512–516

Doherty, D. G., Donaldston, P. T., Whitehouse, D. B., Mieli-Vergani, G., Duthie, A., Hopkinson, D. A. and Mowat, A. P. HLA phenotypes and gene polymorphisms in juvenile liver disease associated with α_1-antitrypsin deficiency. *Hepatology* 12 (1990) 218–223

Eriksson, S., Carlson, J. and Velez, R. The risk of cirrhosis and primary liver cancer in α_1-antitrypsin deficiency. *N. Engl. J. Med.* 314 (1986) 736–739

Freier, E., Sharp, H. L. and Bridges, R. A. α_1-antitrypsin deficiency associated with familial infantile liver disease. *Clin. Chem.* 14 (1968) 782

George, P. M., Travis, J., Vissers, M. C. M., Winterbourn, C. C. and Carrell, R. W. A genetically engineered mutant of α_1-antitrypsin protects connective tissue from neutrophil damage and may be useful in lung disease. *Lancet* 2 (1984) 1426–1428

Ghishan, F. K., Greene, H. L. Liver disease in children with PIZZ α_1-antitrypsin deficiency. *Hepatology* 8 (1988) 307–310

Ghishan, F. K., Gray, G. F. and Greene, H. L. α_1-antitrypsin deficiency presenting with ascites and cirrhosis in the neonatal period. *Gastroenterology* 85 (1983) 435–439

Greenough, A., Pool, J. B., Ball, C., Mieli-Vergani, G. and Mowat, A. P. Functional residual capacity related to hepatitic disease. *Arch. Dis. Child.* 63 (1988) 850–852

Hope, P. L., Hall, M. A., Millward-Sadler, G. H. and Normand, I. C. S. α_1-antitrypsin deficiency presenting as a bleeding diathesis in the newborn. *Arch. Dis. Child.* 57 (1982) 68–70

Johnston, D. I., Mowat, A. P., Orr, H. and Kohn, J. Serum alpha-fetoprotein levels in extrahepatic biliary atresia, idiopathic neonatal hepatitis and α_1-antitrypsin PIZZ. *Acta Paediatr. Scand.* 65 (1976) 623–628

Kelly, C. P., Tyrell, D. N. M., McDonald, G. S. A., Whitehouse, D. B. and Prichard, J. S. Heterozygous FZ α_1-antitrypsin deficiency associated with severe emphysema and hepatic disease: case report and family study. *Thorax* 44 (1989)758–759

Krivit, W., Miller, J., Nowicki, M. and Freier, E. Contribution of monocyte-macrophage system to serum α_1-antitrypsin. *J. Lab. Clin. Med.* 112 (1988) 437–442

Labrune, P., Odievre, M. and Alagille, D. Influence of sex and breastfeeding on liver disease in α_1-antitrypsin deficiency. *Hepatology* 10 (1989) 122

Levy, M. Severe deficiency of α_1-antitrypsin associated with cutaneous vasculitis, rapidly progressive glomerular nephritis and colitis. *Am. J. Med.* 81 (1986) 363

Malone, M., Mieli-Vergani, G., Mowat, A. P. and Portmann, B. The fetal liver in PIZZ α_1-antitrypsin deficiency: A report of 5 cases. *Pediatr. Pathol.* 9 (1989) 623–631

Mondelli, M., Mieli-Vergani, G., Eddleston, A. L. W. F., Williams, R. and Mowat, A. P. Lymphocyte cytotoxicity to autologous hepatocytes in α_1-antitrypsin deficiency. *Gut* 25 (1984) 1044–1049

Mowat, A. P. α_1-antitrypsin deficiency in liver disease. In: Williams, R. and Madre, W. C. (eds.), *Gastroenterology*, Volume 4, 1 (*Butterworths International Medical Reviews*), Butterworths, London, 1984, pp. 57–75

Mowat, A. P. *Liver Disorders in Childhood*, 2nd edn., Butterworths, London, 1987

Nebbia, G., Hadchouel, M. and Alagille, D. Early assessment of evolution of liver disease associated with α_1-antitrypsin deficiency in childhood. *Pediatr.* 102 (1983) 661–668

Noble-Jamieson, G., Barnes, N., Thiru, S. and Mowat, A. P. Severe hypertension after liver transplantation in children with α_1-antitrypsin deficiency. *Arch. Dis. Child.* 65 (1990) 1217–1221

Parham, D. M., Paterson, J. R., Gunn, A. and Guthrie, W. Cholangiocarcinoma in two siblings with emphysema and α_1-antitrypsin deficiency. *Q.J. Med.* 71 (1989) 359–367

Perlmutter, D. H., Schlesinger, M. J., Pierce, J. A., Punsal, P. I. and Schwartz, A. L. Synthesis of stress proteins is increased in individuals with PIZZ α_1-antitrypsin deficiency and liver disease. *J. Clin. Invest.* 84 (1989) 1551–1561

Peters, R. L. Early development of the liver: a review. In: Fischer, M. and Roy, C. C. (eds.), *Paediatric Liver Disorders*, Plenum Press, New York, 1983, pp. 1–19

Povey, S. The genetics of α_1-antitrypsin deficiency in relation to neonatal liver disease. *Mol. Biol. Med.* 7 (1990) 161–172

Psacharopoulos, H. T. and Mowat, A. P. Incidence and early history of obstructive jaundice in infancy in SE England. In: *Neonatal Hepatitis and Biliary Atresia*, DHEW Publication (NIH) 79; 1296, US Government Printing Office, Washington, 1979, pp. 167–171

Psacharopoulos, H. T., Mowat, A. P., Cooke, P. J. L., Carlile, P. A., Portmann, B. and Rodeck, C. H. Outcome of liver disease associated with α_1-antitrypsin deficiency. Implications for genetic counselling and antenatal diagnosis. *Arch. Dis. Child.* 58 (1983) 882–887

Ruoslahti, E. and Pierschbacher, M. D. Molecular basis of cell-extracellular matrix interactions. In: Arias, I. M., Jakoby, W.P., Popper, H., Schachter, D. and Shafritz, D. A. (eds.), *The Liver: Biology and Pathobiology*, 2nd edn., Raven Press, New York, pp. 739–745

Schultz, H. E., Gollner, I., Heide, K., Schonberger, M. and Schwick, G. Zur Kenntis der alpha globuline des menschlichen normalserums. *Z. Naturforsch.* 10 (1955) 463–469

Schwarzenberg, S. J. and Sharp, H. L. Pathogenesis of α_1-antitrypsin deficiency associated liver disease. *J. Pediatr. Gastroenterol. Nutr.* 10 (1990) 5–12

Sharp, H. L., Bridges, R. A., Krivit, W. and Friere, E. R. Cirrhosis associated with α_1-antitrypsin deficiency: a previously unrecognized disorder. *J. Lab. Clin. Med.* 73 (1969) 934–939

Sokal, E., Trivedi, P., Portmann, B. and Mowat, A. P. Developmental changes in the intra-acinar distribution of succinate dehydrogenase, glutamate dehydrogenase, glucose-6-phosphatase and NADPH dehydrogenase in rat liver. *J. Pediatr. Gastroenterol. Nutr.* 8 (1989) 522–527

Starzyl, T. E., Demetris, J. and Van Thield, D. Medical progress: liver transplantation. *N. Engl. J. Med.* 321 (1989) 1014–1022, 1092–1099

Strife, C. F., Hug, G., Chuck, G., McAdams, A. J., Davis, C. A. and Kline, J. J. Membranoproliferative glomerulonephritis and α_1-antitrypsin deficiency in children. *Pediatrics* 71 (1983) 88–92

Sveger, T. The natural history of liver disease in α_1-antitrypsin deficient children. *Acta Paediatr. Scand.* 77 (1988) 847–51

Talbot, I. C. and Mowat, A. P. Liver disease in infancy: Histological features in relationship to α_1-antitrypsin phenotype. *J. Clin. Pathol.* 28 (1975) 559–63

Travis, J. Structure, function and control of neutrophil proteinases. *Am. J. Med.* 84 (1988) 37–42

Trivedi, P., Hindmarsh, P., Risteli, J., Risteli, L., Mowat, A. P. and Brook, C. G. D. Growth velocity, growth hormone therapy and serum concentrations of the aminoterminal propeptide of type III procollagen. *J. Pediatr.* 114 (1989) 225–230

Udall, I. N., Dixon, M., Newman, A. P., Wright, J. A., James, B. and Block, K. I. Liver disease in α_1-antitrypsin deficiency. A retrospective analysis of the influence of early breast versus bottle feeding. *J. Am. Med. Assoc.* 253 (1985) 2679–2682

Wall, M., Moe, E., Eisenberg, J., Powers, M., Buist, N. and Buist, S. Long-term follow-up of a cohort of children with α_1-antitrypsin deficiency. *J. Pediatr.* 116 (1990) 248–251

Wewers, M. Pathogenesis of emphysema. *Chest* 95 (1989) 190–195

Whitehouse, D. B., Abbott, C. M., Lovegrove, J. U., McIntosh, I., McMahon, C. J., Mieli-Vergani, G., Mowat, A. P. and Hopkinson, D. A. Genetic studies on a new deficiency gene (PI* Ztun) at the PI locus. *J. Med. Genet.* 26 (1989) 744–749

Whitehouse, D. B., Lovegrove, J. U., Mieli-Vergani, G., Mowat, A. P. and Hopkinson, D. A. 'SZ-like' α_1-antitrypsin phenotypes in PIZZ children with cirrhosis. Submitted for publication

Wu, W. J., Wilson, J. M. and Wu, C. H. Targeting genes: detection of targeted human albumin gene expression in genetically analbuminaemic rats. *Hepatology* 10 (1989) 618

J. Inher. Metab. Dis. 14 (1991) 512–525
© SSIEM and Kluwer Academic Publishers.

α1-Antitrypsin Deficiency and Liver Disease

P. BIRRER, N. G. MCELVANEY, L. M. CHANG-STROMAN and R. G. CRYSTAL
Pulmonary Branch, National Heart, Lung, and Blood Institute, National Institutes of Health, Bethesda, Maryland, USA

Summary: α_1-Antitrypsin (α_1AT) deficiency, one of the most common lethal hereditary disorders among Caucasians, is associated with emphysema in adults, while in children it is associated with liver disease. Produced in the liver and released into the plasma, α_1AT serves as the body's major inhibitor of neutrophil elastase, a powerful proteolytic enzyme capable of degrading extracellular structural proteins. The pathogenesis of the liver disease associated with α_1AT deficiency is not as well understood, but is clearly linked to specific mutations in coding exons of the α_1AT gene, and the resulting accumulation of α_1AT within hepatocytes. At present, therapy for the liver disease associated with α_1AT deficiency is symptomatic, with liver transplantation as a last resort. New strategies are being developed to suppress the accumulation of α_1AT by transferring the normal gene into the liver.

α_1-Antitrypsin (α_1AT) deficiency (McKusick 20740) is a lethal hereditary disorder characterized by serum concentrations of α_1AT below 11 μmol/L (Brantly *et al.*, 1988a; Cox, 1989; Crystal *et al.*, 1989, Crystal, 1990). The α_1AT deficiency state is one of the most common hereditary disorders in Europe and the USA, occurring in approximately 1 in 2000 Caucasians of northern European descent. In adults, α_1AT deficiency is most frequently associated with emphysema, while in children it is associated with liver disease (Sveger, 1976, 1988; Cox, 1989; Crystal, 1990).

The clinical manifestations of α_1AT deficiency relate to the function of the α_1AT molecule and where it is synthesized. α_1AT is a 52-kDa glycosylated antiprotease produced mainly in the liver (Brantly *et al.*, 1988a; Cox, 1989; Crystal *et al.*, 1989; Crystal, 1990). It serves as the body's major inhibitor of neutrophil elastase, a powerful proteolytic enzyme stored in the primary granules of neutrophils and released with neutrophil activation or disintegration. α_1AT is secreted by hepatocytes into plasma where it is available to diffuse into organs to protect them from neutrophil elastase. The lower respiratory tract is particularly vulnerable to neutrophil elastase; when serum α_1AT concentrations are $< 11\,\mu$mol/L there is insufficient protection for the lung from its burden of neutrophil elastase, with consequent degradation of structural extracellular proteins, leading to emphysema. In contrast to the lung disease, the pathogenesis of the liver disease associated with α_1AT deficiency is not well

---

Reprint requests: Building 10, Room 6D03, National Institutes of Health, Bethesda, Maryland 20892, USA

understood. The goal of this paper is to review the current concepts of liver disease associated with α_1AT deficiency in children and adults. For the lung-related disorders, several reviews are available (Brantly *et al.*, 1988a; Cox, 1989; Crystal, 1989; Crystal *et al.*, 1989; Wewers, 1989; Crystal, 1990; Hubbard and Crystal, 1991a,b).

The α_1AT gene is very pleomorphic, with more than 75 allelic variants known (Crystal, 1989; Crystal *et al.*, 1989; Crystal, 1990; Hubbard and Crystal, 1991a,b). These α_1AT alleles can be conveniently categorized as 'normal' and 'at risk'. A 'normal' allele is one that, in homozygous expression, is associated with serum concentrations of 20–53 μmol/L. At-risk alleles place the individual at risk for lung and/or liver disease and include the 'deficiency' alleles (i.e. α_1AT is detectable in serum, but at reduced levels) and the 'null' alleles (no α_1AT is detectable in serum attributable to that allele). Two at-risk alleles must be inherited for an individual to be at risk for disease. However, of the more than 20 'at risk' α_1AT alleles for which the sequence is known, liver disease has been observed in association with only two, Z and M_{malton} (Table 1). This concept will be discussed in more detail below in regard to pathogenesis of the liver disease. In regard to the clinical manifestations of the liver disease, almost all information relates to the Z gene, as all but a few reports in the literature concern the Z homozygous state. Interestingly, although the Z gene is also responsible for almost all cases of emphysema as well, lung and liver disease are rarely present in the same individual (Crystal, 1989, 1990).

CLINICAL ASPECTS OF THE LIVER DISEASE

The association between α_1AT deficiency and liver disease was first reported by Sharp and colleagues in 1969. All of the initial cases were in children, but it soon became apparent that the liver disease could also affect adults (Eriksson *et al.*, 1986, Cox, 1989). α_1AT deficiency is the most common hereditary cause of liver disease, but only a minority of individuals with α_1AT deficiency actually develop this problem. Although the characteristics of the liver disease are different for children and adults, the one common denominator is the accumulation of α_1AT within hepatocytes (Crystal, 1989, 1990; Crystal *et al.*, 1989). Histologically, this is observed as intracyto-plasmic inclusion bodies found predominantly in periportal hepatocytes (DeLellis *et al.*, 1972; Feldmann *et al.*, 1974; Palmer *et al.*, 1974; Talbot and Mowat, 1975; Roberts *et al.*, 1984). With haematoxylin and eosin staining the inclusion bodies appear as oval globules. The globules are periodic acid–Schiff positive and diastase resistant. Their size and shape vary. The content of the inclusions is demonstrated to be α_1AT by immunohistochemical evaluation with an anti-α_1AT antibody. Electron microscopy shows the inclusions within single membranes, with most of the accumulation of α_1AT in the rough endoplasmic reticulum (RER).

Liver disease in children

Liver disease occurs in about 10% of all neonates with the Z homozygous form of α_1AT deficiency (Sveger, 1976, 1988). It usually presents as a neonatal hepatitis syndrome with cholestasis, but hepatomegaly without jaundice has been reported.

Table 1 Categorization of α_1-antitrypsin alleles by disease risk[a]

No risk[b]	Risk for emphysema[c]	Risk for emphysema and liver disease[d]
M1(Ala^{213})	S	Z
M1(Val^{213})	M$_{heerlen}$	M$_{malton}$
M3	M$_{mineral\ springs}$	
M2	M$_{procida}$	
M4	M$_{nechinian}$	
B$_{alhambra}$	I	
F	P$_{lowell}$	
P$_{saint\ albans}$	W$_{bethesda}$	
V$_{munich}$	Null$_{granite\ falls}$	
X	Null$_{bellingham}$	
X$_{christchurch}$	Null$_{mattawa}$	
	Null$_{isola\ di\ procida}$	
	Null$_{hong\ kong}$[e]	
	Null$_{devon}$	
	Null$_{ludwigshafen}$	
	Null$_{bolton}$	

[a]List includes α_1AT alleles for which a partial or complete sequence is known at the gene or protein levels (see Crystal, 1989 and 1990 for details)
[b]If one of the two parental α_1AT alleles is in the 'no-risk' category, there is no conclusive evidence that the individual is at risk for emphysema or liver disease (see text)
[c]The 'at risk for emphysema' allele must be inherited with another 'at risk for emphysema' allele or an 'at risk for emphysema and liver disease' allele to be at risk for emphysema; the only exception to this rule are the 'mild' at-risk alleles S and I; these alleles must be inherited with a different 'at risk' allele to put the individual at risk (see Crystal, 1989 and 1990 for discussion)
[d]Alleles in this group must be inherited in a homozygous form, or with an allele in the 'risk for emphysema' category to put the individual at risk for either emphysema or liver disease
[e]The Null$_{hong\ kong}$ allele has been described in a single case with emphysema (Sifers et al., 1988); it is not known whether liver disease was also present

Blood studies typically demonstrate conjugated hyperbilirubinaemia and elevated serum aminotransferases. Hepatosplenomegaly is common. About 45% of affected neonates are small for their gestational age, suggesting there may be intrauterine effects of the α_1AT deficiency state (Sveger, 1988; Cox, 1989). Signs of cholestasis begin between 4 days and 2 months after birth and can persist from weeks up to 8 months. Cholestasis can be severe enough to cause acholic stools, and the disease can be confused with hepatic biliary atresia (Cox, 1989). Spontaneous clinical regression is common and usually occurs before 6 months of age, although mild biochemical abnormalities can persist.

In a minority of the neonates who develop liver disease in association with α_1AT deficiency, the disease does not subside but goes on to cirrhosis and liver failure (Sveger, 1976, 1988; Psacharopoulos et al., 1983). Overall, cirrhosis occurs in approximately 3% of individuals born with α_1AT deficiency, representing about 20–30% of the neonates who develop cholestasis. In most of these children, there is progressive liver failure, resulting in death unless corrected by liver transplantation.

Liver disease in adults

The spectrum of liver disease associated with α_1AT deficiency in adults ranges from mild to severe (Eriksson *et al.*, 1986). Initially, there are liver function test abnormalities and histological evidence of hepatitis and fibrosis. This can progress to cirrhosis and hepatic failure with portal hypertension. Often the diagnosis of α_1AT deficiency is unsuspected at the time of histological and immunochemical evaluation of liver disease. Interestingly, cirrhosis in adults in association with α_1AT deficiency can occur without preceding history of childhood liver disease. In adults, once the cirrhosis develops there is frequently rapid progression to death within 2 years of diagnosis (Eriksson *et al.*, 1986).

Adults with α_1AT deficiency are also at increased risk for hepatocellular carcinoma, a relationship that exists both with and without concomitant cirrhosis (Eriksson *et al.*, 1974, 1986; Govindarajan *et al.*, 1981; Sparos *et al.*, 1984). However, the number of cases is small and α_1AT deficiency represents a very small proportion of all cases of primary liver cancer; in studies of primary liver cancer, no increase in the frequency of α_1AT deficiency has been observed (Govindarajan *et al.*, 1981; Sparos *et al.*, 1984).

The incidence of liver disease in adults in association with α_1AT deficiency is unclear. In one study of autopsy records from over 35 000 recorded autopsies, 17 patients with α_1AT deficiency were found (Eriksson *et al.*, 1986). Of these, 8 had cirrhosis and 5 had primary liver cancer. When compared to controls and stratified by sex, there was a higher prevalence of cirrhosis and primary liver cancer in men, an observation also observed in other studies (Cox and Smyth, 1983).

PATHOGENESIS OF THE LIVER DISEASE

The pathogenesis of the liver disease associated with α_1AT deficiency is directly related to where the α_1AT gene is expressed, and the consequences of specific mutations within the coding exons of the α_1AT gene.

The α_1AT gene and its expression

α_1AT is coded for by a single 12.2-kb gene located on chromosome 14 at q31-32.3 (Long *et al.*, 1984; Crystal, 1989, 1990; Hubbard and Crystal, 1991a). The gene consists of three non-coding exons (IA, IB, IC) and four coding exons (II–V). The major site of α_1AT gene expression is the liver, but in humans the α_1AT gene is also expressed in mononuclear phagocytes and neutrophils (Perlmutter *et al.*, 1985; Mornex *et al.*, 1986; du Bois *et al.*, 1989). Despite this, there is no 'disease' of mononuclear phagocytes or neutrophils in association with any α_1AT allele, including the Z allele. One explanation for this may be that related to the level of α_1AT gene expression. In this regard, hepatocytes have at least 200-fold more α_1AT mRNA transcripts than do mononuclear phagocytes, and thus are likely to produce much more α_1AT per cell than do mononuclear phagocytes (Mornex *et al.*, 1986). Evidence in transgenic mice suggests that the gene may also be expressed in kidney and intestinal cells (Carlson *et al.*, 1988), and cultured colon carcinoma cells produce α_1AT (Perlmutter *et al.*, 1989a).

Although the processes that control α_1AT expression are not fully understood, it is known that hepatocyte expression can be modulated, and the expression of α_1AT in hepatocytes is directed by structural elements within a 750-nucleotide region upstream of the hepatocyte transcriptional start site in exon 1C (Crystal, 1989, 1990).

α_1AT biosynthesis

The α_1AT mRNA translation product includes a 24-amino acid N-terminal, hydrophobic signal peptide that is removed during entry of the protein into the rough endoplasmic reticulum (RER) (Lodish, 1988). Here the α_1AT protein is glycosylated with three asparaginyl-linked carbohydrate side-chains. The protein then folds into its three-dimensional structure and is translocated to the Golgi apparatus, where the carbohydrate side-chains undergo modification, after which the final 394-residue 52-kDa mature α_1AT protein is secreted.

Concepts of pathogenesis

In contrast to the pathogenesis of the emphysema in association with α_1AT deficiency, where disease is clearly related to the decreased levels of α_1AT, the pathogenesis of the liver disease is less clear. There are two major hypotheses to explain the liver disease: (1) 'external attack'; and (2) 'internal damage' (Figure 1). The 'external attack' hypothesis is the liver equivalent of the pathogenesis of the emphysema, i.e. that the liver damage is the result of proteolytic attack, probably by neutrophil elastase but possibly by proteolytic enzymes released by bacteria in the gastrointestinal tract that are normally inhibited by α_1AT. The 'internal damage' hypothesis is related to the observation that all patients with α_1AT deficiency who develop liver disease have intracellular accumulation of α_1AT in the RER of hepatocytes (Liebermann *et al.*,

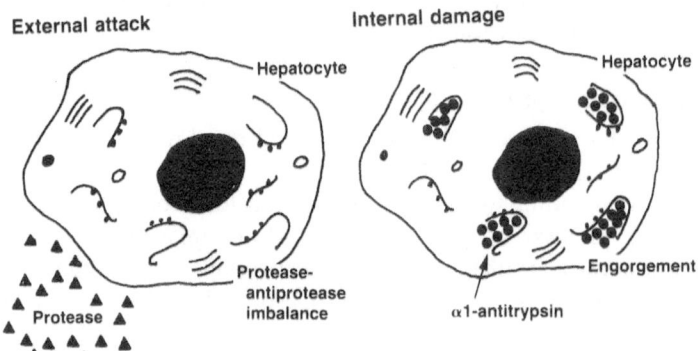

Figure 1   Major hypotheses concerning the mechanism of hepatocyte injury in α_1-antitrypsin (α_1AT) deficiency. *Left*: The 'external attack' hypothesis suggests that the injury is similar to that responsible for emphysema in the lung in α_1AT deficiency, i.e. proteases external to the hepatocyte injure the liver because there is a local deficiency of antiproteases secondary to the α_1AT deficiency state. *Right*: The 'internal damage' hypothesis suggests that accumulation of α_1AT in the rough endoplasmic reticulum of the hepatocytes causes engorgement of the rough endoplasmic reticulum, and subsequent intracellular damage

1972; Jeppsson et al., 1974). In this context, it is hypothesized that the engorged RER, in some (as yet undefined) fashion, results in injury of the hepatocytes. In this regard, the 'internal damage' hypothesis suggests that the liver disease associated with α_1AT deficiency is equivalent to the cellular damage of the general class of metabolic storage disorders.

All available evidence suggests the 'internal damage' hypothesis is the most likely. Most importantly, if the 'external attack' hypothesis is correct, it predicts that all of the different α_1AT alleles causing α_1AT deficiency would be associated with an increased risk for liver disease. However, this is not the case (Table 2). The only proven α_1AT 'at risk' alleles associated with liver disease are the Z and M_{malton} alleles (Brantly et al., 1988b; Perlmutter et al., 1985; Mornex et al., 1986; Carlson et al., 1989; Cox, 1989; Crystal, 1989, 1990; Curiel et al., 1989; Fraizer et al., 1989; Graham et al., 1990; Sifers et al., 1989a). Most importantly, individuals with the null–null α_1AT phenotype have no liver disease, despite the fact that these individuals have no α_1AT in serum and thus would be expected to be at very high risk for the development of liver disease if the 'external attack' hypothesis were correct. In contrast, strikingly, the Z and M_{malton} alleles are associated with intracellular accumulation of α_1AT. That only these two alleles are clearly associated with an increased risk for liver disease strongly argues for the 'internal damage' hypothesis.

There is no question that the Z gene itself is associated with the primary liver abnormalities, since transgenic mice in which the Z gene has been inserted have hepatocyte intracellular α_1AT accumulation and liver inflammation (Carlson et al., 1989). However, the fact that liver disease is not universal in Z homozygotes suggests a complex pathogenesis, possibly involving other genetic and environmental factors. For example, it is unexplained why males develop liver disease in association with

Table 2 Association of disease risk and the molecular mechanism causing the α_1-antitrypsin deficiency state

Dominant molecular mechanism	Allele	α_1AT serum level	Risk for disease[a] Emphysema	Risk for disease[a] Liver
Gene deletion	$\text{Null}_{isola\ di\ procida}$	Low	Yes	No
mRNA degradation	$\text{Null}_{bellingham}$	Low	Yes	No
	$\text{Null}_{granite\ falls}$	Low	Yes	No
α_1AT intracellular accumulation	Z	Low	Yes	Yes
	M_{malton}	Low	Yes	Yes
	$\text{Null}_{hong\ kong}$	Low	Yes	?[b]
α_1AT intracellular degradation	S	Intermediate	No	No
	$\text{Null}_{mattawa}$	Low	Yes	No
	Null_{bolton}	Low	Yes	No
	P_{lowell}	Low	Yes	No
	$W_{bethesda}$	Low	Yes	No
α_1AT function incompetent	$M_{mineral\ springs}$	Low	Yes	No

[a]For the basis of comparison, the assumption is that the allele is inherited in a homozygous fashion, although for some rare alleles such individuals have not been described
[b]It is not known whether $\text{Null}_{hong\ kong}$ is associated with liver disease, although it does cause α_1AT intracellular accumulation in hepatocytes (Sifers et al., 1988)

α_1AT deficiency more often than females (Eriksson *et al.*, 1986), or why breast feeding in the neonatal period seems to offer protection against development of liver injury in infants (Udall *et al.*, 1985). In regard to genetic factors, there are data suggesting that the major histocompatibility locus antigen B5 seems to confer protection against liver disease, while DR3 seems to increase susceptibility (Doherty *et al.*, 1990). Further, if liver disease occurs in association with α_1AT deficiency, there seems to be a higher risk for a second child to develop liver disease beyond that expected from chance alone (Cox and Mansfield, 1987).

While the association of Z and M_{malton} alleles with liver disease is clear, the mechanisms responsible for intracellular accumulation of α_1AT in association with Z and M_{malton} alleles are not fully understood. Most information available relates to the Z mutation, a $Glu^{342} \rightarrow Lys$ mutation that causes a loss of a normal internal salt bridge between Glu^{342} and Lys^{290} (Loebermann *et al.*, 1984). Site-directed mutagenesis studies have demonstrated that although the integrity of the Glu^{342}–Lys^{290} salt bridge is important, it is not completely mandatory for the secretion of α_1AT to occur (Brantly *et al.*, 1988b; McCracken *et al.*, 1989; Sifers *et al.*, 1989a). There is increasing evidence that the presence of the positively charged Lys at the 342 position, independent of salt bridge function, plays a major role in modulating the secretion defect in the Z protein (Sifers *et al.*, 1989a). It has been suggested, but not proved, that the $Glu^{342} \rightarrow Lys$ mutation results in a slowing of the rate of folding of the α_1AT polypeptide and/or a change in the tertiary structure of the α_1AT molecule within the RER (Brantly *et al.*, 1988b; McCracken *et al.*, 1989; Sifers *et al.*, 1989a). In contrast to the substitution of an amino acid that characterizes the Z mutation the M_{malton} allele is characterized by deletion of one residue (Phe^{52}) (Curiel *et al.*, 1989; Fraizer *et al.*, 1989). Like the Z allele, the M_{malton} allele is associated with accumulation of α_1AT in the liver, although it has not been proved that M_{malton} accumulates in the RER of hepatocytes (Curiel *et al.*, 1989). Studies with retroviral transfer of a M_{malton} cDNA into fibroblasts have shown it is the Phe^{52} deletion, *per se*, that causes the α_1AT accumulation (Curiel *et al.*, 1989). It is assumed, but not proved, that like the Z mutation, the accumulation of M_{malton} in the cell results from an abnormal rate of folding and/or change in tertiary structure. Theoretically, there are several ways in which abnormal rate of folding and/or tertiary structure of the Z or M_{malton} α_1AT proteins might affect their secretion and subsequently cause accumulation in the RER.

First, abnormal folding might expose a site on the molecule that is recognized (or not recognized) by a protein in the RER. This interaction may cause the specific intracellular retention of the molecule. For example, resident RER proteins such as BiP recognize and bind to incorrectly folded proteins, thereby preventing their exit from RER (Kozutsumi *et al.*, 1988). However, to date, no association between BiP (or other proteins in this class) and accumulated α_1AT proteins has been proved (Cresteil *et al.*, 1990; Graham *et al.*, 1990).

Second, improperly folded α_1AT may alter the affinity of α_1AT for a 'receptor' that is involved in the normal translocation of the α_1AT from the RER to the Golgi apparatus, with consequent trapping and accumulation of α_1AT in the RER. While no such receptors relevant to α_1AT have been identified, recent studies suggest that improperly folded proteins may be retained in the RER following interaction with members of the heat-shock protein family (Kozutsumi *et al.*, 1988). Consistent with this concept, synthesis of heat-shock protein is increased in the presence of abnormally folded proteins and expression of HSP 70 is induced in *Xenopus* oocytes by injections of denatured proteins but not by injection of proteins in their native form (Ananthan *et al.*, 1986). Members of the heat-shock protein family bind to secretory proteins until they are completely folded; once the folding is completed, secretory proteins dissociate to permit transport (Pelham, 1986). If this is not achieved, as may occur with the Z mutation, the Z form of α_1AT might remain in the RER. Consistent with the possibility that heat-shock protein may be involved in the pathogenesis of the Z protein accumulation, there is evidence that stress proteins (HSP 70, HSP 90 and ubiquitin) are increased in monocytes of homozygous Z individuals, but not in those of normal individuals (Perlmutter *et al.*, 1989b).

Third, specific intracellular systems have been identified in the RER that degrade improperly folded proteins (Kozutsumi *et al.*, 1988; Graham *et al.*, 1990; Le *et al.*, 1990). One such system is the ubiquitin pathway, in which selectivity for degradation depends on the conjugation of the protein to ubiquitin (Parag *et al.*, 1987; Ganoth *et al.*, 1988). Interestingly, ubiquitin levels are increased in monocytes and hepatocytes of Z homozygotes suggesting that the ubiquitin pathway may be involved, i.e. accumulation of the Z form of α_1AT in hepatocytes may be due to a combination of a relative increase in binding to heat-shock proteins and/or a malfunctioning degrading system (Perlmutter *et al.*, 1988).

Finally, the Z and M_{malton} proteins may accumulate because a slow rate of folding in the RER permits usually 'hidden' hydrophobic residues within the α_1AT molecule to interact with like molecules, resulting in the formation of α_1AT aggregates that cannot be translocated to the Golgi (Loebermann *et al.*, 1984; Sifers *et al.*, 1989b).

While the mechanism of the intracellular α_1AT accumulation is unclear, even less is known about the mechanism of the hepatocyte damage associated with the α_1AT accumulation. It is assumed, but not proved, to result from the engorgement of the RER, perhaps by sheer 'mass effect'. Alternatively, the engorgement may cause the release of lysosomal enzymes, as suggested by studies in which Z mRNA transcripts were injected into *Xenopus* oocytes (Bathurst *et al.*, 1985).

THERAPY

While there is good evidence of biochemical efficacy for augmentation therapy with α_1AT for the emphysema associated with α_1AT deficiency, there is no specific therapy available for the liver disease, either in neonates or adults (Crystal, 1990; Povey, 1990). In this regard, other than standard symptomatic therapy for liver cirrhosis and portal hypertension, the only therapy currently available is liver transplantation. As long as the exact pathophysiology is unknown, strategies for therapeutic approaches cannot be definitive.

Liver transplantation

Liver transplantation has been used successfully to treat the liver diseases in α_1AT-deficient children, with 5-year survival rates exceeding 70% (Esquivel *et al.*, 1987, 1988a). α_1AT deficiency is the most common hereditary disorder for which liver transplantation is used and is the second (next to biliary atresia) overall most common indication for liver transplantation in children (Esquivel *et al.*, 1988b). The long-term survival for liver transplantation in the adult group with α_1AT deficiency and liver disease is good but slightly lower (60%) than for children (Esquivel *et al.*, 1988b). In liver transplants performed in Z homozygotes with α_1AT deficiency, conversion of serum α_1AT to the α_1AT phenotype of the transplanted liver occurs together with normalization of serum α_1AT levels (Putnam *et al.*, 1977; Van Furth *et al.*, 1986), i.e. not only does liver transplantation 'cure' the liver disease, but presumably also will protect the lung against the development of emphysema. However, despite its being the definitive therapy for α_1AT deficiency, there are still many problems associated with liver transplantation, including the lack of donor organs, the need for long-term immunosuppressive therapy, and the significant mortality rate (Putnam *et al.*, 1977; Van Furth *et al.*, 1986; Esquivel *et al.*, 1987, 1988a,b; Dindzans *et al.*, 1988).

Augmentation of liver α_1AT secretion

If the liver could be induced to secrete α_1AT without increasing synthesis, the accumulation of the Z or M_{malton} proteins would decrease, and there would probably be less liver damage. Various attempts have been made to increase serum α_1AT levels in Z homozygotes by modifying liver production and/or secretion, including administration of typhoid vaccine, oestrogen–progesterone combinations, danazol and tamoxifen (Laurell *et al.*, 1967; Gadek *et al.*, 1980; Eriksson, 1983; Wewers *et al.*, 1986, 1987). However, the increases of α_1AT levels in serum are small, and it is theoretically possible that they could cause the liver problems to worsen by increasing synthesis and accumulation. To date no specific α_1AT-releasing agents are available.

Augmentation therapy with α_1-antitrypsin

Theoretically, it might be possible to suppress α_1AT synthesis by hepatocytes so that the amount of α_1AT that accumulates in the RER would be less. For example, if hepatocytes had receptors for α_1AT, raising levels might suppress α_1AT gene expression by negatively feeding back on the α_1AT promoter, or by down-regulating α_1AT synthesis at sites distal to transcription but prior to the RER (Figure 2). Although a receptor has been identified on hepatocytes for a portion of the α_1AT molecule that is exposed following the α_1AT–neutrophil elastase interaction (Perlmutter *et al.*, 1990), free α_1AT does not have the ligand for this receptor exposed, and it is not known whether triggering this receptor will decrease Z-homozygote hepatocyte α_1AT synthesis. Thus, at least for now, there is no known way to suppress α_1AT synthesis in hepatocytes of α_1AT-deficient individuals. Further, in our anecdotal experience of treating adults with α_1AT deficiency with emphysema and mild liver function abnormalities, augmentation of serum α_1AT levels does not alter serum markers of liver injury.

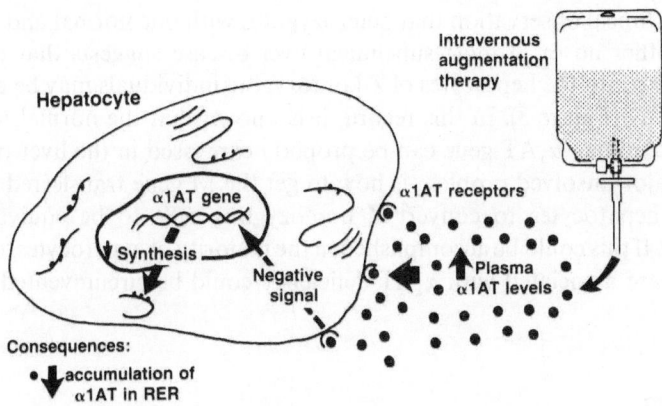

Figure 2 Strategy of treatment of the liver disease associated with α_1-AT deficiency using intravenous α_1AT augmentation therapy. This strategy assumes that the hepatocyte injury results from accumulation of α_1AT in the rough endoplasmic reticulum (RER), and that the hepatocyte has receptors for α_1AT. If so, it is theoretically possible that increased plasma α_1AT levels consequent to augmentation therapy might send a negative feedback signal to suppress α_1AT gene expression. The result would be decrease in α_1AT synthesis, and less liver injury secondarily to decreased accumulation of α_1AT in the RER.

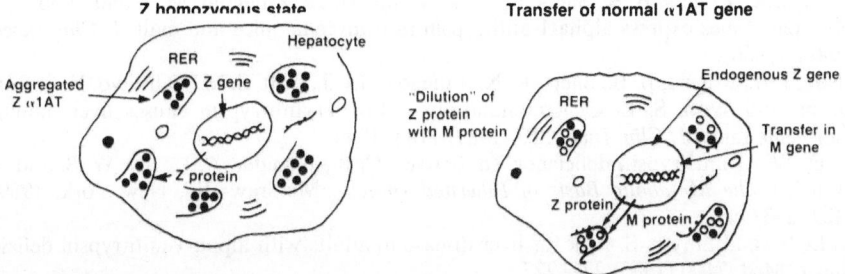

Figure 3 Strategy of treatment of the liver disease associated with α_1-AT deficiency by transferring the normal α_1AT gene to hepatocytes. *Left*: In hepatocytes of individuals with the Z homozygous form of α_1AT deficiency, expression of the two parental Z alleles of the α_1AT gene results in aggregation of the Z form of α_1AT protein in the rough endoplasmic reticulum (RER) and consequent injury to the hepatocyte. *Right*: Theoretically, transfer of a normal α_1AT gene to the hepatocyte could convert the hepatocyte to one that expressed both the Z and M forms of the α_1AT gene. If expression of the newly transformed M gene is sufficient, there should be enough M protein produced to 'dilute' the amount of Z protein in RER sufficiently to prevent hepatocyte damage.

Gene therapy

Several strategies have been devised that utilize gene transfer technology to augment the α_1AT levels in the lung, making gene therapy an attractive approach to treating the pulmonary problems associated with α_1AT deficiency (Crystal, 1989). However, approaches that specifically increase the anti-neutrophil elastase screen without changes in liver α_1AT secretion and/or synthesis are not likely to help the liver disease. The clinical observation that heterozygotes with one normal and one Z α_1AT allele have either no or at most subclinical liver disease suggests that transfer of a normal M gene into the heptocytes of Z homozygote individuals may be an attractive form of therapy (Figure 3). In this regard, it is known that the normal M as well as the mutant Z human α_1AT gene can be properly expressed in the liver of transgenic mice. The major unsolved problem is how to get the M gene transferred to sufficient numbers of hepatocytes to convert Z homozygous cells to be equivalent to the heterozygote. If this could be accomplished in the majority of hepatocytes, theoretically the liver disease associated with α_1AT deficiency could be circumvented.

REFERENCES

Ananthan, J., Goldberg, A. L. and Voellmy, R. Abnormal proteins serve as eukaryotic stress signals and trigger the activation of heat shock genes. *Science* 232 (1986) 522–524

Bathurst, I. C., Errington, D. M., Foreman, R. C., Judah, J. D. and Carrell, R. W. Human Z α1-antitrypsin accumulates intracellularly and stimulates lysosomal activity when synthesized in the xenopus qocyte. *FEBS Lett.* 183 (1985) 304–308

Brantly, M., Toshihiro, N. and Crystal, R. G. Molecular basis of alpha-1-anti-trypsin deficiency. *Am. J. Med.* 84 (6A) (1988a) 13–31

Brantly, M., Courtney, M. and Crystal, R. G. Repair of the secretion defect in the Z form of α1-antitrypsin by addition of a second mutation. *Science* 242 (1988b) 1700–1702

Carlson, J. A., Rogers, B. B., Sifers, R. N., Hawkins, H. K., Finegold, M. J. and Woo, S. L. C. Multiple tissues express alpha-1-antitrypsin in transgenic mice and man. *J. Clin. Invest.* 82 (1988) 26–36

Carlson, J. A., Rogers, B. B., Sifers, R. N., Finegold, M. J., Clift, S. M., DeMayo, F. J., Bullock, D. W. and Woo, S. L. C. Accumulation of PiZ α1-antitrypsin causes liver damage in transgenic mice. *J. Clin. Invest.* 83 (1989) 1183–1190

Cox, D. W. α1-antitrypsin deficiency. In: Scriver, C. R., Beaudet, A. L., Sly, W. S. and Valle, D. (eds.) *The Metabolic Basis of Inherited Disease.* McGraw-Hill, New York, 1989, pp. 2409–2437

Cox, D. W. and Smyth, S. Risk for liver disease in adults with alpha-1-antitrypsin deficiency. *Am. J. Med.* 74(2) (1983) 221–227

Cox, D. W., Mansfield, T. Prenatal diagnosis of alpha-1-antitrypsin deficiency and estimates of fetal risk for disease. *J. Med. Genet.* 24 (1987) 52

Cresteil, D., Ciccarelli, E., Soni, T., Alonso, M. A., Jacobs, P., Bollen, P. and Alvarez, F. BiP expression is not increased by accumulation of PiZ α1-antitrypsin in the endoplasmic reticulum. *FEBS Lett.* 267(2) (1990) 277–280

Crystal, R. G. The α1-antitrypsin gene and its deficiency states. *Trends Genet.* 5(12) (1989) 411–417

Crystal, R. G. α1-antitrypsin deficiency, emphysema, and liver disease. Genetic basis and strategies for therapy. *J. Clin. Invest.* 85 (1990) 1343–1352

Crystal, R. G., Brantly, M. L., Hubbard, R. C., Curiel, D. T., States, D. J. and Holmes, M. The alpha-1-antitrypsin gene and its mutations. Clinical consequences and strategies for therapy. *Chest* 95 (1989) 196–208

Curiel, D. T., Holmes, M. D., Okayama, H., Brantly, M. L., Vogelmeier, C., Travis, W. D., Stier, L. E., Perks, W. H. and Crystal, R. G. Molecular basis of the liver and lung disease associated with the α1-antitrypsin deficiency allele M_{malton}. *J. Biol. Chem.* 264 (23) (1989) 13938–13945

DeLellis, R., Balogh, K., Merk, F. and Chirife, A. Distinctive hepatic cell globules in adult α1-antitrypsin deficiency. *Arch. Pathol.* 94 (1972) 308–316

Dindzans, V. J., Schade, R. R. and Van Thiel, D. H. Medical problems before and after transplantation. *Gastroenterol. Clin. N. Am.* 17(1) (1988) 19–32

Doherty, D. G., Donaldson, P. T., Whitehouse, D. B., Mieli-Vergani, G., Duthie, A., Hopkinson, D. A. and Mowat, A. P. HLA phenotypes and gene polymorphisms in juvenile liver disease associated with α1-antitrypsin deficiency. *Hepatology* 12 (1990) 218–223

du Bois, R. M., Bernaudin, J.-F., Paakko, P., Takahashi, T., Curiel, D., Ferrans, V. J. and Crystal, R. G. Human neutrophils express the α1-antitrypsin gene and synthesize and secrete α1-antitrypsin. *Clin. Res.* 37(2) (1989) 611A

Eriksson, S. The effect of tamoxifen in intermediate alpha-1-antitrypsin deficiency associated with phenotype PiSZ. *Ann. Clin. Res.* 15 (1983) 95–98

Eriksson, S. and Haegerstrand, I. Cirrhosis and malignant hepatoma in α1-antitrypsin deficiency. *Acta Med. Scand.* 195 (1974) 451–458

Eriksson, S., Carlson, S. and Velez, R. Risk of cirrhosis and primary liver cancer in alpha-1-antitrypsin deficiency. *N. Engl. J. Med.* 314 (1986) 736–739

Esquivel, C. O., Vicente, E., Van Thiel, D., Gordon, R., Marsh, W., Makowka, L., Koneru, B., Iwatsuki, S., Madrigal, M., Delgado Milan, M. A., Todo, S., Tzakis, A. and Starzl, T. E. Orthotopic liver transplantation for alpha-1-antitrypsin deficiency: an experience in 29 children and 10 adults. *Transplant. Proc.* 19 (1987) 3798–3802

Esquivel, C. O., Marino, I. R., Fioravanti, V. and Van Thiel, D. H. Liver transplantation for metabolic disease of the liver. *Gastroenterol. Clin. N. Am.* 17(1) (1988a) 167–177

Esquivel, C. O., Mash, J. W. and Van Thiel, D. H. Liver transplantation for chronic cholestatic liver disease in adults and children. *Gastroenterol. Clin. N. Am.* 17(1) (1988b) 145–155

Feldmann, G., Bignon, J., Chahinian, P., Degott, C. and Benhamou, J. Hepatocyte ultrastructural changes in α1-antitrypsin deficiency. *Gastroenterology* 74 (1974) 1214–1224

Fraizer, G. C., Harrold, T. R., Hokfer, M. H. and Cox, D. W. In-frame single codon deletion in the Mmalton deficiency allele of α1-antitrypsin. *Am. J. Hum. Genet.* 44(6) (1989) 894–902

Gadek, J. E., Fulmer, J. D., Gelfand, J. A., Frank, M. M., Petty, T. L. and Crystal, R. G. Danazol-induced augmentation of serum α1-antitrypsin levels in individuals with marked deficiency of this antiprotease. *J. Clin. Invest.* 66 (1980) 82–87

Ganoth, D., Leshinsky, E., Eytan, E. and Hershko, A. A multicomponent system degrades proteins conjugated to ubiquitin. *J. Biol. Chem.* 263(25) (1988) 12412–12419

Govindarajan, S., Ashcavai, M. and Peters, R. L. α-1-antitrypsin phenotypes in hepatocellular carcinoma. *Hepatology* 1(6) (1981) 628–631

Graham, K. S., Le, A., Sifers, R. N. Accumulation of the insoluble PiZ variant of human α1-antitrypsin within the hepatic endoplasmatic reticulum does not elevate the steady-state level of grp78/BiP. *J. Biol. Chem.* 265(33) (1990) 20463–20468

Hubbard, R. C. and Crystal, R. G. Antiproteases. In: Crystal, R. G. and West, J. B. (eds.) *The Lung.* Raven Press, New York, 1991a, pp. 1775–1788

Hubbard, R. C. and Crystal, R. G. Susceptibility of the lung to proteolytic injury. In: Crystal, R. G. and West, J. B. (eds.) *The Lung.* Raven Press, New York, 1991b, pp. 2059–2072

Jeppsson, J.-O., Larsson, C. and Eriksson, S. Characterization of α1-antitrypsin in the inclusion bodies from the liver in α1-antitrypsin deficiency. *N. Engl. J. Med.* 293 (1974) 576–579

Kozutsumi, Y., Segal, M., Normington, K., Gething, M.-J. and Sambrook, J. The presence of malfolded proteins in the endoplasmic reticulum signals the induction of glucose-regulated proteins. *Nature* 332 (1988) 462–464

Laurell, C. B., Kullander, S. and Thorell, J. Effect of administration of a combined estrogen-progestin contraceptive on the level of individual plasma proteins. *Scand. J. Clin. Lab. Invest.* 21 (1967) 337–343

Le, A., Graham, K. S. and Sifers, R. N. Intracellular degradation of the transport-impaired human PiZ α1-antitrypsin variant. *J. Biol. Chem.* 265(23) (1990) 14001–14007

Liebermann, J., Mittmann, C. and Gordon, H. W. Alpha-1-antitrypsin in the livers of patients with emphysema. *Science* 175 (1972) 63–65

Loebermann, H., Tokuoka, R., Deisenhofer, J. and Huber, R. Human α1-proteinase inhibitor crystal structure analysis of two crystal modifications, molecular model and preliminary analysis of the implications for function. *J. Mol. Biol.* 177 (1984) 531–556

Lodish, H. F. Transport of secretory and membrane glycoproteins from the rough endoplasmic reticulum to the Golgi. *J. Biol. Chem.* 263(5) (1988) 2107–2110

Long, G. L., Chandra, T., Woo, S. L. C., Davie, E. W. and Kurachi, K. Complete sequence of the cDNA for human α1-antitrypsin and the gene for the S variant. *Biochemistry* 23 (1984) 4828–4837

McCracken, A. A., Kruse, K. B. and Brown, J. L. Molecular basis for defective secretion of the Z variant of human alpha-1-proteinase inhibitor: Secretion of variants having altered potential for salt bridge formation between amino acids 290 and 342. *Mol. Cell. Biol.* 9(4) (1989) 1406–1414

Mornex, J. F., Chytil-Weir, A., Martinet, Y., Courtney, M., LeCoq, J. P. and Crystal, R. G. Expression of the alpha-1-antitrypsin gene in mononuclear phagocytes of normal and alpha-1-antitrypsin-deficient individuals. *J. Clin. Invest.* 77 (1986) 1952–1961

Palmer, P. E., DeLellis, R. A. and Wolfe, H. J. Immunohistochemistry of liver in α1-antitrypsin deficiency. *Am. J. Clin. Pathol.* 64 (1974) 350–354

Parag, H. A., Raboy, B. and Kulka, R. G. Effect of heat shock on protein degradation in mammalian cells: involvement of the ubiquitin system. *EMBO J.* 6(1) (1987) 55–61

Pelham, H. R. B. Speculations on the functions of the major heat shock and glucose-regulated proteins. *Cell* 46 (1986) 959–961

Perlmutter, D. H., Kay, R. M., Cole, F. S., Rossing, T. H., Van Thiel, D., Colten, H. R. The cellular defect in α1-proteinase inhibitor (α1-PI) deficiency is expressed in human monocytes and in xenopus oocytes injected with human liver mRNA. *Proc. Natl. Acad. Sci. USA* 82 (1985) 6918–6921

Perlmutter, D. H., Daniels, J. D., Auerbach, H. S., De Schryver-Kecskemeti, K., Winter, H. S. and David, H. A. The alpha-1-antitrypsin gene expressed in a human intestinal epithelial cell line. *J. Biol. Chem.* 264(16) (1989a) 9485–9490

Perlmutter, D. H., Schlesinger, M. J., Pierce, J. A., Punsal, P. I. and Schwartz, A. L. Synthesis of stress proteins is increased in individuals with homozygous PiZZ α1-antitrypsin deficiency and liver disease. *J. Clin. Invest.* 84 (1989b) 1555–1561

Perlmutter, D. H., Schlesinger, M. J., Pierce, J. A., Campbell, E. J., Rothbaum, R. J. and Schwartz, A. L. Induction of the stress response in α1-antitrypsin deficiency. *Trans. Assoc. Am. Phys.* 101 (1988) 33–41

Perlmutter, D. H., Glover, G. I., Rivetna, M., Schasteen, C. S. and Fallon, R. J. Identification of a serpin-enzyme complex receptor on human hepatoma cells and human monocytes. *Proc. Natl. Acad. Sci. USA* 87 (1990) 3753–3757

Povey, S. Genetics of alpha-1-antitrypsin deficiency in relation to neonatal liver disease. *Mol. Biol. Med.* 7(2) (1990) 161–172

Psacharopoulos, H. T., Mowat, A. P., Cook, P. J. L., Carlile, P. A., Portmann, B. and Rodeck, C. H. Outcome of liver disease associated with α1-antitrypsin deficiency (PiZ). *Arch. Dis. Child.* 58 (1983) 882–887

Putnam, C. W., Porter, K. A., Peters, R. L., Ashcavai, M., Redeker, A. G. and Starzl, T. E. Liver replacement for alpha 1-antitrypsin deficiency. *Surgery* 81(3) (1977) 258–261

Roberts, E. A., Cox, D. W., Medline, A. and Wanless, I. R. Occurrence of alpha-1-antitrypsin deficiency in 155 patients with alcoholic liver disease. *Am. J. Clin. Pathol.* 82 (1984) 424–427

Sharp, H. L., Bridges, R. A., Krivit, W. and Freier, E. F. Cirrhosis associated with alpha-1-antitrypsin deficiency: a previously unrecognized inherited disorder. *J. Lab. Clin. Med.* 73(6) (1969) 934–939

Sifers, R. N., Hardick, C. P., Woo, S. L. C. Disruption of the 290-342 salt bridge is not responsible for the secretory defect of the PiZ α1-antitrypsin variant. *J. Biol. Chem.* 264(5) (1989a) 2997–3001

Sifers, R. N., Finegold, M. J. and Woo, S. L. C. Alpha-1-antitrypsin deficiency: Accumulation or degradation of mutant variants within the hepatic endoplasmatic reticulum. *Am. J. Respir. Cell. Mol. Biol.* 1 (1989b) 341–345

Sifers, R. N., Brashears-Macatee, S., Kidd, V. J., Muensch, H. and Woo, S. L. C. A frameshift mutation results in a truncated α1-antitrypsin that is retained within the rough endoplasmic reticulum. *J. Biol. Chem.* 263(15) (1988) 7330–7335

Sparos, L., Tountas, Y., Chapuis-Cellier, C., Theodoropoulos, G. and Trichopoulos, D. Alpha-1-antitrypsin levels and phenotypes and hepatitis B serology in liver cancer. *Br. J. Cancer,* 49 (1984) 567–570

Sveger, T. Liver disease in alpha-1-antitrypsin deficiency detected by screening of 200,000 infants. *N. Engl. J. Med.* 294 (1976) 1316–1321

Sveger, T. The natural history of liver disease in α1-antitrypsin deficient children. *Acta Paediatr. Scand.* 77 (1988) 847–851

Talbot, I. C. and Mowat, A. P. Liver disease in infancy: histological features and relationship to α1-antitrypsin phenotype. *J. Clin. Pathol.* 28 (1975) 559–563

Udall, J. N., Dixon, M., Newman, A. P., Wright, J. A., James, B., Bloch, K. J. Liver disease in α1-antitrypsin deficiency. *J. Am. Med. Assoc.* 253 (1985) 2679–2682

Van Furth, R., Kramps, J. A., Van der Putten, A. B., Krom, R. A., Gips, C. H. Change in alpha-1-antitrypsin phenotype after orthotopic liver transplant. *Clin. Exp. Immunol.* 66 (3) (1986) 669–672

Wewers, M. Pathogenesis of emphysema. *Chest* 95 (1989) 190–195

Wewers, M. D., Brantly, M. L., Casolaro, M. A. and Crystal, R. G. Evaluation of Tamoxifen as a therapy to augment alpha-1-antitrypsin concentrations in Z homozygous alpha-1-antitrypsin-deficient subjects. *Am. Rev. Respir. Dis.* 135 (1987) 401–402

Wewers, M., Gadek, J. E., Keogh, B. A., Fells, G. A. and Crystal, R. G. Evaluation of danazol therapy for patients with PiZZ alpha-1-antitrypsin deficiency. *Am. Rev. Respir. Dis.* 134 (1986) 476–480

J. Inher. Metab. Dis. 14 (1991) 526–530

Clinical Presentation of Metabolic Liver Disease

M. ODIEVRE

Service de Pédiatrie, Hôpital Antoine Beclere, 157 rue de la Porte de Trivaux, 92 141 Clamart Cedex, France

Summary: Some clinical clues should alert paediatricians to the possibility of metabolic liver diseases. They can be classified into three categories:

(i)   Manifestations due to hepatocellular necrosis, acute or subacute, which can reveal galactosaemia, hereditary fructose intolerance, tyrosinaemia type I, Wilson disease and α_1-antitrypsin deficiency. Symptoms and signs suggestive of Reye syndrome should lead to a study of fatty acid oxidation and urea cycle enzymes. All these manifestations may necessitate a rapid diagnosis and treatment when liver dysfunction is severe.

(ii)   Cholestatic jaundice can reveal α_1-antitrypsin deficiency, Byler's disease, cystic fibrosis, Niemann–Pick disease and some disorders of peroxisome biogenesis.

(iii)   Hepatomegaly can reveal disorders with liver damage but also storage diseases such as glycogen storage diseases, cholesteryl ester storage disease and, when associated with splenomegaly, lysosomal storage diseases.

Appropriate investigations for recognizing all these entities are proposed.

The purpose of this paper is to present a clinical approach to the treatment of patients with metabolic liver diseases. The first step in the evaluation is a thorough clinical assessment including history; as many of the metabolic disorders are recessively inherited, the familial history (consanguinity, previous death of one sibling of undetermined cause) is critical.

Clinical manifestations of liver involvement which should lead to suspicion of inborn errors of metabolism can be separated into three categories: manifestations due to hepatocellular necrosis, cholestatic conditions and hepatomegaly.

MANIFESTATIONS DUE TO HEPATOCELLULAR NECROSIS

The situation, acute or subacute, is characterized by some degree of jaundice and/or oedema, ascites, bleeding tendency and sometimes hepatic encephalopathy. The clinical picture can be similar to septicaemia and it is not uncommon for an intercurrent sepsis to unmask an inborn error of metabolism (Burton, 1987).

Laboratory studies can show elevated serum transaminases, hypoprothrombinaemia, hypofibrinogenaemia, hypoglycaemia and elevated blood ammonia concentration indistinguishable from the results of liver function tests seen in severe viral hepatitis. The liver size should help to distinguish between the two conditions: in metabolic diseases, the liver remains enlarged while a rapid atrophy is seen in acute liver failure of viral origin (Alagille and Odievre, 1979).

A rapid diagnosis of these diseases is essential since many of the patients have a potentially treatable liver dysfunction. The age at which hepatic failure becomes apparent provides an important clue to the aetiology.

Onset in infancy: Three disorders have to be discussed:

(i) Galactosaemia is an early cause of metabolic liver dysfunction. Manifestations, essentially jaundice and bleeding tendency, typically appear at the end of the first or during the second week of life. Other circumstances suggesting galactosaemia are sepsis due to *Escherichia coli* (Levy *et al.*, 1977) and exceptionally pseudotumour cerebri. Suspicion of this diagnosis requires examination of the lens, immediate suppression of galactose-containing foods and appropriate enzyme assays in erythrocytes, galactosuria being unspecific in an infant with liver failure.

(ii) Hereditary fructose intolerance should be considered when symptoms appear as soon as fructose is introduced into the diet. Vomiting is a constant finding while other postprandial symptoms due to hypoglycaemia are in our experience less frequent (Odievre *et al.*, 1978). A distaste for sweet foods represents a good index of suspicion but it occurs later. Any suspicion of fructose intolerance must lead to the immediate withdrawal of sucrose and fructose from the diet. As seen also in galactosaemia, the beneficial effect of withdrawal of the toxic substrates is seen within 2 or 3 days and can be considered as the first positive element of diagnosis before specific investigation can be made.

(iii) The acute form of tyrosinaemia type I should be considered in all infants presenting with liver failure in whom galactosaemia and hereditary fructose intolerance have been excluded by specific investigations or when a galactose or fructose-free diet remains ineffective. A boiled cabbage odour of the urine is an index of suspicion. The chronic form is usually diagnosed when vitamin D-resistant rickets associated with liver disease by the age of 6 months to 1 year is discovered.

Onset in the older child: Two disorders can be responsible for severe hepatocellular necrosis: Wilson disease and α_1-antitrypsin deficiency.

(i) The clinical manifestations of Wilson disease are highly variable, but in children are predominantly hepatic (Odievre *et al.*, 1974). Most often the liver disease is subacute or chronic, ranging from a persistent increase in serum transaminases to chronic active hepatitis and/or cirrhosis with progressive development of liver failure. However, some patients present with fulminant liver failure associated with intravascular haemolysis and renal failure. This association is highly suggestive of the disease and has a very high mortality rate. In fact, any type of liver disease of unknown aetiology in children above the age of 6 years must be considered to be Wilson disease until proven otherwise. Evidence of renal tubular abnormalities, haemolysis and, from 10 years of age, neurological abnormalities are helpful for diagnosis. Suspicion of Wilson's disease must immediately lead to a search for corneal Kayser–Fleisher rings, even in those patients with overwhelming symptoms. Establishing the diagnosis on the basis of a study of copper metabolism poses a problem in fulminant liver failure, since blood ceruloplasmin level can be non-specifically decreased; in this case, an elevated serum copper level has been shown to be useful in separating patients with Wilson disease from others (Rakela *et al.*, 1986). Patients with fulminant liver failure have to be transferred to the transplantation centre as soon as possible (Sternlieb, 1984).

(ii) α_1-Antitrypsin deficiency: this disorder is among the most common of all inherited metabolic diseases. Some children develop cirrhosis which can be revealed by unpredictable and unexplained fulminant liver failure (Odievre, 1989). Because a history of prolonged neonatal cholestasis suggesting the aetiology may be absent, the search for absence of an α_1-globulin peak on the serum protein electrophoresis is mandatory in all patients with unexplained overwhelming liver disease.

Onset in infancy or childhood: At any age, any infant or child presenting with findings suggestive of Reye syndrome or with atypical or recurrent Reye-like episodes should be evaluated for the possibility of disorders of fatty acid oxidation and urea cycle defects (Burton, 1987).

DISEASES REVEALED BY CHOLESTATIC JAUNDICE

Affected patients have jaundice, dark urine, light or acholic stools and hepatomegaly.
   α_1-Antitrypsin deficiency is one of the most frequent causes of neonatal cholestasis, 10 to 20% of infants with the phenotype PIZZ developing this type of manifestation. Cholestasis is sometimes so complete that extrahepatic biliary atresia is considered (Odievre *et al.*, 1976). The absence of an α_1-globulin peak permits a rapid diagnosis. Cholestasis usually disappears before the 6th month of age; when it persists, an associated hypoplasia of interlobular bile ducts must be considered. About half of the patients having neonatal cholestasis will develop cirrhosis within the first two or three years of life.
   Byler disease is considered by some authors to be metabolic in origin. Cholestasis, including pruritus, appears during the first year of life and initially occurs intermittently, often being provoked by infection. Between attacks lasting a few days to several months, remission is never complete and this severe familial intrahepatic cholestasis progresses to cirrhosis and death before 15 years of age. The underlying biochemical abnormality remains to be defined.
   Other inborn errors of metabolism are rarely associated with neonatal cholestasis. However, some infants with galactosaemia, hereditary fructose intolerance, tyrosinaemia type I or cystic fibrosis can also present with cholestasis.
   Neonatal cholestasis is a possible presenting manifestation of Niemann–Pick

disease type C (several cases of this entity have been published as giant cell hepatitis) and of disorders of peroxisome biogenesis such as Zellweger syndrome and infantile Refsum disease (Lazarow and Moser, 1989). In this last condition, dysmorphic features, hypotonia and sensorineural dysfunction should orient the diagnosis.

DISEASES REVEALED BY HEPATOMEGALY

Metabolic diseases revealed by hepatomegaly fall into two general categories: disorders with liver damage and storage diseases. An important clue to the diagnosis is the consistency of the liver and characteristic of its surface. The differential diagnosis of a firm or rock-hard liver must include the difference causes of cirrhosis, whether associated with liver dysfunction or not. Galactosaemia, hereditary fructose intolerance and tyrosinaemia type I below 1 year of age, α_1-antitrypsin deficiency above this age, and Wilson disease and cystic fibrosis in school age children are instances of metabolic cirrhosis. In a few patients, intestinal haemorrhage due to portal hypertension is the presenting manifestation. Wilson disease must be recognized in order to avoid surgical portosystemic shunt which is invariably followed by severe encephalopathy (Alagille and Odievre, 1979). Glycogen storage disease type IV (brancher deficiency) is another exceptional cause of cirrhosis during the first years of life. Glycogen storage disease type III (debrancher deficiency) can be complicated by the progressive development of portal fibrosis, sometimes responsible for portal hypertension in late childhood.

In other metabolic diseases the consistency of the enlarged liver is normal or soft. Documenting the presence or absence of splenomegaly allows one to distinguish between two categories of patients:

(i) In those with isolated hepatomegaly, some additional findings can suggest a diagnosis (Table 1). Sometimes a mild hepatomegaly is the only finding, as seen in some cases of cholesteryl ester storage disease and glycogen storage diseases due to phosphorylase or phosphorylase kinase deficiency. If erythrocyte and leukocyte assays show normal enzyme activity of the phosphorylase system, a liver biopsy is often the only way to progress to aetiology.

Table 1 Clinical diagnostic aids in evaluating a patient with isolated hepatomegaly

Findings	Metabolic disorder
Liver extending to the iliac crest	GSD types IA, IB
Doll-like appearance and short stature	GSD of any type
Enlarged kidneys at X-ray and/or ultrasonography	GSD type IA
Cardiomegaly	GSD type II
Muscular involvement	GSD types II, III
Fasting intolerance	GSD types IA, IB, III Fructose-1,6-diphosphatase deficiency
Chronic diarrhoea and malnutrition	Cystic fibrosis
Repeated infections	GSD type IB (with granulopenia)

GSD: Glycogen storage disease

(ii) Hepatomegaly and splenomegaly can reflect storage of substances in endothelial and/or parenchymal cells (Sharp, 1978). This is characteristic of lysosomal metabolic defects in which massive enlargement of the spleen is more often seen in storage diseases than in portal hypertension.

Many of these diseases are accompanied by a history of slow development or of regression, coarse facial appearance and ocular and skeletal abnormalities. A detailed discussion of each entity is beyond the scope of this paper. Examination of peripheral blood for vacuolated white cells and bone marrow for storage cells and pertinent X-rays are mandatory. When the diagnosis still remains obscure, a liver biopsy should be performed for light and electron microscopy, and additional tissue should be frozen for future biochemical determinations. In rare cases, diagnosis has to be discussed when the history reveals a hydrops fetalis (Gillan, 1984).

In summary, we have attempted to present some clinical clues which should alert paediatricians to the possibility of metabolic liver diseases. Some of the diseases are complicated by a severe liver dysfunction which necessitates a rapid diagnosis and treatment while others, not currently amenable to effective treatment, permit time for correct diagnosis and genetic counselling.

REFERENCES

Alagille, D. and Odievre, M. *Liver and Biliary Tract Disease in Children*, Wiley Flammarion, New York and Paris, 1979

Burton, B. K. Inborn errors of metabolism: the clinical diagnosis in early infancy. *Pediatrics* 79 (1987) 359–369

Gillan, J. E., Lowden, J. A., Gaskin, K. and Cutz, E. Congenital ascites as a presenting sign of lysosomal storage disease. *J. Pediatr.* 104 (1984) 225–231

Lazarow, P. B. and Moser, H. W. Disorders of peroxisome biogenesis. In Scriver, C. R., Beaudet, A. L., Sly, W. S. and Valle, D. (eds.) *The Metabolic Basis of Inherited Disease*, McGraw-Hill, New York, 1989, pp. 1479–1509

Levy, H. L., Sepe, S. J., Shih, V. E., Vawter, G. F. and Klein, J. O. Sepsis due to *Escherichia coli* in neonates with galactosemia. *N. Engl. J. Med.* 297 (1977) 823–825

Odievre, M. Liver transplantation for inborn errors of metabolism. In Vis, H., Van Hoof, F. and Schaub, J. (eds.) *Inborn Errors of Metabolism*. Nestlé Nutrition Workshop Series Vol. 24. New York, Raven Press, 1991

Odievre, M., Vedrenne, J., Landrieu, P. and Alagille, D. Les formes hépatiques 'pures' de la maladie de Wilson chez l'enfant. A propos de 10 observations. *Arch. Fr. Pediatr.* 31 (1974) 215–222

Odievre, M., Martin, J. P., Hadchouel, M. and Alagille, D. Alpha-1-antitrypsin deficiency and liver diseases in children: phenotypes, manifestations and prognosis. *Pediatrics* 57 (1976) 226–231

Odievre, M., Gentil, C., Gautier, M. and Alagille, D. Hereditary fructose intolerance in childhood: diagnosis, management and course in 55 patients. *Am. J. Dis. Child.* 132 (1978) 605–608

Rakela, J., Kurtz, S. B., McCarthy, J. T., Ludwig, J., Ascher, N. L., Bloomer, J. R. and Claus, P. L. Fulminant Wilson's disease treated with postdilution hemofiltration and orthotopic liver transplantation. *Gastroenterology* 90 (1986) 2004–2007

Sharp, N. L. Metabolic liver disease. In Lebenthal, E. (ed.), *Digestive Diseases in Children*, Grune and Stratton, New York, 1978, pp. 589–610

Sternlieb, I. Wilson's disease. Indications for liver transplants. *Hepatology* 4 (1984) 15s–17s

J. Inher. Metab. Dis. 14 (1991) 531–537

Investigation of Paediatric Liver Disease

D. KELLY[1] and A. GREEN[2]
[1]*The Liver Unit and* [2]*Department of Clinical Chemistry, The Children's Hospital, Birmingham B16 8ET, UK*

Summary: The investigation of children with liver disease falls into two categories: the investigation of the cholestatic baby and the investigation of the older child (over 2 years) with hepatomegaly. The approach to investigation is directed by the clinical features and employs many different investigational methods including biochemistry, haematology, radiology, electrophysiology and histology. As the clinical presentation of many diseases is similar, it is appropriate to perform a variety of first-line tests, proceeding to more complex investigations only as indicated.

Investigation of paediatric liver disease can be divided into the investigation of the neonate or infant with cholestasis and the investigation of older children (over 2 years) with hepatomegaly.

NEONATAL LIVER DISEASE

The majority of children with liver disease will present in infancy with cholestasis. The main differential diagnosis is between extrahepatic biliary atresia, neonatal hepatitis or other disorders involving the biliary tree (Odievre, 1990).

A number of clinical clues will be evident from the clinical or family history and physical examination (Odievre, 1990) and the series of investigation will be directed by this information.

The first step in investigating any jaundiced baby is to establish whether there is significant conjugated hyperbilirubinaemia (> 15% of total bilirubin) (Mowat, 1987). Standard liver function tests are unlikely to be helpful in the differential diagnosis between biliary obstruction and 'neonatal hepatitis' (Table 1) but some information about hepatic synthesis and the chronicity of liver disease may be implied by low albumin concentration and prolonged coagulation times that are unresponsive to vitamin K therapy. Poor hepatic function at birth suggests that the disease process has existed *in utero* and may be either an inborn error of metabolism or an infection.

As most neonatal liver disease presents in a similar way, it is usual to perform a series of first-line tests in order to exclude the known causes of intrauterine infection and certain inborn errors of metabolism (Table 2 and Figures 1 and 2) and to establish the patency of the extrahepatic biliary tree. More specialized investigations for specific metabolic disorders are only performed if clinical suspicion is high or the first-line tests suggest an inborn error of metabolism (Table 2).

Table 1 Liver function tests in the diagnosis of neonatal liver disease

	Extrahepatic biliary disorder	'Neonatal' hepatitis
Bilirubin, $< 20\,\mu mol/L$	↑Conjugated	↑Conjugated
Aminotransferases		
aspartate $< 50\,u/L$	↑	↑↑
alanine		
Alkaline phosphatase, $< 600\,u/L$	↑↑	↑
Albumin, $> 30\,g/L$	N	Low/N
Cholesterol, $1-4\,mmol/L$	N	N/High
Bicarbonate, $21-25\,mmol/L$	N	N/Low
Prothrombin (PT), 12 s	N	N/Abn
Partial thromboplastin (PTT) 35 s	N	N/Abn

Table 2 First line investigations for paediatric liver disease

Bacterial culture of blood and urine
TORCH
Hepatitis A, B, C + HIV
Chromosomes
Sweat test
Plasma glucose and lactate
Free T_4 and TSH
Serum iron and ferritin
α_1-Antitrypsin level and phenotype
Galactose-1-phosphate UDT
Plasma amino acids
Urine:
  Reducing sugars
  Amino acids
  Organic acids

It is essential to exclude associated infection by performing bacterial culture of blood and urine. Serological tests are performed to identify: toxoplasma, rubella, herpes simplex and parvo virus B19 (PHLS Working Party, 1990). IgM antibodies to cytomegalovirus (CMV) imply active infection (although not necessarily hepatitis), particularly if associated with CMV early antigen in urine, or positive throat and urine CMV cultures (Best, 1987). Hepatitis A, B or C are rare causes of neonatal hepatitis.

Chromosome studies should be performed because of the association between neonatal hepatitis and trisomy 13 and 18. A sweat test is carried out to exclude cystic fibrosis, which occasionally presents with neonatal hepatitis. Hypothyroidism is usually associated with unconjugated hyperbilirubinaemia, but it may exacerbate underlying hepatitis. All babies should have been screened for congenital hypothyroidism as part of a neonatal screening programme; however, this cannot be assumed. If there is any doubt, free T4 and TSH should be measured.

It is important to exclude extrahepatic biliary atresia or a choledocal cyst at an

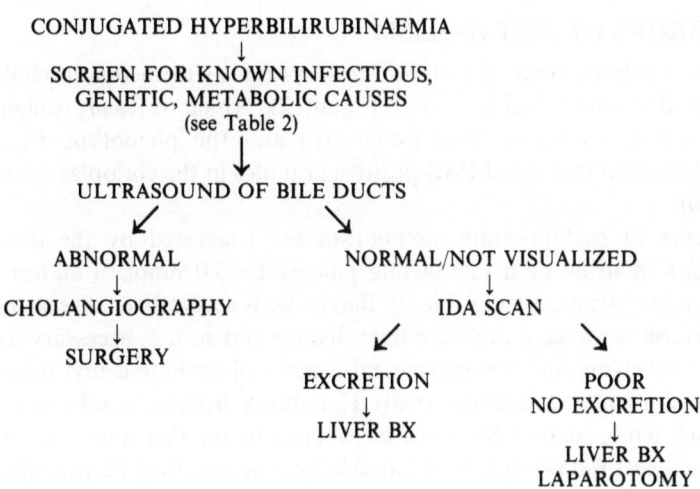

CONJUGATED HYPERBILIRUBINAEMIA
↓
SCREEN FOR KNOWN INFECTIOUS,
GENETIC, METABOLIC CAUSES
(see Table 2)
↓
ULTRASOUND OF BILE DUCTS
↙   ↘
ABNORMAL   NORMAL/NOT VISUALIZED
↓   ↓
CHOLANGIOGRAPHY   IDA SCAN
↓   ↙   ↘
SURGERY   EXCRETION   POOR
↓   NO EXCRETION
LIVER BX   ↓
LIVER BX
LAPAROTOMY

Figure 1 Evaluation of liver disease in childhood

early stage as corrective or palliative surgery is possible if performed early enough (Ohi *et al.*, 1985). The most useful investigation is an abdominal ultrasound, which may demonstrate a choledocal cyst or an absent gallbladder. If the ultrasound is normal or equivocal it is necessary to perform a radioisotope scan using technetium-IDA (iminodiacetic acid) to demonstrate hepatic uptake of isotope and excretion into the bowel. There is usually poor uptake but good excretion of isotope in neonatal hepatitis syndromes, whereas good uptake but no excretion into bowel suggests either extrahepatic biliary atresia or severe intrahepatic cholestasis.

Liver histology may differentiate between intra- and extrahepatic disorders, but there is considerable overlap in the pathological features. Classically, neonatal hepatitis of any aetiology will show giant cell transformation and rosette formation of hepatocytes with an inflammatory cell infiltrate. Excessive fat deposition is suggestive (but not diagnostic) of a metabolic disease. In extrahepatic biliary obstruction of any kind there will be fibrous expansion of the portal tracts with proliferation of bile ducts, but features of each disorder may be present and it may be necessary to perform a laparotomy and an operative cholangiogram to outline the extrahepatic biliary tree before the diagnosis is secure.

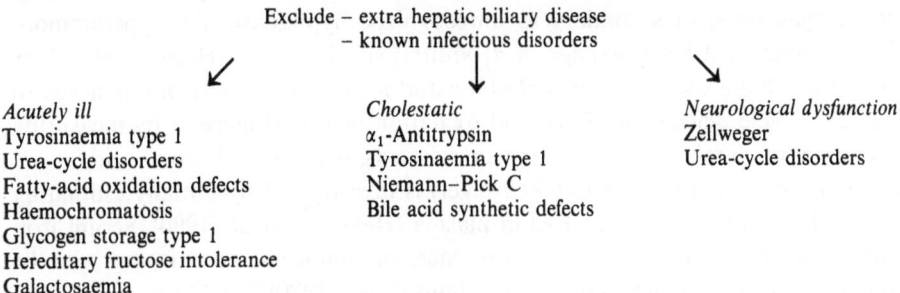

Exclude – extra hepatic biliary disease
– known infectious disorders
↙   ↓   ↘

Acutely ill   *Cholestatic*   *Neurological dysfunction*
Tyrosinaemia type 1 α_1-Antitrypsin   Zellweger
Urea-cycle disorders   Tyrosinaemia type 1   Urea-cycle disorders
Fatty-acid oxidation defects   Niemann–Pick C
Haemochromatosis   Bile acid synthetic defects
Glycogen storage type 1
Hereditary fructose intolerance
Galactosaemia

Figure 2 Differential diagnosis of metabolic liver disease in infants

INBORN ERRORS OF METABOLISM

The commonest inborn error of metabolism to present with neonatal cholestasis is α_1-antitrypsin deficiency (Table 2 and Figure 2), which is easily diagnosed by establishing a reduced serum level ($< 0.8\,g/L$) and the phenotype PIZZ. Liver histology will confirm storage of PAS-positive granules in the endoplasmic reticulum (Mowat, 1990).

Inborn errors of carbohydrate metabolism are suggested by the detection of reducing sugars in urine or a low fasting glucose ($< 3.0\,mmol/L$) and/or a raised plasma lactate ($> 3.0\,mmol/L$) (Table 2). Babies with severe liver disease may have gross galactosuria secondary to severe liver disease and so it is necessary to exclude galactosaemia by estimating the enzyme galactose-1-phosphate uridyl transferase in red cells (Gitzelmann and Hansen, 1980). Hereditary fructose intolerance presents later in infancy when sucrose has been introduced to the diet and is confirmed by measuring fructose-1,6-diphosphate aldolase in liver or intestinal biopsies (Steinmann and Gitzelmann, 1981).

Glycogen storage disease does not present with neonatal cholestasis but with hepatomegaly and in some variants hypoglycaemia and a raised plasma lactate. It can be confirmed by measuring the appropriate enzymes in liver, leukocytes or muscle (Fernandes, 1990).

In patients with liver disease, tyrosinaemia type I is the commonest disorder of amino-acid metabolism and is suggested by the finding of elevated tyrosine and methionine in plasma and urine. A non-specific increase of tyrosine and methionine can occur in severe liver disease from any cause and therefore measurement of urinary succinyl-acetone is essential as this is elevated in tyrosinaemia type I. The diagnosis is then confirmed by demonstrating a deficiency of fumaryl-acetoacetate in leukocytes or cultured skin fibroblasts (Kvittingen, 1990). An elevated alpha-fetoprotein ($> 800\,IU/L$) is additional suggestive evidence of tyrosinaemia and may indicate early malignant change in the liver, which can be confirmed by abdominal ultrasound, computed tomography or liver histology.

Niemann–Pick C is the commonest lipid storage disease to present with neonatal hepatitis. There is no screening test but the diagnosis must be excluded by looking for the characteristic storage cells in liver, in bone marrow and in ganglion cells on rectal biopsy (Lake, 1990).

Neurological problems in babies with neonatal liver disease may be primary (e.g. Zellweger syndrome) or secondary to unrecognized hypoglycaemia, hyperammonaemia or intracranial haemorrhage in α_1-antitrypsin deficiency (Hope *et al.*, 1982). Many of these babies will not be cholestatic and if they are acutely ill one needs to exclude urea-cycle defects and fatty-acid oxidation defects (Figure 2) by measuring plasma ammonia, amino acids, urinary amino acids, organic and orotic acid.

A peroxisomal disorder (such as Zellweger) is investigated by initially estimating very-long-chain fatty acids (VLCFA) in plasma (Heymans *et al.*, 1990). Serum iron is usually elevated. The absence, or presence, of abnormal peroxisomes can be demonstrated in liver tissue using special stains (Lake, 1990).

Patients with persisting cholestasis in whom all other investigations for inborn errors of metabolism are negative should have urine screened for inborn errors of bile acid synthesis using FAB-MS (Clayton, 1990).

LIVER DISEASE IN CHILDREN OVER 2 YEARS

The commonest form of liver disease in this age group is acute or chronic hepatitis secondary to viral infection (Table 3). It is important to exclude the other diseases mentioned in Table 3 as they have a different clinical course and therapy.

Standard biochemical tests may show a hepatitis (raised transaminases 4–10 times upper limit of normal) or evidence of poor hepatocellular function (low albumin and abnormal coagulation). Abdominal ultrasound may show a small liver and an enlarged spleen, suggesting cirrhosis and portal hypertension from any cause. Evidence of chronic liver disease may be gained from X-rays of the wrist, which may show osteopenia or rickets. Severe rickets suggests a renal tubular disorder that is usually secondary to an inborn error of metabolism, e.g. Wilson disease, hereditary fructose intolerance, tyrosinaemia type I. As the most common diagnosis in this age group is acute or chronic viral hepatitis, a viral aetiology must be excluded at all times.

Autoimmune liver disease presents in either sex, although the incidence is higher in girls (3:1). Non-organ-specific autoantibodies may be demonstrated in 70% of children and there is always an increase in IgG ($> 20 \text{g/L}$).

As Wilson disease may present with almost any form of liver disease it must always be considered in children over 3 years old. Classically the diagnosis is established by detecting a reduced serum copper ($< 10 \mu\text{mol/L}$), ceruloplasmin ($< 200 \text{mg/L}$) and excess urine copper ($> 1.0 \mu\text{mol/24 h}$). Approximately 24% of children presenting with hepatic disease may have normal or borderline ceruloplasmin but all should have elevated urinary copper excretion, particularly after treatment with penicillamine (20 mg/kg) (Werlin *et al.*, 1978). There will be increased hepatic copper on liver histology ($> 250 \text{mg/g}$ dry weight) which is higher than the amount detected in chronic cholestasis.

In equivocal cases, radioactive copper studies using either ^{64}Cu or [67]Cu will demonstrate reduced incorporation into ceruloplasmin compared to normals.

Table 3 Causes of chronic liver disease in children

Chronic persistent/active hepatitis
  Post-viral hepatitis B, C, undefined
  Autoimmune hepatitis
  Drugs (nitrofurantrin, α-methyldopa)

Wilson disease (> 3 years)

α_1-Antitrypsin deficiency

Cystic fibrosis secondary to
  Neonatal liver disease
  Bile duct lesions

Table 4   Causes of acute liver failure in
children

Infection
  Viral hepatitis A, B, C, undefined

Poisons/drugs
  Paracetamol, isoniazide
  Halothane
  Amanita phalloides

Metabolic
  Wilson disease
  Tyrosinaemia type 1
  Fatty-acid oxidation defects

Autoimmune hepatitis

Reye syndrome

ACUTE LIVER FAILURE

Acute liver failure may present at any age. The clinical features are varied. Jaundice is not universally present, but there is always hypoglycaemia, encephalopathy and abnormal coagulation. The commonest cause is fulminant viral hepatitis (usually an unidentified virus) but a search for other aetiologies is mandatory (Table 4). It is important to perform a toxological screen for paracetamol as a history of drug ingestion is not always available.

Biochemical evidence of acute hepatitis with raised transaminases (10–100 times upper limit of normal) is always present in the early stages. Falling transaminases with a rising bilirubin and increasing coagulation times implies a poor prognosis.

An elevated ammonia is non-specific, but may suggest an inborn error of metabolism that should be excluded as described earlier. Encephalopathy can be monitored using an electroencephalogram (EEG), which correlates with the clinical state. The appearance of triphasic waves is characteristic of hepatic encephalopathy and the development of diffuse slow activity suggests a poor prognosis. Computed tomography of the brain may demonstrate cerebral oedema in acute fulminant viral hepatitis or Reye syndrome, which is important for management but not diagnosis. Liver biopsy to confirm the diagnosis is usually impossible because of coagulation abnormalities.

A Reye-like syndrome with acute liver failure and convulsions may be due to an underlying metabolic disorder, in particular fatty-acid oxidation defects. These disorders should be excluded by measuring plasma ammonia and amino acids, urinary amino acids and organic acids in the urine. A liver biopsy demonstrating microvesicular fatty deposition in the hepatocytes (Ballistreri, 1990) occurs both in Reye syndrome and fatty-acid oxidation defects and is not diagnostic.

REFERENCES

Ballistreri, W. F. Idiopathic Reye's syndrome and its metabolic mimickers. In: Ballistreri, W. F. and Stocker, J. T. (eds.) *Pediatric Hepatology*. Hemisphere, New York, 1990, pp. 183–198

Best, J.M. Congenital cytomegalovirus infection. *Br. Med. J.* 294 (1987) 1440–1441

Clayton, P. T. Inherited errors of bile acid metabolism. *J. Inher. Metab. Dis.* 14 (1991) 478–496

Fernandes, J. The glycogen storage diseases. In: Fernandes, J., Saudubray, J. M. and Tada, K. (eds.) *Inborn Metabolic Diseases.* Springer-Verlag, Heidelberg, 1990, pp. 69–88

Gitzelmann, R. and Hansen, R. G. Galactose metabolism, hereditary defects and their clinical significance. In: Burman, D., Holton, J. B. and Pennock, G. A. (eds.) *Inherited Disorders of Carbohydrate Metabolism.* MTP Press, Lancaster, 1980, pp. 61–101

Heymans, H. S. A., Wanders, R. J. A. and Schutgens, R. B. H. Peroximal disorders. In: Fernandes, J., Saudubray, J. M. and Tada, K. (eds.) *Inborn Metabolic Diseases.* Springer-Verlag, Heidelberg, 1990, pp. 421–436

Hope, P. L., Hall, M. A., Millward-Sadler, G. H. and Normand, I. C. S. Alpha-1-Antitrypsin deficiency presenting as a bleeding diathesis in the newborn. *Arch. Dis. Child.* 57 (1982) 68–79

Kvittingen, E. A. Tyrosinemia type I. *J. Inher. Metab. Dis.* 14 (1991) 554–562

Lake, B. D. The role of histochemical investigation in the diagnosis of inherited metabolic disorders. *J. Inher. Metab. Dis.* 14 (1991) 538–545

Mowat, A. P. Unconjugated hyperbilirubinemia. In: *Liver Disorders in Childhood.* Butterworths, London, 1987, p. 24

Hussain, M., Mieli-Vergani, G. and Mowat, A. P. α_1-Antitrypsin deficiency and liver disease. *J. Inher. Metab. Dis.* 14 (1991) 497–511

Odievre, M. Clinical presentation of metabolic liver disease. *J. Inher. Metab. Dis.* 14 (1991) 526–530

Ohi, R., Hanamatsu, M. and Mochizuki, I. Progress in the treatment of biliary atresia. *Surgery* 9 (1985) 285–290

Public Health Laboratories Service Working Party on Fifth Disease. Prospective study of human parvo virus (B19) infection in pregnancy. *Br. Med. J.* 300 (1990) 1166–1170

Steinmann, B. and Gitzelmann, R. Diagnosis of hereditary fructose intolerance. *Helv. Paediatr. Acta* 36 (1981) 297–316

Werlin, S. L., Grand, R. J., Perman, J. A. and Watkins, J. B. Diagnostic dilemmas of Wilson's disease: diagnosis and treatment. *Pediatrics* 62 (1978) 47–51

J. Inher. Metab. Dis. 14 (1991) 538–545
© SSIEM and Kluwer Academic Publishers.

The Role of Histochemical Investigations in Metabolic Disorders Affecting the Liver

B. D. LAKE

Department of Histopathology, Hospital for Sick Children and Institute of Child Health, Great Ormond Street, London WC1N 3JH, UK

Summary: The application of histochemical techniques to the study of metabolic disorders affecting the liver can yield considerable information, provided the methods used are sound and the interpretation is not over-enthusiastic. The appropriate methods can give insight into liver function and can identify and localize a wide variety of carbohydrates, lipids, proteins and enzyme activities. It is often thought that tissue taken for histochemical analysis cannot be used for morphology, but properly prepared tissue will provide the architectural and cytological detail necessary for histological assessment. There are several advantages to the histochemical approach, the main ones being economy of use of the valuable tissue sample (in theory about 100 sections and tests can be done on a 1 mm depth of tissue) and that the results of the tests can be assessed in relation to the structure of the liver.

There are two areas in which histochemical investigations are used: firstly, to detect cellular constituents, structures and cells not otherwise visible by routine methods. In this mode, histochemistry is an extension of the histological approach and constitutes a 'super haematoxylin and eosin' stain. Secondly, it is possible to assess enzyme activities and their localization, and in some well-defined instances to offer reliable indications of whether there is deficient activity, normal activity or enhanced activity.

Although there is a body of opinion which believes that quantitative enzyme histochemistry is possible and reliable, the author has not found the data, in particular on lysosomal enzymes, to be reliable and remains unconvinced that this technique has a place in the study of pathological tissue.

This review outlines a simple approach to the study of metabolic liver disease and illustrates the findings in a range of disorders of glycogen and lipid metabolism.

GENERAL APPROACH TO THE INVESTIGATION OF THE LIVER BIOPSY

Ideally, the investigation of metabolic liver disease is a team effort and when a biopsy is considered each member of the team (physician, biochemist and pathologist) should be aware of the aims of the biopsy and of the strengths and limitations of the methods used in its assessment. However, this ideal situation does not always exist, even in recognized centres of excellence, and a biopsy may arrive unexpectedly. Fortunately what should be done does not differ materially from the ideal approach, provided the sample arrives fresh and without fixative.

The decision to biopsy the liver is made having carried out the important clinical assessment of the patient, and having performed the appropriate range of biochemical tests on blood, urine, etc. At this stage there should be a clear indication of the type of disorder to be diagnosed or excluded, and the liver biopsy sample can be appropriately divided for histology, histochemistry, electron microscopy and biochemistry. The necessary information can readily be obtained from an adequate needle sample provided there is forward planning and that the people involved in the division and handling of the specimen are present when the biopsy is taken (Figure 1). The proportions taken for each investigation will vary depending on the index of suspicion. In some instances routine histology may be an unnecessary luxury and the bulk of the sample is best directed for biochemistry. However, even in these circumstances a small (2–3 mm) portion should always be reserved for histochemistry study and electron microscopy. The problem must also be faced of what should be done if a sample of only 2 mm is obtained. In this instance the sample is best snap frozen for histochemical examination which will give the most information. Such small samples cannot be divided and are quite inadequate for histology or biochemistry.

The need for structural assessment

Some histology or structural assessment is important. This can be done either on routine paraffin sections of fixed tissue, or perfectly adequately on cryostat sections

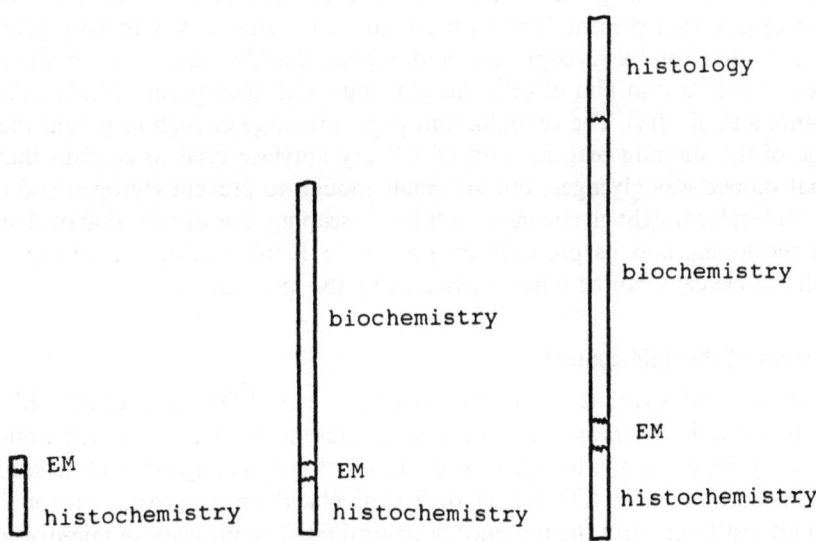

Figure 1 Division of a core of liver biopsy depending on the amount of tissue obtained. A good core will provide adequate material for histology, biochemistry, electron microscopy (EM) and histochemistry. An inadequate sample should allow histochemical studies and electron microscopy.

of the snap frozen sample taken for histochemistry. Assessment of structure and cytological detail will confirm that the tissue is indeed liver and not skeletal muscle, kidney, jejunum, adipose tissue, or lung. Each of these tissues has been known to comprise part or all of the sample, and on at least one occasion the sample was found to be neuroblastoma rather than liver. Thus the first role of the microscopist is to establish that the tissue is liver. Structural examination will also give an indication of the amount of hepatocytic tissue in relation to connective tissue so that account may be taken in cases where low activities of enzymes are recorded in a tissue homogenate. Any disease-specific features can also be noted. Bile pigment is preserved in cryostat sections while much is removed on fixation and processing.

Assessment of the glycogen content

The solubility of glycogen depends mainly on the length of the outer chains, being higher with shorter outer chain length and lower with longer outer chain length. Since patients undergoing liver biopsy have generally been fasted, the outer chains will have been eroded to variable extents and this will influence the amount of glycogen preserved in routine histological preparations. Glycogen is not fixed by formalin (there is never any justification for the wasteful practice of fixation in alcohol or other special fixatives for the demonstration of glycogen) but is trapped by the cell proteins which are rendered insoluble by the fixation. However, considerable amounts of glycogen can escape from the tissue during fixation. Such constraints do not apply to cryostat sections of snap frozen tissue. All glycogen is preserved on freezing and provided the cut section is suitably treated to prevent any escape of glycogen during staining, the intensity of the PAS reaction is proportional to the amount of glycogen present. The most suitable and reliable way to keep glycogen (and other water-soluble glycoproteins and oligosaccharides) in the section is to cover the section with a thin film of celloidin (dip slide with section into 0.25% celloidin in ethanol and air dry). The celloidin film pores are large enough to permit the free passage of the staining reagents and of salivary amylase used to confirm that the material stained was glycogen, but are small enough to prevent glycogen and other higher molecular weight glycocompounds from escaping. The distribution of glycogen within the lobule and its presence or absence in Kupffer cells, macrophages and smooth muscle cells can be reliably assessed by this procedure.

Assessment of the lipid content

Vacuoles in hepatocytes are generally filled with neutral fat (triglyceride), although there are some disorders in which no lipid is present in vacuoles, which would be regarded by most histopathologists as evidence of fatty change in routine sections. Thus a simple fat stain (Oil red O or Sudan black) on a cryostat section is an important test to confirm the presence of neutral fat. The presence of microvesicular fat, an indication of an acute rather than chronic condition, may not always be apparent in routine histological preparations but is always clearly demonstrated in cryostat sections stained with Oil red O. Examination of the stained section by polarizing microscopy shows no birefringence if the lipid is triglyceride but if cholesteryl esters are present there is marked birefringence of the crystallized esters. There are numerous histochemical methods for the detection of a wide range of lipids. While many of the methods may be applicable in theory, in practice under the constraints of the amount of tissue available only two are routinely useful. These are the ferric haematoxylin method (Elleder and Lojda, 1973), which stains phospholipids in general and can be used specifically for sphingomyelin, and the Schultz or PAN method for cholesterol (including esters) (Filipe and Lake, 1990).

Assessment of the activity of acid phosphatase

The method (or methods) for the demonstration of acid phosphatase activity are useful to detect the presence of macrophages, the number and shapes of Kupffer cells and to assess the state of the hepatocyte. The intensity of staining does not appear to relate to the amount of enzyme activity detected by conventional biochemical means (Lake and Ellis, 1974), but reflects the physiological state of the cell by revealing lysosomal activity (actual rather than potential) at the time the sample was frozen. Normal hepatocytes have a few active lysosomes in a pericanalicular distribution, but with liver cell damage or with lysosomal storage disorders the hepatocyte shows strong activity. Involvement of the perisinusoidal lining cells or of bile duct epithelium in a storage process is highlighted by increased activity or by activity where none is normally found.

Other methods of assessment

The foregoing methods are helpful in the general assessment of the state of the liver and are the first steps (which would also include a standard haematoxylin and eosin stain) in the investigation of unknown liver disease. Where the preliminary biochemical tests have indicated a particular disease or disorder of a particular organelle, the relevant areas can also be investigated. These can include the glycogenoses, α_1-antitrypsin deficiency, the urea cycle defects and mitochondrial and peroxisomal disorders. For these areas tissue may need to be preserved in different ways and for this to be done advance planning is necessary.

DISORDERS OF GLYCOGEN METABOLISM

The glycogen storage disorders (Hers *et al.*, 1989; Shin, 1990) affecting the liver can be broadly distinguished from each other by application of the aforementioned staining methods and a method to detect glucose-6-phosphatase activity. Although there are methods published which are designed to detect the activities of liver phosphorylase, liver phosphorylase kinase, branching and debranching enzymes and glycogen synthetase, they are based on the formation of newly synthesized glycogen and its colour reaction with iodine, which may or may not be valid in normal tissue. However, in pathological liver tissue these methods are not reliable and give results which may be at complete variance with biochemical assays. For example, a 'good' reaction for liver phosphorylase indicates normal activity, but a weak reaction may correspond to normal or deficient activity defined biochemically. By contrast, the method for myophosphorylase is consistently reliable and will readily detect the complete deficiency in McArdle's disease in the presence of normal smooth muscle phosphorylase.

Glycogen synthetase deficiency (McKusick 24060):   This deficiency is characterized by absent or very low glycogen levels and abundant neutral fat. Glucose-6-phosphatase activity should be present. Few cases are recorded and the histochemical profile is probably identical to long chain fatty acid coenzyme A dehydrogenase deficiency.

Glucose-6-phosphatase deficiency and its subtypes (McKusick 23220, 23222, 23224):   These conditions all show mildly to markedly increased glycogen contents and abundant neutral fat with a prominent periportal accentuation of the panlobular macroglobular change. In type IA the activity of glucose-6-phosphatase is undetectable, while in all other disorders of glycogen metabolism at least some activity may be found with the correct localization (diffuse in the hepatocyte with a paranuclear ring of activity corresponding to the endoplasmic reticulum; no activity in Kupffer cells or macrophages). The presence of nuclear glycogen is a feature of type I glycogen storage diseases and is more prominent in the older cases.

Acid maltase deficiency (McKusick 23230):   Liver biopsy in this case is unlikely to be an investigation undertaken by design. Massive glycogen deposition in hepatocytes and Kupffer cells and markedly enhanced activity of acid phosphatase are the characteristic features.

Debranching enzyme deficiency (McKusick 23240):   This results in the massive deposition of the very soluble limit dextrin in hepatocytes which appear as plant-like cells in routine sections. Glycogen may be undetectable in routine histopathological sections due to its extreme solubility, but in protected cryostat sections the distension of the hepatocytes can be seen to be due entirely to glycogen. Very little neutral fat is found but a mildly fibrotic reaction occasionally leading to cirrhosis is always present. Glucose-6-phosphatase activity is reduced but present.

Branching enzyme deficiency (McKusick 23250):   This is one of the easier diagnoses to make due to the indigestible nature of the amylopectin in hepatocytes and macrophages. The intensity of PAS positivity is only marginally diminished after digestion by salivary amylase and the amylopectin has a lilac-purple-brown colour with Lugol's iodine. There is portal fibrosis leading to cirrhosis and bile pigment is usually present.

Phosphorylase and phosphorylase kinase deficiencies (McKusick 23270, 30600):   These result in marked glycogen deposition and moderate neutral fat without fibrosis. Glucose-6-phosphatase activity is reduced but present.

Fructrose intolerance (McKusick 22960):   In fructose intolerance with fructose-1-phosphate aldolase deficiency the liver shows normal glycogen with marked panlobular macroglobular fatty change characteristic of a chronic disorder. The fatty change is present even in patients on a well-controlled diet. In some cases it is possible to see a marked increase in glucose-6-phosphatase activity, and this may be a helpful pointer.

DISORDERS OF LIPID METABOLISM

Many disorders affecting the liver result in neutral fat accumulation (Table 1), and on its own a fatty liver is not a helpful diagnostic finding. When lipid deposition also occurs in muscle and kidney then a generalized disorder of lipid metabolism can be suspected. Medium and long chain coenzyme A dehydrogenase deficiencies (MCAD and LCAD respectively, McKusick 20145 and 20146) and glutaric aciduria type 2 (McKusick 23168) are examples of these disorders. MCAD can be reliably differentiated from Reye syndrome by showing succinate dehydrogenase activity in the former (none is found in the early stages of Reye syndrome). The glycogen content of the liver in MCAD and LCAD may be very low despite intravenous dextrose therapy given to combat the hypoglycaemia encountered in these conditions. In other circumstances the glycogen content may be markedly increased by this treatment.

Triglycerides and cholesterol esters occur in acid esterase deficiency (Wolman disease and cholesteryl ester storage disease, McKusick 27800 and 21500) and these are strongly stained (Sudanophilic) by Oil red O or Sudan black. In both clinical phenotypes the Kupffer cells are also involved in storage. Increased acid phosphatase

Table 1 Fatty change in the liver

Some metabolic disorders with markedly fatty livers:
  Glycogen storage diseases type IA, IB and IC
  Glycogen synthetase deficiency
  Fructose intolerance
  Fructose-1,6-diphosphatase deficiency
  Galactosaemia
  Wolman disease
  Cholesteryl ester storage disease
  Fatty acid CoA dehydrogenase deficiencies
  Multiple CoA dehydrogenase deficiency
  Organic acidaemias
  Glutaric aciduria type 2
  Cytochrome oxidase deficiency
  Alpers disease
  Hypo- and a-β-lipoproteinaemia
  Hyperlipoproteinaemias

Fatty livers also occur with:
  Reye syndrome
  Malnutrition (protein)
  Total parenteral nutrition
  Drugs and toxins
  Chronic inflammatory bowel disease

activity outlining the lipid droplets in both hepatocytes and Kupffer cells, a positive cholesterol stain and marked birefringence of crystalline lipid deposits in sections mounted in glycerine jelly are the most striking features. The detection of acid esterase deficiency in cryostat sections is unreliable due to the very low activity demonstrable in the normal liver under these conditions. Special techniques (semipermeable membrane methods) may be more reliable, but tissue taken for separate fixation is necessary for the convincing demonstration of plentiful activity in the normal with none in affected tissues (Lake and Patrick, 1970).

The ferric haematoxylin method will detect the sphingomyelin deposition in the hepatocytes and enlarged Kupffer cells of Niemann–Pick disease types A and B (McKusick 25720). However, Niemann–Pick disease type C (McKusick 25722) presents a much more difficult diagnostic problem. The majority of patients present with a clinical picture of neonatal hepatitis, and a liver biopsy will be almost indistinguishable from other causes of neonatal hepatitis. Histochemical studies under these conditions are unhelpful and ultrastructural examination is needed. However, if a diagnosis of Niemann–Pick disease type C is suspected, the best and most reliable diagnostic route by microscopy is by bone marrow aspirate and rectal biopsy. Older patients do not present with liver disease or hepatomegaly and liver biopsy is not indicated, although it would be diagnostically helpful.

In all cases where vacuolated liver cells are found it is important to confirm that lipid is present. Absence of lipid staining in such cases could indicate infantile sialic acid storage disease, GM1-gangliosidosis type 1, or a mucopolysaccharidosis.

Urea cycle defects

There are no specific features which assist in the diagnosis. Demonstration of ornithine carbamoyl transferase activity requires specially fixed tissue, which if taken can show the deficiency in the male, and random staining of some cells due to lyonization in the female (Wareham et al., 1983).

Peroxisomal disorders

In suspected cases of a peroxisomal enzyme defect there are two possible approaches. Firstly, the demonstration of the presence (or absence) of the peroxisome itself can be accomplished in sections of specially fixed tissue processed to show the activity of catalase. This is done in the presence of 1 mmol/L cyanide to suppress the cytochrome oxidase of mitochondria which would otherwise cause problems in interpretation. This approach, useful in the early days of peroxisomal disorders, is helpful mainly in the syndromes which have absent peroxisomes, but may also give useful ultrastructural information in the conditions in which peroxisomes have variable shape and size. Immunohistochemistry using antisera to the various components of the peroxisomal β-oxidation system and to catalase can be successful. Not only are the peroxisomes shown in routine histopathological and cryostat sections by this approach, but the presence of the enzyme protein is also demonstrated (Espeel et al., 1990). While this yields results which would mirror those of Western blotting, the functional capacity of the enzyme protein cannot be implied (Wanders et al., 1990).

SUMMARY AND CONCLUSIONS

The main functions of the histochemical study of liver in liver disorders are:

1. To establish the identity of the tissue under study.
2. To develop a staining profile of the liver and to assess the morphology which can be used as a guide to subsequent areas of biochemical investigation.
3. To make specific diagnoses in certain circumstances which can then be confirmed with minimal biochemical effort.

The benefits of the histochemical approach are that structure can be assessed and that the staining profile can be accomplished with economical use of the valuable tissue sample.

ACKNOWLEDGEMENTS

My thanks are due to Professor A. D. Patrick and staff of the Enzyme Laboratory of the Institute of Child Health, London with whom I have had the opportunity to collaborate and with whom I have been able to compare the biochemical and histochemical results on which the approach outlined in this review has been based.

REFERENCES

Elleder, M. and Lojda, Z. Studies in lipid histochemistry. XI. New simple, rapid and selective method for the demonstration of phospholipids. *Histochemie* 36 (1973) 149–166

Espeel, M., Hashimoto, T., De Craemer, D. and Roels, F. Immunocytochemical detection of peroxisomal β-oxidation enzymes in cryostat and paraffin sections of human post mortem liver. *Histochem. J.* 22 (1990) 57–62

Filipe, M. I. and Lake, B. D. (eds.) *Histochemistry in Pathology*, 2nd edn., Churchill Livingstone, Edinburgh, 1990

Hers, H-G., Van Hoof, F. and De Barsy, T. Glycogen storage diseases. In Scriver, C. R., Beaudet, A. L., Sly, W. S. and Valle, D. (eds.) *The Metabolic Basis of Inherited Disease*, 6th edn., McGraw-Hill, New York, 1989, pp. 425–452

Lake, B. D. and Ellis, R. B. What do you think you are quantifying? An appraisal of histochemical methods in the measurement of the activities of lysosomal enzymes. *Histochem. J.* 8 (1976) 357–366

Lake, B. D. and Patrick, A. D. Wolman's disease. Deficiency of E-600 resistant acid esterase activity with storage of lipids in lysosomes. *J. Pediatr.* 76 (1970) 262–266

Shin, Y. S. Diagnosis of glycogen storage disease. *J. Inher. Metab. Dis.* 13 (1990) 419–434

Wanders, R. J. A., van Roermund, C. W. T., Schelen, A., Schutgens, R. B. H., Tager, J. M., Stephenson, J. P. B. and Clayton, P. T. A bifunctional protein with deficient enzyme activity. Identification of a new peroxisomal disorder using novel methods to measure the peroxisomal β-oxidation enzyme activities. *J. Inher. Metab. Dis.* 13 (1990) 375–379

Wareham, K. A., Howell, S., Williams, D. and Williams, E. D. Studies of X-chromosome inactivation with an improved technique for ornithine carbamoyl transferase. *Histochem. J.* 15 (1983) 363–371

J. Inher. Metab. Dis. 14 (1991) 546–553

Techniques for Studying Hepatic Metabolism *in vivo*

J. V. LEONARD[1] and G. N. THOMPSON[2]
[1]*The Institute of Child Health, London, WC1N 1EH, UK;* [2]*The Murdoch Institute, The Royal Children's Hospital, Parkville, Victoria, Australia*

Summary: Techniques for studying metabolic events *in vivo* in patients with inborn errors are reviewed. Loading or provocation tests that have been used widely are insensitive and frequently non-specific. Compounds labelled with stable isotopes can be used to study enzyme kinetics and substrate turnover, providing more detailed and specific information. Intracellular events may be studied using nuclear magnetic resonance spectroscopy.

The results using these techniques to study patients with selected inborn errors are discussed, namely phenylketonuria, glycogen storage disease type I and propionic acidaemia.

INTRODUCTION

A wide range of tests have been developed to study hepatic metabolism *in vivo*. In this short review only those techniques that have been applied to study patients with inborn errors will be considered. Many of the early tests were developed to assist with the diagnosis of inborn errors and are relatively non-specific, but it is now possible to measure enzyme activity, substrate kinetics and changes in the intracellular metabolite concentrations *in vivo*.

The methods that have been used to study metabolism *in vivo* are

Loading tests
Stimulation or other provocative tests
Studies using isotopically labelled compounds
Nuclear magnetic resonance spectroscopy

and each will be considered briefly. Most of these investigations measure the sum of activity of all tissues but, as for many compounds, the liver is the principal site of metabolism and the results largely represent hepatic metabolism.

INVESTIGATIVE TECHNIQUES

Loading tests

Loading tests can be used for two purposes; first to probe the integrity of biochemical pathways and secondly as a non-specific test of the overall function of the liver.

546

The response to loading tests is usually assessed by following secondary changes in the blood and urine. For example, an intravenous fructose load can be used to substantiate the diagnosis of fructosaemia. In the patient with fructosaemia there is a fall in blood glucose and plasma phosphate with a rise in the plasma concentration of urate and magnesium (Baerlocher *et al.*, 1980). None of the changes are found in controls, but this test is relatively insensitive, requiring a fructose load of 0.25 g/kg and is not specific as similar changes may be seen in patients with fructose-1,6-bisphosphatase deficiency (Baerlocher *et al.*, 1980).

A galactose load may be used in patients with suspected glycogen storage disease to help establish a diagnosis. In normal individuals there is a rise in blood glucose following an intravenous load of galactose that is not seen if there is a defect in the glucose-6-phosphatase complex (Cornblath and Schwartz, 1976). A brisk rise in blood glucose is seen in patients with debrancher deficiency and defects in phosphorylase cascade (Fernandes *et al.*, 1974). However, there is considerable variation in these responses, which may overlap those of normals.

The results of these tests may depend not just on inborn biochemical defects but also on overall hepatic function. Some loading tests have been used as liver function tests, for example galactose (Tengstrom *et al.*, 1967). With many of these loading tests erroneous results are, therefore, likely in patients with generalized liver disease whether acquired or secondary to a metabolic disorder.

Stimulation and other provocation tests

The glucagon stimulation test has been used for many years to diagnose patients with glycogen storage disease (Cornblath and Schwartz, 1976). However, there is a wide range of response, even in patients with type I glycogen storage disease (Dunger and Leonard, 1982). Patients with mild variants of glucose-6-phosphatase deficiency (glycogen storage disease type I) may have a normal rise in blood glucose and in those with phosphorylase and phosphorylase kinase deficiency the response is almost invariably normal. In addition, false positive tests are common in patients with severe liver disease (Cornblath and Schwartz, 1976) regardless of its cause, in some inborn errors such as disorders of long-chain fatty-acid oxidation and occasionally in organic acidaemias such as methylmalonic acidaemia (J.V. Leonard, unpublished observations).

Studying the metabolic response to fasting is a useful investigation to establish the diagnosis in those with recurrent hypoglycaemia and those in whom disorders of fatty-acid oxidation and of ketone-body metabolism are suspected. However, it is potentially hazardous and should only be used under close supervision. In those with defective β-oxidation there is a reduced rise in ketones relative to the increase in plasma free fatty acids concentration (Bonnefont *et al.*, 1991). The results of the fast in a patient with medium-chain acyl-CoA dehydrogenase deficiency are shown in Figure 1A. There is no ketone body response during the fast despite the rise in free fatty acids. However, the interpretation of the results is not always as straightforward. Figure 1B shows the result of a fast in another patient. He had an acute encephalopathy with a dicarboxylic aciduria that was labelled 'Reye syndrome'. On fasting there was a modest rise in the concentration of 3-hydroxybutyrate. When the plasma

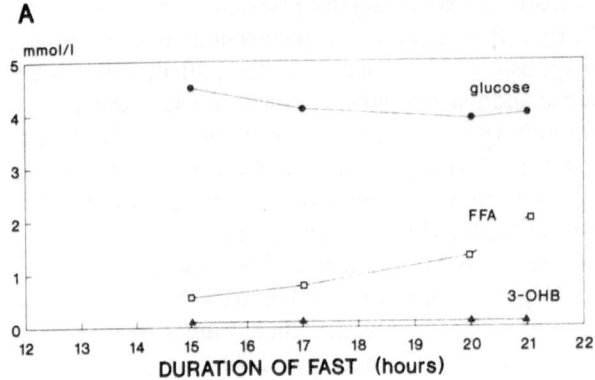

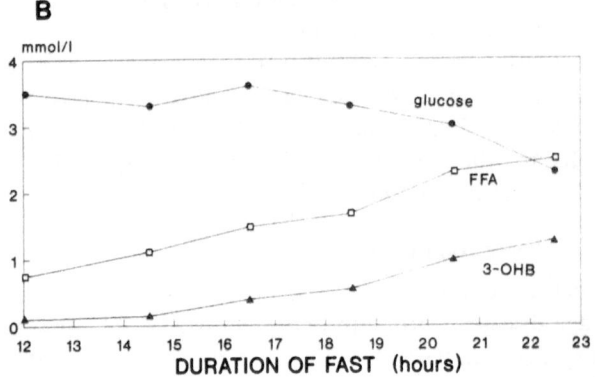

Figure 1 Blood glucose, 3-hydroxybutyrate and plasma free fatty acid concentrations during fasting. (A) Medium-chain CoA dehydrogenase deficiency (confirmed by ETF assay on cultured skin fibroblasts — Drs D. Hale and P. Coates). (B) Undiagnosed fatty-acid oxidation defect

concentrations of free fatty acids and 3-hydroxybutyrate are plotted using the data of Bartlett and colleagues (1991) the results are clearly abnormal (Figure 2). A repeat fast gave a similar result but no enzyme diagnosis has yet been made.

In both these tests the plasma metabolite concentrations reflects the net balance between production and disposal, but does not, of course, give any information about individual rates.

Isotope studies

Isotopes can be used to label compounds so that their metabolism can be studied, investigating pathways and both substrate and enzyme kinetics. In early studies radioactive isotopes were used, but with a wider availability of mass spectrometry and of compounds labelled with stable isotopes these are now used almost exclusively, avoiding the use of ionizing radiation.

The concept of using labelled compounds to investigate pathways and their kinetics is simple and, with careful choice of the appropriate substrate, the site and nature of

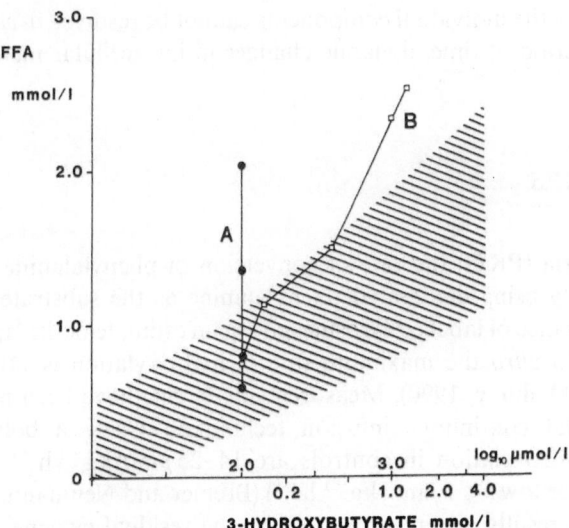

Figure 2 Plasma free fatty acid and blood 3-hydroxybutyrate concentrations during a prolonged fast. The data shown in Figure 1 have been replotted. **A** represents the patient with medium-chain acyl CoA dehydrogenase deficiency. **B** represents the patient with the undiagnosed fatty-acid oxidation disorder. Shaded area represents the results of the control patients. (Bartlett *et al.*, 1991)

the label, as well as the product that is assayed, it is possible to use stable isotopes to study substrate kinetics and enzyme activity *in vivo*. However, in practice the assumptions that have to be made and the analysis of the results can be complex and sometimes difficult to validate. Detailed discussion of these aspects is beyond the scope of this review; the reader is referred to other reviews (for example, Wolfe, 1984). Secondly, almost all studies measure whole-body turnover, but if the pathway or enzyme being studied is largely confined to the liver the results can be regarded as representing hepatic activity.

Nuclear magnetic resonance spectroscopy

Nuclear magnetic resonance spectroscopy (NMRS) can be used to study intracellular metabolite concentrations *in vivo*. For details of the theory and practice of NMRS the subject is reviewed in detail elsewhere (for example, Gadian, 1982). Although many atomic nuclei could be used for NMRS, in practice only a small number are likely to be widely used for the study of inborn errors, namely isotopes of hydrogen, carbon and phosphorus.

It is difficult to study hepatic metabolism in adults using proton NMRS because of paramagnetic material stored in the liver. It may be possible to study younger patients, but this has received little attention.

In ^{13}C spectra the major peaks are glycogen, fatty acids and triglyceride (Jue *et al.*, 1989). The peaks that are clearly identifiable in ^{31}P spectra are phosphomono- and diesters (PME, PDE respectively), inorganic phosphate and the three phosphate groups in ATP (Taylor, 1990). The phosphomono-ester and phosphodiester peaks are compound and the individual components cannot be resolved *in vivo*. By collecting spectra over a period of time, dynamic changes in intracellular metabolism may be followed.

INBORN ERRORS

Phenylketonuria

In phenylketonuria (PKU) the rate of conversion of phenylalanine to tyrosine can be studied directly using deuterated phenylalanine as the substrate and measuring the rate of appearance of labelled tyrosine, giving an estimate of the 'apparent' enzyme activity *in vivo*. *In vitro* the maximum rate of hydroxylation is $110 \mu mol\, kg^{-1} h^{-1}$ (Thompson and Halliday, 1990). Measurements *in vivo* have been made using both a fixed bolus and continuous infusion techniques. Using a bolus the rates of phenylalanine hydroxylation in controls are $14-25 \mu mol\, kg^{-1} h^{-1}$ and in patients with PKU they are low ($< 1 \mu mol\, kg^{-1} h^{-1}$) (Bremer and Neumann, 1966; Lehmann *et al.*, 1984). The results are in proportion to the residual enzyme activity in liver. However, using a primed continuous infusion technique the results in controls are lower than those obtained using the bolus ($3-8 \mu mol\, kg^{-1} h^{-1}$) but much higher values are obtained in PKU ($1-8 \mu mol\, kg^{-1} h^{-1}$) (Clarke and Bier, 1982; Thompson and Halliday, 1990). The explanation for these results is illustrated graphically in Figure 3. Using a fixed bolus the label is diluted in the expanded pool in the PKU patients and therefore even if the rate of hydroxylation were the same in the controls and PKU patients the rate of appearance of labelled tyrosine and hence the apparent hydroxylation rate would be greatly reduced. Using the continuous infusion technique, the hydroxylation rate is calculated from isotope enrichment in the steady state so that the effect of the pool is eliminated. The rates of phenylalanine hydroxylation in

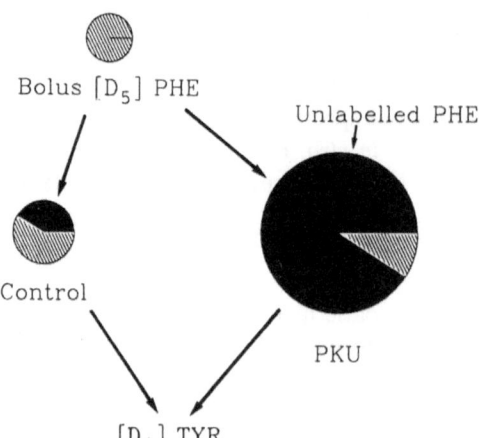

Bolus $[D_5]$ PHE

Unlabelled PHE

Control

PKU

$[D_4]$ TYR

Figure 3   Measurement of phenylalanine activity *in vivo* using a fixed bolus of $[D^5]$phenylalanine. For explanation see text. Redrawn from Thompson and Halliday (1990)

PKU are unexpectedly high because, at increased high substrate concentrations, there is probably conversion of phenylalanine to tyrosine by tyrosine and tryptophan hydroxylase since these enzymes are known to have some activity towards phenylalanine.

Glycogen storage disease type I

In the severe forms of glycogen storage disease the blood glucose concentrations usually fall rapidly on fasting and during a glucagon test may also fall, suggesting that glucose production is markedly reduced. It was rather surprising, therefore, to find that glucose production rates in patients with glycogen storage disease type I were between 30% and 100% of the predicted normal rates (Kalhan *et al.*, 1982; Schwenk and Haymond, 1986; Kalderon *et al.*, 1989; Collins *et al.*, 1990). Glucagon increases the rate of production (Collins *et al.*, 1990), but if there is a fall in blood glucose concentration this must be matched by a greater increase in the rate of disposal.

Earlier studies suggested that in glycogen storage disease type I hepatic glucose-6-phosphate concentrations were low (Hers, 1980). By contrast, direct measurement of glucose-6-phosphate concentrations *in vivo* using ^{31}P NMRS demonstrated that the concentration of glucose-6-phosphate rose on fasting and decreased after a glucose load (Oberhaensli *et al.*, 1988). However, the mechanism by which glucose-6-phosphate was then converted to free glucose was not clear. Three possibilities have been suggested: firstly that there was residual activity of glucose-6-phosphatase; secondly that glucose was produced by non-specific hydrolysis of glucose-6-phosphate; and thirdly that glucose was produced not from glucose-6-phosphate directly but from the hydrolysis $\alpha(1-6)$ bonds of branch points of glycogen by the debrancher enzyme. Using stable isotope and nuclear magnetic resonance techniques, Lapidot and her colleagues have shown that although glucose is converted to lactate there is no recycling of the label in lactate into free glucose. From this they deduced that the activity of glucose-6-phosphatase must be very low, so the third alternative is the most likely one (Kalderon *et al.*, 1989).

Propionic and methylmalonic acidaemia

The prognosis of an inborn error is often closely related to the residual enzyme activity, but it can be difficult to assess this. Many conventional biochemical markers are of limited prognostic value, and it may also be difficult to judge the response to pharmacological doses of the cofactor or precursor vitamin, particularly if other therapy is given simultaneously. Stable isotope techniques can also be used to assess this and to evaluate the effect of therapy. In propionic acidaemia the rate of propionate oxidation *in vivo* is a useful prognostic indicator and can also be used to measure the response to biotin (Thompson *et al.*, 1990a,b). This type of investigation could be extended to the study of many other inborn errors.

CONCLUSIONS

Earlier tests *in vivo* gave only rather crude data, often deduced from the secondary metabolic consequences after relatively large doses of substrates or unphysiological stimuli. However, using isotopically labelled substrates, accurate measurements of kinetic data and even enzyme activity can be obtained. Nevertheless, care must be taken to understand all aspects of the technique being used.

NMRS can be used to measure intracellular changes in the liver but it remains a relatively insensitive technique. However, future developments of proton emission tomography and related techniques may give both kinetic data and localization.

REFERENCES

Baerlocher, K., Gitzelmann, R. and Steinmann, B. Clinical and Genetic Studies of disorders in fructose metabolism. In: Burman, D., Holton, J. B. and Pennock, C. A. (eds.) *Inherited Disorders of Carbohydrate Metabolism*. MTP Press, Lancaster, 1980, pp. 163–190

Bartlett, K., Aynsley-Green, A., Leonard, J. V. and Turnbull, D. M. Inherited disorders of mitochondrial β-oxidation. In: Vis, H., Van Hoof, F. and Schaub, J. (eds.) *Inborn Errors of Metabolism*. Nestlé Nutrition Workshop Series Vol. 24. Raven Press, New York, 1991, pp. 19–41

Bonnefont, J.-P., Specola, N. B., Bassault, A., Lombes, A., Ogier, H., de Klerk, J. B. C., Munnich, A., Coude, M., Paturneau-Jouas, M. and Saudubray, J.-M. The fasting test in paediatrics. *Eur. J. Pediatr.* 150 (1991) 80–85

Bremer, H. J. and Neumann, W. Tolerance of phenylalanine after intravenous administration in phenylketonurias, heterozygous carriers and normal adults. *Nature* 209 (1966) 148–1149

Clarke, J. T. R. and Bier, D. M. The conversion of phenylalanine to tyrosine in man. Direct measurement by continuous intravenous tracer infusions of L-[^{2}H5]phenylalanine and L-[1-^{13}C]tyrosine in the post absorbtive state. *Metab. Clin. Exp.* 31 (1982) 999–1005

Collins, J. E., Bartlett, K., Leonard, J. V. and Aynsley-Green, A. Glucose production rates in type I glycogen storage disease. *J. Inher. Metab. Dis.* 13 (1990) 195–206

Cornblath, M. and Schwartz, R. *Disorders of Carbohydrate Metabolism*. W. B. Saunders, Philadelphia, 1976

Dunger, D. B. and Leonard, J. V. Value of the glucagon test in screening for hepatic glycogen storage disese. *Arch. Dis. Child.* 57 (1982) 384–389

Fernandes, J., Koster, J. F., Grose, W. F. A. and Sorgedrager, N. Hepatic phosphorylase deficiency: Its differentiation from other hepatic glycogenoses. *Arch. Dis. Child.* 49 (1974) 186–191

Gadian, D. G. *Nuclear Magnetic Research and Its Application to Living Systems*. Oxford University Press, Oxford, 1982

Hers, H. G. Carboydrate metabolism and its regulation. In: Burman, P., Holton, J. B. and Pennock, C. A. (eds.) *Inherited Disorders of Carbohydrate Metabolism*. MTP Press, Lancaster, 1980, pp. 3–18

Jue, T., Rothman, D. L., Tavitian, B. A. and Shulman, R. G. Natural abundance ^{13}C NMR study of glycogen repletion in human liver and muscle. *Proc. Natl. Acad. Sci. USA* 86 (1989) 1439–1442

Kalderon B., Korman, S. H., Gutman, A. and Lapidot, A. Estimation of glucose carbon recycling in children with glycogen storage disease: A ^{13}C NMR study using [U-^{13}C]glucose. *Proc. Natl. Acad. Sci. USA* 86 (1989) 4690–4694

Kalhan, S. C., Gilfillan, C., Tseng, K.-Y. and Savin, S. M. Glucose production in type 1 glycogen storage disease. *J. Pediatr.* 101 (1982) 159–160

Lehmann, W. D., Theobald, N., Heinrich, H. C., Clemens, P. and Gruttner, R. Detection of heterozygous carriers for phenylketonuria by a L-[^{2}H$_5$]phenylalanine stable isotope loading test. *Clin. Chim. Acta* 138 (1984) 59–71

Oberhaensli, R., Rajagopalan, B., Taylor, D. J., Radda, G., Collins, J. E. and Leonard, J. V. Study of liver metabolism in glucose-6-phosphatase deficiency by ^{31}P magnetic resonance spectroscopy. *Pediatr. Res.* 23 (1988) 375–380

Schwenk, W. F. and Haymond, M. W. Optimal rate of enteral glucose administration in children with glycogen storage disease type 1. *N. Engl. J. Med.* 314 (1986) 682–685

Taylor, D. J. Nuclear magnetic resonance spectroscopy. In: Fernandes, J., Saudubray, J.-M. and Tada, K. (eds.). *Inborn Metabolic Diseases.* Springer-Verlag, Berlin, 1990, pp. 55–65

Tengstrom, B., Hjelm, M., de Verdier, C. H. and Werner, I. Intravenous galactose tolerance test with the use of an enzymatic method for the determination of galactose. *Am. J. Dig. Dis.* 12 (1967) 853–861

Thompson, G. N. and Halliday, D. Significant phenylalanine hydroxylation in vivo in patients with classical phenylketonuria. *J. Clin. Invest.* 86 (1990) 317–322

Thompson, G. N., Bresson, J. L., Bonnefont, J. P., Walter, J. H., Read, M. A., Saudubray, J. M., Leonard, J. V. and Halliday, D. A simple isotopic technique for assessing vitamin responsiveness in vivo in propionic acidaemia. *J. Inher. Metab. Dis.* 13 (1990a) 349–351

Thompson, G. N., Walter, J. H., Bresson, J.-L., Bonnefont, J.-P., Saudubray, J.-M., Leonard, J. V. and Halliday, D. In vivo propionate oxidation as a prognostic indicator in disorders of propionate metabolism. *Eur. J. Pediatr.* 149 (1990b) 408–411

Wolfe, R. R. *Tracers in Metabolic Research: Radio Isotopes and Stable Isotope/Mass Spectrometry Methods.* Alan Liss, New York, 1984

J. Inher. Metab. Dis. 14 (1991) 554–562

Tyrosinaemia Type I – an Update

E. A. KVITTINGEN

Institute of Clinical Biochemistry, Rikshospitalet, 0027 Oslo 1, Norway

Summary: Tyrosinaemia type I is a recessively inherited disorder caused by a deficiency of fumarylacetoacetase (FAH), the last enzyme in tyrosine degradation. The presumed toxic agents are fumaryl- and maleylacetoacetate which are converted to succinylacetone (SA), a metabolite found in increased amounts in urine and plasma of the patients. The major clinical features are progressive liver damage and renal tubular defects with hypophosphataemic rickets. Renal tubular dysfunctions with secondary rickets may be lacking altogether, even in chronic patients. Hepatocellular carcinoma is a major cause of death in the chronic form. Diagnosis of the disorder is made by assay of SA in urine and serum and by determination of FAH in lymphocytes or fibroblasts. Prenatal diagnosis is performed by SA assay in amniotic fluid supernatant and FAH analysis in cultured amniotic fluid cells or chorionic villus material. Presence of a 'pseudodeficiency' gene for FAH prevents prenatal diagnosis by enzyme analysis in some families, and this gene also precludes identification of heterozygotes outside tyrosinaemia families. Immunoblot analyses show that acute patients and some chronic patients lack immunoreactive FAH protein. cDNA probes for FAH have been developed and several polymorphisms related to the FAH gene have been reported, which may allow prenatal diagnosis in families with complex genotypes. The gene for FAH has been mapped to chromosome 15 q23-q25. Liver transplantation is the ultimate treatment; most patients continue to excrete SA in urine after liver transplantation and therefore there is a possibility of kidney disease after transplantation.

The hallmarks of tyrosinaemia type I, elevated blood tyrosine, liver cirrhosis and renal tubular defects, are found in a number of liver diseases in childhood. Before the identification of succinylacetone (SA), no specific laboratory parameters were associated with tyrosinaemia, and a number of patients have presumably been erroneously diagnosed as having tyrosinaemia type I. The discovery of SA in tyrosinaemia patients and the suggestion that fumarylacetoacetase (FAH) was the primary defect in tyrosinaemia was a breakthrough in the understanding of the disorder (Lindblad *et al.*, 1977). Deficiency of FAH in tyrosinaemia patients was soon confirmed by several groups.

The essential biochemistry of tyrosinaemia is illustrated in Figure 1. A deficiency of FAH leads to accumulation of fumaryl- and possibly maleylacetoacetate, which are presumed to be converted to SA by reduction and decarboxylation. An important feature of SA is the strong inhibitory effect on the enzyme δ-aminolevulinate dehydratase (δ-ALA DH), which explains the elevated levels of δ-ALA found in tyrosinaemia patients. Fumarylacetoacetate also inhibits δ-ALA DH and this compound furthermore inhibits adenosylmethionine synthase, which may explain the elevation of methionine found in many patients (Berger *et al.*, 1983). Tyrosinaemia patients have low levels of *p*-hydroxy-phenylpyruvate dioxygenase in liver tissue resulting in hypertyrosinaemia and increased excretion of phenolic acids. Fumarylacetoacetate and SA have not been found to inhibit the dioxygenase directly (Berger *et al.*, 1983). It is still plausible that this enzyme is depressed through some mechanisms secondary to the primary block at the FAH level.

The disorder occurs worldwide with the highest frequency in Quebec, Canada, where in some regions 1 child in 700 is born with the disease (Goldsmith and Laberge, 1989).

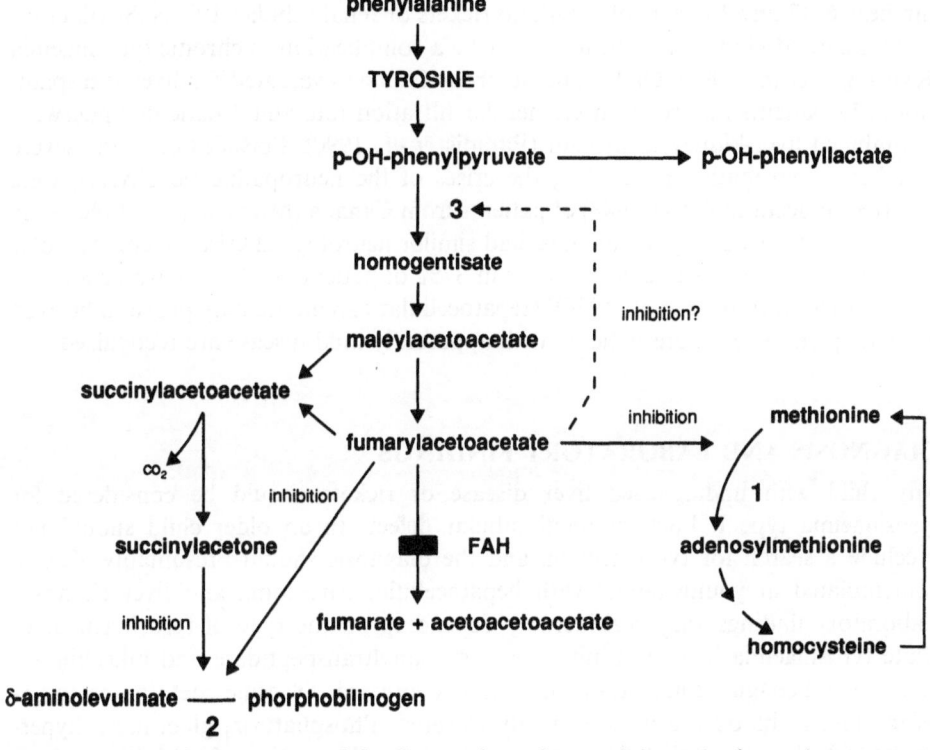

Figure 1 The primary enzyme defect in tyrosinaemia type I is at the fumarylacetoacetase (FAH) step of tyrosine degradation. Due to the enzyme block fumaryl- and possibly maleylacetoacetate accumulate, being reduced and decarboxylated to succinylacetone, a potent inhibitor of the enzyme δ-aminolevulinate dehydratase (2). This enzyme is also inhibited by fumarylacetoacetate which furthermore inhibits adenosylmethionine synthase (1). Fumarylacetoacetate and succinylacetone have not been shown to directly inhibit *p*-hydroxy-phenylpyruvate dioxygenase (3), which has low activity in liver tissue from tyrosinaemia patients, but presumably the enzyme is depressed due to some mechanisms secondary to the primary defect

CLINICAL ASPECTS

The clinical variation of tyrosinaemia is considerable. Since the disorder is now diagnosed by specific parameters, new clinical presentations are recognized. The disorder can be divided into acute and chronic forms but both presentations have been found within one family. In the acute form the patients show signs of liver failure from the first months of life. Ascites, a bleeding tendency and hypoglycaemia are found, and proximal renal tubular defects with acidosis and hypophosphataemic rickets may be present at an early stage. Cardiomyopathy has been reported in two patients (Edwards et al., 1987). The patients usually die within the first year of life. The chronic form of the disorder is generally described as similar to but milder than the acute form. Often the patients present at about one year of age with rickets and moderate hepatosplenomegaly, but may present at school age with only the symptoms of rickets. These patients have few, if any, laboratory findings of liver disease. Renal tubular defects with hypophosphataemic rickets have been considered obligatory for the chronic form of tyrosinaemia, but we recently reported three patients (in two families), 6, 13 and 15 years old, with no rickets or renal tubular defects (Søvik et al., 1990). Reduced glomerular filtration may be a complication in chronic tyrosinaemia (Kvittingen et al., 1991). Of 19 patients from Canada evaluated for liver transplantation, 12 patients had reduced glomerular filtration rate and 2 patients underwent a combined liver-kidney transplant (Paradis et al., 1990). Episodes of acute, severe peripheral neuropathy, resembling the crises of the neuropathic porphyrias, were reported to occur in 42% (20/48) of patients from Canada (Mitchell et al., 1990); only 1 out of 15 Norwegian patients have had similar neurological crises. Hepatocellular carcinoma has been estimated to occur in 37% of patients with the chronic form of the disorder (Weinberg et al., 1976). Hepatocellular carcinoma may prove to be even more frequent when more patients with apparently mild disease are recognized.

DIAGNOSIS AND LABORATORY FINDINGS

Any child with undiagnosed liver disease or rickets should be considered for tyrosinaemia type I. Lack of renal tubular defects in an older child should not preclude a search for tyrosinaemia, and the diagnosis should presumably also be contemplated in young adults with hepatocellular carcinoma and liver cirrhosis. Laboratory findings vary considerably depending on the type of tyrosinaemia. In acute tyrosinaemia liver transaminases, γ-glutamyltranspeptidase and bilirubin are elevated and coagulation factors are severely depressed. Tyrosine, methionine and α-fetoprotein in blood are usually highly elevated. Phosphaturia, glucosuria, hyperaminoaciduria and renal acidosis may be present and excretion of δ-ALA and phenolic acids is elevated. In chronic tyrosinaemia liver transaminases and methionine may be normal. Usually γ-glutamyltranspeptidase is slightly elevated and vitamin K-dependent coagulation factors are somewhat depressed. Findings of proximal renal tubular defects are prominent in most cases, but may be totally absent; even excretion of β_2-microglobulin is normal (Søvik et al., 1990). Plasma tyrosine, although usually high, is sometimes only slightly elevated and has also been reported to be normal

(Goulden *et al.*, 1987; De Almeida *et al.*, 1990). α_1-Fetoprotein can be completely normal. Phenolic acid excretion is elevated.

The diagnosis of both acute and chronic tyrosinaemia relies entirely on the demonstration of increased levels of SA or the precursors, accompanied by a deficiency of FAH. To the author's knowledge there is no convincing report of an elevated SA level in any patient for whom a diagnosis other than tyrosinaemia has been established. SA has been claimed not to be elevated in some cases of tyrosinaemia. Reduction of fumaryl- and maleylacetoacetate to SA requires an enzymatic activity which could be lacking in certain individuals. If SA is not demonstrable by direct methods (GC–MS), it should still be possible to demonstrate the precursors by the δ-ALA DH inhibition assay. The method for SA determination should preferably be sufficiently sensitive to allow SA quantitation in healthy individuals, and such methods have been reported (Jakobs *et al.*, 1988; Schierbeek and Berger, 1989). According to the author's experience SA is not consistently stable and material for SA determination should be stored at $-70°C$.

FAH deficiency can be demonstrated in lymphocytes, fibroblasts and possibly also in erythrocytes (Kvittingen and Brodtkorb, 1986; Lindblad *et al.*, 1986). FAH activity may be severely depressed in liver tissue from patients with various liver diseases (unpublished results and personal communication, Dr Berger, Utrecht). Thus liver tissue is not an optimal tissue for demonstration of the primary enzyme defect in suspected tyrosinaemia patients. Due to the existence of a 'pseudodeficiency' gene for FAH, as discussed below, demonstration of FAH deficiency alone (in any tissue) may not be conclusive for a diagnosis of tyrosinaemia.

PRENATAL DIAGNOSIS AND CARRIER DETECTION

Prenatal diagnosis of tyrosinaemia is performed by determination of SA in amniotic fluid supernatant (Jakobs *et al.*, 1988) and by assay of FAH in cultured amniotic fluid cells or in chorionic villus material (Kvittingen and Brodtkorb, 1986). It is important to realize the impact of the 'pseudodeficiency' gene for FAH on prenatal diagnosis by enzyme analysis. The 'pseudodeficiency' gene for FAH results in enzyme activity nearly as low *in vitro* as the tyrosinaemia gene, but apparently does not give the disease. Of 94 obligate heterozygotes for tyrosinaemia (in 49 families) 4 individuals (in 3 families) had enzyme activities (in lymphocytes or fibroblasts) compatible with a compound heterozygous genotype for the tyrosinaemia and 'pseudodeficiency' genes. In any tyrosinaemia family in which one parent is a compound heterozygote, only a healthy child can be predicted with certainty. If both parents are compound heterozygotes then prenatal diagnosis by FAH determination is not feasible at all. In approximately 1 out of 16 tyrosinaemia families one parent will be compound heterozygote; therefore before embarking on prenatal diagnosis the FAH activity of both parents should be determined.

It is not yet known if determination of SA in amniotic fluid will distinguish between a homozygote for tyrosinaemia and a compound heterozygote. Investigation in one individual with compound heterozygote genotype did not reveal elevated levels of SA in urine under ordinary conditions, but δ-ALA DH activity in erythrocytes was depressed, and after the injection of homogentisic acid there was a significant excretion of SA (Kvittingen *et al.*, 1985). This indicates that the FAH activity of this individual is also reduced *in vivo* and the term 'pseudodeficiency' is not truly appropriate.

Recently a cDNA probe for FAH was reported by Agsteribbe and colleagues (1990). In collaboration with this group we have searched for DNA polymorphisms related to the FAH gene. With three restriction enzymes six polymorphisms have been found. These were informative in two tyrosinaemia families with complex genotypes and could be useful in prenatal diagnosis in such families. The results have been briefly reported (Rootwelt *et al.*, 1990).

Since carriers of the 'pseudodeficiency' gene have FAH activities near the range of obligate carriers of tyrosinaemia, positive identification of heterozygotes for tyrosin-aemia, outside tyrosinaemia families, cannot be achieved by FAH determination. The FAH values in fibroblasts from 72 obligate carriers, excluding compound heterozygotes, were from 0.9 to 2.2 U/g protein (mean activity 1.45). Controls have values from 2.2 to 3.9 U/g protein; therefore enzyme values well above 2.2 U/g protein presumably exclude a carrier state for tyrosinaemia. Lymphocyte FAH values correspond closely to fibroblast values.

THE MOLECULAR BASIS OF TYROSINAEMIA

Recently antibodies towards FAH were produced and immunoblots showed lack of cross-reactive material in acute patients and reduced but present immunoreactivity in chronic patients (Tanguay *et al.*, 1984; Berger *et al.*, 1987). By pulse label pulse chase experiments, Berger and colleagues (1988) have shown that immunoreactive material could be detected in both an acute and a chronic patient. The difference in immunoreactivity between the patients was due to varying stability of FAH protein. In the acute patient, cross-reactive material disappeared after a chase of one day compared to four days in the chronic patient and seven days in controls. Very few chronic patients were investigated in the first reports on Western blotting. In collaboration with Berger's group we have therefore performed immunoblotting in 28 tyrosinaemia patients with variable clinical phenotypes. We found no consistent relationship between clinical findings and the amount of cross-reactive material; most chronic patients had no immunreactive material in fibroblast extract. Also, the 'pseudodeficiency' gene product did not appear to give definite immunoreactivity in fibroblasts. The results have been briefly reported (Kvittingen *et al.*, 1990).

A well-founded classification of tyrosinaemia patients must await identification of the DNA mutations causing the defective protein. The recently published cDNA probes for FAH will be helpful in elucidating the molecular genetics of tyrosinaemia. FAH mRNA from rat liver has been purified and the relative abundance of this mRNA was found to be 0.14% (Nicole *et al.*, 1986). The FAH gene has been mapped to chromosome 15 q23-q25 by *in situ* hybridization with a cDNA probe designated phFAH HA2 (Berube *et al.*, 1989).

TREATMENT OF TYROSINAEMIA

Restriction of phenylalanine and tyrosine intake has been the standard treatment of tyrosinaemia; this ameliorates the renal tubular defects, but the effect on the liver disease has been difficult to evaluate. Dietary treatment reduced the SA excretion by 50–70% in three Norwegian patients (unpublished observations). This possibly reflects reduced production of the primary metabolites, and it seems reasonable to keep the intake of phenylalanine and tyrosine as low as possible whilst allowing for continuous growth of the patient. Diet does not cure tyrosinaemia patients and liver transplantation is the ultimate treatment.

A number of reports on liver transplantation in tyrosinaemia patients have emerged (Kvittingen *et al.*, 1986; Tuchmann *et al.*, 1987; Van Spronsen *et al.*, 1989; Flye *et al.*, 1990; Mieles *et al.*, 1990). Liver transplantation would be expected to cure the liver disease in tyrosinaemia since the transplant retains the karyotype of the donor and thus produces normal FAH enzyme. Rather surprisingly, liver transplantation also has a marked beneficial effect on the kidney disease. The need for dietary restriction after liver transplantation has not been reported. Three patients reported by Tuchman and colleagues (1987) had persistence of some renal tubular dysfunctions after liver transplantation. This indicates that the renal tubular defects are at least not immediately resolved by liver transplantation. Most patients reported have had continuous urinary excretion of SA after liver transplantation, but in highly variable amounts. Presumably the kidneys are the only extrahepatic organs producing the metabolite, since the SA level in blood after liver transplantation is not elevated as determined by the activity of δ-ALA DH in erythrocytes.

Tyrosine loading after liver transplantation increases urinary excretion of SA but the blood SA level does not rise, further substantiating the theory that SA is produced only in the kidneys after transplantation (Kvittingen *et al.*, 1986; Tuchman *et al.*, 1987). The increase in SA excretion after tyrosine loading was not accompanied by a deterioration of the renal tubular function in one transplanted patient (Kvittingen *et al.*, 1986). The SA concentration in the urine of one of the patients reported by Tuchman and colleagues (1987) was reduced by more than 99%, from 128.4 μg/mg creatinine to less than 0.5 μg/mg creatinine (the detection limit), after liver transplantation. This indicates that tyrosine degradation in the kidneys may be low in some patients, and the possible risk of kidney disease as a late complication of the disorder is presumably variable.

While liver transplantation has been, and will be, life-saving for many tyrosinaemic patients, the timing of the liver transplantation is a matter for concern. In the acute patient with severe symptoms timing may not be optional, but for patients with mild disease it is a difficult question. All chronic patients are threatened by hepatocellular carcinoma, and at present α_1-fetoprotein determination and liver ultrasound/CT are the only non-invasive investigations which can indicate cancer development. Tumour detection by imaging techniques is difficult (Day *et al.*, 1987) and the α-fetoprotein level may be normal when a tumour is evident by imaging techniques (Kvittingen *et al.*, 1991). Mieles and colleagues (1990) report that two of their transplanted patients, 3 and 3.5 years old, had multifocal hepatocellular carcinoma not detected by the preoperative ultrasound examination. The levels of α-fetoprotein were not reported in these patients. Some patients with malignancy have died due to recurrence of the cancer after transplantation. On the other hand, a number of patients with hepatocellular carcinoma have been successfully transplanted (Mieles *et al.*, 1990), contrasting with the statement of Dehner and colleagues (1989) that the outlook is extremely dismal if not futile if transplantation is postponed until cancer has developed. Since many patients with mild disease are living good lives on dietary treatment or vitamin D supplementation, a more balanced discussion is called for; liver transplantation has a definite mortality and there is postoperative morbidity due to the immunosuppressive treatment. A close follow-up and careful evaluation of each patient on individual terms must be the basis for timing the liver transplantation in chronic patients.

REFERENCES

Agsteribbe, E., van Faassen, H., Hartog, M. V., Reversma, T., Taanman, J.-W., Pannekoek, H., Evers, R. F., Welling, G. M. and Berger, R. Nucleotide sequence of cDNA encoding human fumarylacetoacetase. *Nucleic Acids Res.* 18 (1990) 1887

Berger, R., van Faassen, H. and Smith, G. P. A. Biochemical studies on the enzymatic deficiencies of hereditary tyrosinemia. *Clin. Chim. Acta* 134 (1983) 129–141

Berger, R., van Faassen, H., Taanman, J. W., de Vries, H. and Agsteribbe, E. Type I tyrosinemia: lack of immunologically detectable fumarylacetoacetase enzyme protein in tissues and cell extracts. *Pediatr. Res.* 22 (1987) 394–398

Berger, B., van Faassen, H., van der Berg, I., Agsteribbe, E. and Wiemer, E. Different types of mutation in the chronic and acute forms of type I tyrosinemia. *Pediatr. Res.* 24 (1988) 266 (abstract)

Berube, D., Phaneuf, D., Tanguay, R. M. and Gagne, R. Assignment of the fumarylacetoacetate hydrolase gene to chromosome 15q23-15q25. *Cytogenet. Cell Genet.* 51 (1989) 962 (abstract)

Day, D. L., Letourneau, J. G., Allan, B. T., Sharp, H. L., Ascher, N., Dehner, L. P. and Thompson, W. M. Hepatic regenerating nodules in hereditary tyrosinemia. *Am. J. Roentgenol.* 149 (1987) 391–393

De Almeida, I. T., Leandro, P. P., Silva, M. F. B., Silveira, C., Da Silva, A., Salazar De. Sousa, J. and Duran, M. Tyrosinaemia type I with normal levels of plasma tyrosine. *J. Inher. Metab. Dis.* 13 (1990) 305–307

Dehner, L. P., Snover, D. C., Sharp, H. L., Ascher, N., Nakhleh, R. and Day, D. L. Hereditary tyrosinemia type I (chronic form): pathologic findings in the liver. *Hum. Pathol.* 20 (1989) 149–158

Edwards, M. A., Green, A., Colli, A. and Rylance, G. Tyrosinaemia type I and hyperthrophic obstructive cardiomyopathy. *Lancet* 1 (1987) 1437–1438

Flye, M. W., Riely, C. A., Hainline, B. E., Sassa, S., Gusberg, R. J., Blakemore, K. J., Barwick, K. W. and Horwich, A. L. The effects of early treatment of hereditary tyrosinemia type I in infancy by orthotopic liver transplantation. *Transplantation* 49 (1990) 916–921

Goldsmith, L. A. and Labrege, C. Tyrosinemia and related disorders. In Scriver, C. R., Beaudet, A. L., Sly, W. S. and Valle, D. (eds.) *The Metabolic Basis of Inherited Disease*, McGraw-Hill, New York, 1989, pp. 547–562

Goulden, K. J., Moss, M. A., Cole, D. E. C., Tithecott, G. A. and Crocker, J. F. S. Pitfalls in the initial diagnosis of tyrosinemia: three case reports and a review of the literature. *Clin. Biochem.* 20 (1987) 207–212

Jakobs, C., Lambertus, D., Wikkerink, B., Kok, R. M., de Jong, A. P. J. M. and Wadman, S. K. Stable isotope dilution analysis of succinylacetone using electron capture negative ion mass fragmentography: an accurate approach to the pre- and neonatal diagnosis of hereditary tyrosinemia type I. *Clin. Chim. Acta* 223 (1988) 223–232

Kvittingen, E. A. and Brodtkorb, E. The pre- and post-natal diagnosis of tyrosinemia type I and the detection of the carrier state by assay of fumarylacetoacetase. *Scand. J. Clin. Lab. Invest.* 46 Suppl. 184 (1986) 35–40

Kvittingen, E. A., Leonard, J. V., Pettit, B. R. and King, G. S. Concentrations of succinylacetone after homogentisate and tyrosine loading in healthy individuals with low fumarylacetoacetase activity. *Clin. Chim. Acta* 152 (1985) 271–279

Kvittingen, E. A., Jellum, E., Stokke, O., Flatmark, A., Bergan, A., Sødal, G., Halvorsen, S., Schrumpf, E. and Gjone, E. Liver transplantation in a 23-year-old tyrosinaemia patient: effects on the renal tubular dysfunction. *J. Inher. Metab. Dis.* 9 (1986) 216–224

Kvittingen, E. A., Rootwelt, H., van Dam, T., van Faassen, H. and Berger, R. Hereditary tyrosinemia type I – lack of correlation between clinical findings and amount of immunoreactive fumarylacetoacetase protein. *Vth International Congress on Inborn Errors of Metabolism*, Asilomar, California, 1–5 June 1990

Kvittingen, E. A., Talseth, T., Halvorsen, S., Jakobs, C., Hovig, T. and Flatmark, A. Renal failure in adult patients with hereditary tyrosinaemia type I. *J. Inher. Metab. Dis.* 14 (1991) 53–62

Lindblad, B., Lindstedt, S. and Steen, G. On the enzymic defects in hereditary tyrosinemia. *Proc. Natl. Acad. Sci. USA* 84 (1977) 4641–4645

Lindblad, B., Friden, J., Greter, J., Holme, E., Lindstedt, S. and Sjøsteen, C. Treatment of hereditary tyrosinaemia (fumarylacetoacetase deficiency) by enzyme substitution. *J. Inher. Metab. Dis.* 9 Suppl. 2 (1986) 257–261

Mieles, L. A., Esquivel, C. O., van Thiel, D. H., Koneru, B., Makowka, L., Tzakis, A. G. and Starzl, T. E. Liver transplantation for tyrosinemia. A review of 10 cases from the University of Pittsburgh. *Digest. Dis. Sci.* 35 (1990) 153–157

Mitchell, G., Larochelle, J., Lambert, M., Michaud, J., Grenier, A., Ogier, H., Gauthier, M., Lacroix, J., Vanasse, M., Larbrisseau, A., Paradis, K., Weber, A., Lefevre, Y., Melancon, S. and Dallaire, L. Neurologic crises in hereditary tyrosinemia. *N. Engl. J. Med.* 322 (1990) 432–437

Nicole, L. M., Valet, J. P., Laberge, C. and Tanguay, R. M. Purification of mRNA coding for the enzyme deficient in hereditary tyrosinemia, fumarylacetoacetate hydrolase. *Can. J. Biochem. Cell Biol.* 64 (1986) 489–493

Paradis, K., Weber, A., Seidman, E., Larochelle, J., Lenaerts, C. and Roy, C. C. Evaluation of tyrosinemic children for liver transplantation. *Pediatr. Res.* 27 (1990) 538 (abstract)

Rootwelt, H., Kvittingen, E. A., Agsteribbe, E., Hartog, M. V., van Faassen, H. and Berger, R. The fumarylacetoacetase gene: Characterization of restriction fragment length polymorphisms and identification of haplotypes – possibility for prenatal diagnosis in families with compound genotypes for the tyrosinemia and 'pseudodeficiency' genes. *Vth International Congress on Inborn Errors of Metabolism*, Asilomar, California, 1–5 June 1990

Schierbeek, H. and Berger, R. Determination of succinylacetone and succinylacetoacetate in physiological samples as the common product 5(3)-methyl-3(5)-isoxasole propionic acid using an isotope dilution method and mass spectrometry. *Clin. Chim. Acta* 184 (1989) 243–250

Søvik, O., Kvittingen, E. A., Steen-Johnson, J. and Halvorsen, S. Hereditary tyrosinemia of chronic course without rickets or renal tubular dysfunction. *Acta Paedatr. Scand.* 79 (1990) 1063–1068

Tanguay, R. T., Laberge, C., Lescault, T., Valet, J. P., Duband, J. L. and Quenneville, Y. Molecular basis of hereditary tyrosinemia: Proof of the primary defect by Western blotting. In Scott, W., Amhad, F., Black, S., Schultz, J. and Whelan, W. J. (eds.) *Advances in Gene Technology: Human Genetic Disorders, ICSU Short Reports* 1 (1984) 250–251

Tuchman, M., Freese, D. K., Sharp, H. L., Ramnaraine, M. L. R., Ascher, N. and Bloomer, J. P. Contribution of extrahepatic tissues to biochemical abnormalities in hereditary tyrosinemia type I: study of three patients after liver transplantation. *J. Pediatr.* 110 (1987) 399–403

Van Spronsen, F. J., Berger, R., Smit, G. P. A., De Klerk, J. B. C., Duran, M., Bijleveld, C. M. A., Van Faassen, H., Slooff, M. J. H. and Heymans, H. S. A. Tyrosinaemia type I: Orthotopic liver transplantation as the only definite answer to a metabolic as well as an oncological problem. *J. Inher. Metab. Dis.* 12 Suppl. 2 (1989) 339–342

Weinberg, A. G., Mize, C. E. and Worthen, H. G. The occurrence of hepatoma in the chronic form of hereditary tyrosinemia. *J. Pediatr.* 88 (1976) 434–438

J. Inher. Metab. Dis. 14 (1991) 563–579
© SSIEM and Kluwer Academic Publishers.

Investigation of the Molecular Basis of the Genetic Deficiency of UDP-Glucuronosyltransferase in Crigler–Najjar Syndrome

K. J. ROBERTSON, D. CLARKE, L. SUTHERLAND, R. WOOSTER,
M. W. H. COUGHTRIE and B. BURCHELL
*Department of Biochemical Medicine, Ninewells Hospital and Medical School,
University of Dundee, Dundee DD1 9SY, UK*

Summary: Liver biopsy samples were obtained from eight Crigler–Najjar patients. Bilirubin UDPGT activity, assayed by a microassay with HPLC analysis, was not detectable in type I livers, and low levels (9–26% of controls) of monoglucuronide conjugates only were observed in type II livers. 1-Naphthol UDPGT activity was normal in most patients, where membrane integrity was maintained by correct sample procurement and preparation. Our data on type II livers suggest that a defect in UDPGA transport is an unlikely cause of the hyperbilirubinaemia, but reduced affinity for UDPGA was observed in one sample. Analysis of four patient liver samples by immunoblot analysis revealed the heterogeneous nature of this inherited disease within the patient population, and one sample where 1-naphthol UDPGT activity was considerably reduced appeared to correlate with the non-detection of a phenol UDPGT protein. Progress towards a molecular genetic diagnosis of Crigler–Najjar syndromes is discussed.

INTRODUCTION

Crigler–Najjar syndrome (McKusick 21880) is a severe type of unconjugated hyperbilirubinaemia (Crigler and Najjar, 1952) which has been observed worldwide (Schmid and McDonagh, 1978; Wolkoff *et al.*, 1983). Infants often develop severe neurological damage from bilirubin encephalopathy (kernicterus). Patients have been classified into two types based on (a) the level of unconjugated hyperbilirubinaemia (type I, greater than $340 \, \mu mol/L$ (20 mg/dl) and type II, below this division; Wolkoff *et al.*, 1983) and (b) the dramatic response of type II patients to barbiturate therapy (Arias *et al.*, 1969). This clear difference in response to barbiturate therapy between type I and type II patients suggests a fundamental difference in the molecular basis of the metabolic defect.

Patients with Crigler–Najjar syndrome type I have a complete defect in hepatic bilirubin glucuronidation. However, the genetic lesion has been reported to affect other UDPGT isoenzymes since glucuronidation of other aglycones was reduced (Schmid and McDonagh, 1978). In particular, defects in steroid glucuronidation and in glucuronidation of *N*-acetyl-*p*-aminophenol or menthol have been observed, although there is considerable variation in the results reported (Schmid and McDonagh, 1978; Van Es *et al.*, 1990).

Glucuronidation of bilirubin is significantly decreased in Crigler–Najjar syndrome type II (McKusick 14350) patients due to a greatly reduced or absent bilirubin UDPGT activity in the liver (Schmid and McDonagh, 1978). The low levels of conjugates produced are predominantly in the form of monoglucuronides. The inheritance of this type II syndrome has been difficult to establish, although the most recent study has suggested an autosomal recessive transmission (Labrune *et al.*, 1989). Formation of menthol and salicylamide glucuronides, measured *in vivo*, was reduced in most cases of type II disease.

The glucuronidation of 2-aminophenol, 4-methylumbelliferone and *p*-nitrophenol by hepatic microsomes was apparently reduced (Schmid and McDonagh, 1978), although the extent of the defect in glucuronidation with respect to xenobiotics has yet to be carefully assessed, with good liver preparations and sensitive assay methods.

Assay of UDPGTs

The membrane-bound location of human liver UDPGTs has led to many problems with accurate assay of these enzymes (Burchell *et al.*, 1987). The transferases are deemed to be latent and do not express full potential activity due to the constraints of the endoplasmic reticulum membrane. Damage to the endoplasmic reticulum by slow freezing, poor storage, vigorous homogenization or unwise selection of buffer systems may lead to large differences in microsomal enzyme activities measured. The latency or intactness of individual microsomal preparations should be independently assessed by measurement of mannose-6-phosphate hydrolysis or 1-naphthol UDPGT (Burchell and Coughtrie, 1989), to enable comparison of different preparations obtained from different tissue specimens. Alternatively, maximum levels of UDPGT activity could be used as a basis for data comparison, after release of latent activity by treatment of microsomes with a suitable detergent such as Lubrol PX. Unfortunately, to measure maximal UDPGT activities, detergent must be titrated with microsomes to determine the maximum response (see the results section). The maximal transferase activity will depend on the original intactness of the microsomes and the aglycone substrate used and thus selection of optimal levels of detergent addition should be determined in each case. Further variability in measurements of UDPGT activities may be caused by differential inducibility of the transferases by drugs (Bock *et al.*, 1984; Jackson *et al.*, 1987). Routine treatment of Crigler–Najjar patients in the UK with barbiturates may well affect UDPGT activity levels but also introduce variability for optimal activation of the transferases by detergents in routine assays.

The difficulties encountered in biochemical analysis of the enzymological defects result from problems in obtaining sufficient liver biopsy material in good condition, the sensitivity of the assay procedures and the availability of age-matched controls. Black and colleagues (1970) described a method for the assay of bilirubin UDPGT activity in needle biopsy samples, but required approximately 10 mg of liver per assay, so only very large needle biopsies would provide sufficient tissue for more than one simple assay. This limitation is a problem when a kinetic analysis of the transferases is required. The introduction of HPLC analysis of bilirubin conjugates facilitated an improvement in both the sensitivity and discrimination of product formation in the bilirubin UDPGT assay (Blanckaert *et al.*, 1980; Onishi *et al.*, 1980; Odell *et al.*, 1990).

Glucuronidation is catalysed by a family of enzymes

Hepatic microsomal UDP-glucuronosyltransferases (EC 2.4.2.1.17) are a family of closely related isoenzymes catalysing the conjugation of various endogenous compounds (including bilirubin) and many exogenous compounds with UDP-glucuronic acid, resulting in the formation of more polar, water soluble and readily excreted metabolites (Burchell and Coughtrie, 1989). Anti-rat UDPGT antibodies and rat liver UDPGT cDNAs have been used to clone human liver UDPGT cDNAs.

The seven cDNA clones were separated into two subfamilies on the basis of deduced amino acid sequence homology. Subfamily 1 contained five clones with 65–90% sequence similarity and subfamily 2 contained two clones with 80% sequence similarity. The sequence identity between the two subfamilies was only 44% overall. However, the similarity between the two sequences was concentrated in the C-terminal half of the protein showing 65% identity (Burchell and Coughtrie, 1989).

The UDPGT isoenzymes encoded by the full length cDNAs HLUG25 and HLUGP1 had characteristic N-terminal signal sequences. *In vitro* transcription/translation studies using the clone HLUG25 indicated that this signal sequence was cleaved, and that the UDPGT was glycosylated. Expressing the cDNAs in COS-7 cells confirmed the translational glycosylation (Burchell and Coughtrie, 1989).

The topology of rat liver UDPGTs has been examined using proteases and antibodies complemented by computer-based DNA sequence analysis. A characteristic C-terminal stop transfer signal and a single membrane spanning region retaining the transferases in the endoplasmic reticulum with the majority of the protein including the active site in the endoplasmic reticulum lumen have also been identified with the human liver UDPGTs. The N-terminal portions of the proteins between residues 60–120 show the major dissimilarity between sequences and are believed to provide the specificity of acceptor substrate binding, whereas the common C-terminal portion between residues 350–400 probably binds UDP-glucuronic acid (Burchell and Coughtrie, 1989).

Two full-length human liver cDNAs have been expressed in COS-7 cells to assess their function. The major human phenol UDPGT expressed in COS-7 cells catalysed the glucuronidation of 1-naphthol, 4-methylumbelliferase and 4-nitrophenol. The use of a series of related phenols provided an outline description of the restrictions of substituent and electronic configurations imposed upon phenolic structures accepted as substrates by the enzyme. The glucuronidation of steroids was not catalysed by this cloned UDPGT (Burchell and Coughtrie, 1989).

A second human liver cDNA transiently expressed in COS-7 cells encoded a UDPGT enzyme specifically responsible for the glucuronidation of 6-hydroxy bile acids, which are excreted in human urine. This enzyme does not catalyse the glucuronidation of steroids or other bile acids. A third cloned human liver UDPGT cDNA has been determined to encode a transferase specifically catalysing the glucuronidation of oestriol (Burchell and Coughtrie, 1989).

Possible molecular lesions in Crigler–Najjar syndrome

UDPGTs are latent microsomal membrane-bound enzymes with active sites in the lumen of the endoplasmic reticulum. Evidence has accumulated suggesting the presence of a UDPGA transporter in microsomes, limiting access of substrate to the transferase (Burchell and Coughtrie, 1989). Glycogen storage diseases types 1b and 1c have been shown to be caused by defects in microsomal glucose-6-phosphate and phosphate transporters or permeases (Burchell, 1990). Parallels can be drawn between the glucose-6-phosphatase system and glucuronidation. It is possible that genetic lesions in a UDPGA or bilirubin transport may cause certain hyperbilirubinaemias, such as Crigler–Najjar type II syndrome. However, the more likely common causes are molecular lesions within the regulatory or coding regions of the gene for bilirubin UDP-glucuronosyltransferase.

We have developed microassays for the analysis of bilirubin glucuronide formation utilizing HPLC techniques. Here we describe our recent work examining the molecular basis of the UDPGT defect in liver samples from eight Crigler–Najjar patients, reassessing the biochemical analyses and describing immunochemical analysis. Molecular genetic analysis of this disorder in the near future is discussed.

EXPERIMENTAL PROCEDURES

Materials

Ammonium acetate (Aristar grade) and acetonitrile (HPLC grade) were from BDH Ltd. UDPGA, Lubrol PX and bilirubin were from Sigmal Chemical Company. All other chemicals were of analytical grade obtained from commonly used suppliers.

Patients and liver samples

Crigler–Najjar syndrome type I

Case 1: This boy (MS) is the first child of non-consanguineous parents. The mother is thought to have Gilbert's syndrome but has not yet been investigated. He required exchange transfusion at 4 days of age. He was treated with phenobarbitone (up to 10 mg/kg) but this had no effect on his serum bilirubin. His bilirubin was maintained at around 130 μmol/L by phototherapy. A needle biopsy was obtained at about 8 weeks of age. The tissue was not frozen on arrival.

Case 2: A liver biopsy weighing 3.0 mg was obtained from a girl (SB) aged 9 months in whom a clinical diagnosis of Crigler–Najjar syndrome type I had been made. She had received phototherapy from the first week of life and her serum bilirubin at the time of biopsy was 190 μmol/L. She was also receiving phenobarbitone (30 mg/day).

Case 3: Liver samples obtained from a Belgian infant (B1) with a clinical diagnosis of Crigler–Najjar syndrome type I transplanted with normal liver in 1990. Further clinical details were not available.

Case 4: A liver biopsy from a second Belgian patient (B2). Clinical details were not available.

Case 5: A needle biopsy weighing 9.0 mg was obtained from a male (AA) aged 2 years 9 months who had been jaundiced since birth. He had not responded to phenobarbitone treatment and was managed by daily phototherapy.

Crigler–Najjar type II

Cases 1 and 2: Needle liver biopsies of 14 mg and 18.7 mg were obtained from a brother (MI) and sister (SI) respectively, with clinical diagnoses of Crigler–Najjar syndrome type II. The boy was 8 years 9 months old at the time of biopsy and his sister was 5 years 8 months. Both children were receiving phenobarbitone, which had reduced their serum bilirubin to around 60 μmol/L at the time of biopsy.

Case 3: A 72-year-old man (EM) who clinically has Crigler–Najjar type II. He has been investigated previously with equivocal results (Gollan *et al.*, 1975). No bilirubin UDPGT activity was found after 6 weeks of phenobarbitone therapy, but they had found a low level of activity before commencing therapy (3.1 pmol min^{-1} (mg protein)$^{-1}$).

He had been on phenobarbitone (180 mg/day) from 1973 until the time of his recent operation. He required a cholecystectomy for recurrent cholecystitis and cholestasis secondary to cholelithiasis. His serum bilirubin was 130 μmol/L.

Normal adult human liver samples were used for the kinetic and latency studies as well as for controls when the patient's biopsies were assayed.

Methods

Preparation of liver homogenates: The biopsies were frozen immediately by immersion in liquid nitrogen and stored at $-80°C$ until they were assayed. Homogenates 10% (w/v) of liver in sucrose 0.25 mol/L, HEPES 5 mmol/L, pH 7.4, were prepared by hand using a Teflon-headed homogenizer. The suspension was placed on ice for 10 min to allow the larger debris to settle and the supernatant was then decanted for use in the assays. Homogenates were prepared as above for microassays except that a miniature Teflon homogenizer and an Eppendorf centrifuge tube were used. Homogenates were stored on ice, and all assays were performed within 4 h.

Enzyme assays: All UDPGT assays were performed using established assay procedures in the presence of optimally activated concentrations (determined for each developmental age) of the non-ionic detergent Lubrol PX, in order to counteract any effects of variable latency during development and to allow the measurement of the maximum glucuronidation potential of the liver sample.

Bilirubin UDP-glucuronosyltransferase activity was measured by the method of Van Roy and Heirwegh (1968) or by microincubations (50 μl total volume) and HPLC analysis of glucuronide formation. All assay reactions were linear for 90 min when

using 124 µmol/L bilirubin and 3 or 30 mmol/L UDP-glucuronic acid. Microincubations were stopped with 50 µl of acetonitrile centrifuged at 10 000 g for 5 min and the
entire supernatant was injected onto the HPLC column. HPLC determination of
bilirubin glucuronide formation was by the method of Odell and colleagues (1990).
Bilirubin glucuronide standards were isolated from Wistar rat bile (Muraca and
Blanckaert, 1983).

UDP-glucuronosyltransferase activity towards 1-naphthol was assayed by the
method of Otani and colleagues (1976) and the activity towards morphine by the
method of Svensson and colleagues (1982) as modified by Coughtrie and colleagues
(1989). UDPGT activity towards menthol was measured by the Sep-Pak method of
Puig and Tephly (1986) using 8 mmol/L menthol substrate concentration in the assay.
Activators such as UDP-N-acetylglucosamine and competitive inhibitors such as
menthol were added directly to incubation mixtures.

Anti-UDPGT antibodies: The production and characterization of anti-rat liver
testosterone/4-nitrophenol UDPGT (RAL 1) and anti-rat kidney 1-naphthol/bilirubin
UDPGT (RAK 1) have been described elsewhere (Coughtrie *et al.*, 1988). Rabbit
anti-rat liver testosterone UDPGT and anti-human phenol UDPGT peptide antibodies have recently been obtained by this laboratory (unpublished work).

Electrophoresis and immunoblot analysis: Microsomal samples were resolved on
7.5% polyacrylamide gels in the presence of 0.1% SDS, essentially as described by
Laemmli (1970). For immunoblot analysis of resolved microsomal UDPGTs, proteins
were transferred after electrophoresis to nitrocellulose by the method of Towbin
and colleagues (1979), and chromogenic detection of immunoreactive UDPGT
polypeptides was performed using the alkaline phosphatase linked detection system
(Coughtrie *et al.*, 1988). Protein in microsomal samples was determined by the method
of Lowry and colleagues (1951) on microsomal preparations which had been frozen
and thawed once only. Bovine serum albumin was used to construct standard curves.

RESULTS

Assay of UDP-glucuronosyltransferase

Maximal activation of UDPGTs by optimal levels of the detergent Lubrol PX were
investigated in normal human liver samples to enable comparison with results
obtained when using different patient samples. Detergent activation curves were
performed for two patient samples as illustrated in Figure 1. The results obtained
for normal liver show that the optimal ratio of Lubrol: liver wet weight was different
for bilirubin UDPGT (0.004 mg Lubrol/mg liver) when compared to 1-naphthol
UDPGT (0.01 mg Lubrol/mg liver). The concentration of the donor substrate,
UDPGA, was also examined because difficulties have been encountered in saturating
bilirubin UDPGT (Strebel and Odell, 1971).

The effect of increasing the final concentration of UDPGA on bilirubin UDPGT
activity in human liver homogenates and microsomes was measured. Typical plots,

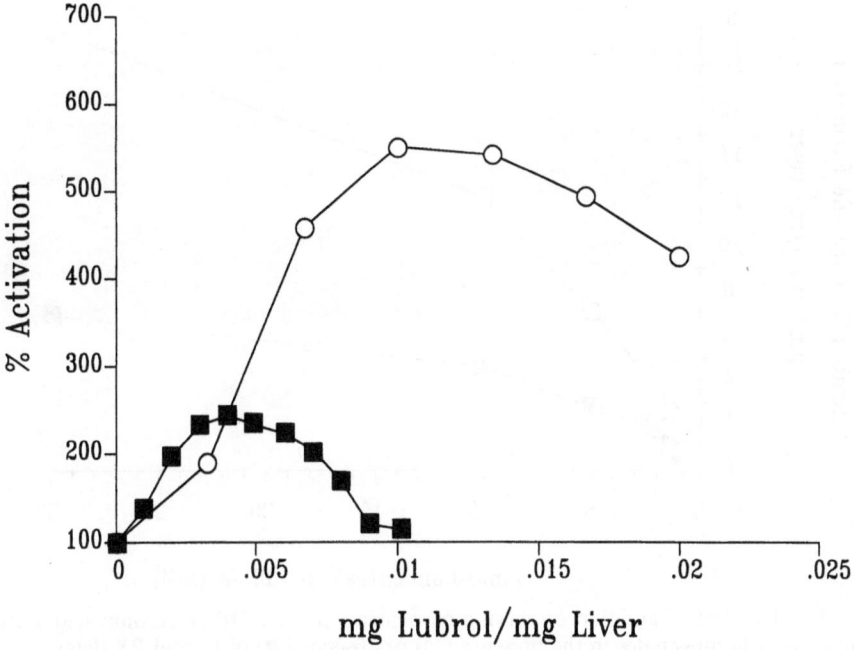

Figure 1 Detergent activation of UDP-glucuronosyltransferase activities in human liver homogenate. Activation curves for 1-naphthol UDPGT (○) and bilirubin UDPGT (■) in response to the non-ionic detergent Lubrol-PX

with and without detergent, are shown in Figure 2 and it was clear that the curves were not asymptotic. The non-asymptotic curves render the calculation of K_m values from double reciprocal plots difficult, but using best fit lines the K_m values for UDPGA were: homogenate, without Lubrol 9 mmol/L, with Lubrol 17 mmol/L; microsomes, without Lubrol 9 mmol/L and with Lubrol 12 mmol/L. The addition of UDPNAG (final concentration 2.26 mmol/L) did not improve saturation (data not shown).

UDP-glucuronosyltransferase activities in Crigler–Najjar syndrome

Assay of 1-naphthol UDPGT activity: The determination of UDPGT isoenzyme activity other than for bilirubin was important in order to confirm the viability of tissues in which bilirubin UDPGT activity was greatly reduced or absent. This also provided information on latency and hence membrane integrity.

Measurement of 1-naphthol UDPGT activity (Table 1) demonstrated that none of the samples were deficient in 1-naphthol glucuronidation compared to the controls. Furthermore, detergent activation was normal in five patient livers and there was apparently no defect in membrane integrity. Lower 1-naphthol UDPGT activities were observed in livers MS and EM; detergent activation was also poor, indicating that the sample collection was not ideal (liver MS not frozen on arrival) and that the age of a patient may be an important parameter (see EM, Table 1).

J. Inher. Metab. Dis. 14 (1991)

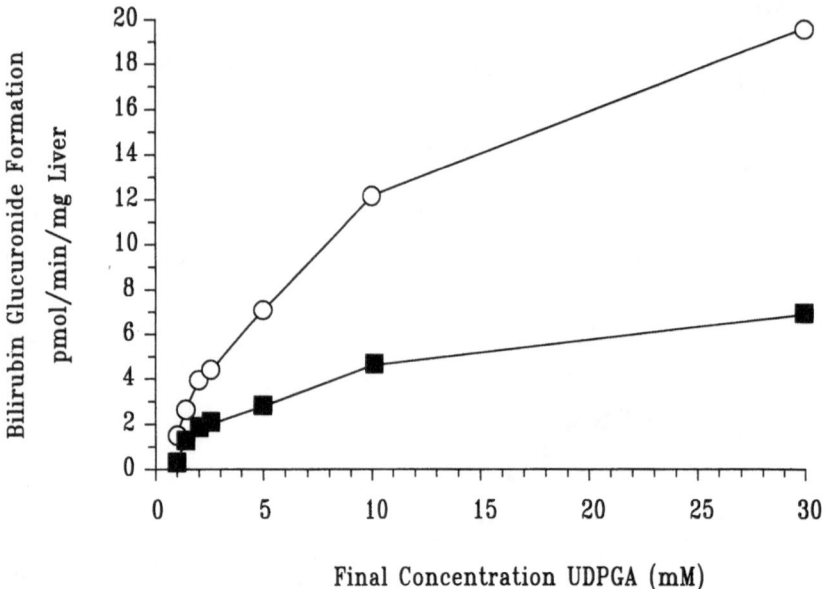

Figure 2 The effect of addition of varying concentrations of UDP-glucuronic acid activity in human liver homogenates in the presence (○) or absence (■) of Lubrol PX detergent

The results obtained with type II patient liver samples also suggested that the molecular cause of the disorder was not due to a defect in substrate transport into the endoplasmic reticulum. Stimulation of the transport of UDP-glucuronic acid by UDP-*N*-acetylglucosamine has been previously proposed (Burchell *et al.*, 1983). 1-Naphthol UDP-glucuronyltransferase activity in liver homogenates was therefore also measured in the presence of 2 mmol/L UDPNAG. The results showed that stimulation of 1-naphthol UDPGT activity in Crigler–Najjar type I and type II samples was up to 2-fold, similar to liver controls (data not shown).

Assay of morphine UDPGT activity: Tissue viability was further tested by assay of morphine UDPGT activity. This assay was performed only for case 3 (type II) due to lack of tissue for the other cases but, consistent with the 1-naphthol results, the activity was 1.7 times the control level (patient, 47 pmol min^{-1} (mg liver)$^{-1}$; control 27 pmol min^{-1} (mg liver)$^{-1}$.

Assay of menthol UDPGT activity: Measurement of menthol UDPGT in a single Crigler–Najjar patient (B1) liver homogenate has indicated that the level of activity (22 pmol min^{-1} (mg liver)$^{-1}$) was similar to control values. Furthermore, menthol was shown to be a poor competitive inhibitor of bilirubin UDPGT, indicating that menthol glucuronidation is catalysed by a different transferase.

Assay of bilirubin UDPGT activities: A diagnostic test for Crigler–Najjar syndrome is assay of bilirubin UDPGT activity; none was demonstrable in liver homogenates

| | | | UDP-glucuronosyltransferase activity | | | | | |
| | | | Bilirubin (pmol min^{-1} (mg liver)$^{-1}$) | | Activation (fold) | 1-Naphthol (nmol min^{-1} (mg liver)$^{-1}$) | | Activation (fold) |
Case	Age (years)	Lubrol	−	+		−	+	
Crigler–Najjar type I								
B1	?		ND	ND	—	0.08	0.36	4.5
B2	?		ND	ND	—	0.09	0.19	2.1
MS	0.15		ND	ND	—	0.08	0.12	1.5
SB	0.58		ND	ND	—	0.07	0.24	3.4
AK	2		ND	ND	—	0.10	0.58	5.8
Crigler–Najjar type II								
MI	9		0.12	ND	—	0.15	0.66	4.4
SI	6	3 mmol/L UDPGA	0.07	0.09	1.3	0.11	0.64	5.8
		30 mmol/L UDPGA	0.54	0.40	0.7	–	–	–
EM	72		0.04	–	–	0.08	0.18	2.3
Adult controls	40–73							
		3 mmol/L UDPGA	0.46 (0.07)	1.57 (0.13)	3.5 (0.8)	0.1 (0.05)	0.46 (0.14)	5.2 (2.4)
		30 mmol/L UDPGA	1.50 (0.58)	4.68 (2.48)	3.1 (0.9)	–	–	–

For adult controls, values represent mean (SD) for five determinations
ND: not detected

from patients with type I syndrome but the Crigler–Najjar type II samples (cases 1, 2 and 3) exhibited 26%, 15% and 9% respectively of control bilirubin UDPGT activity in the absence of detergent (Table 1). The control tissue optimum Lubrol concentration inactivated bilirubin UDPGT in case MI and therefore a limited Lubrol activation curve was performed for case SI. The '+ Lubrol' result in Table 1 (1.3-fold activation) was obtained with 1/10 of the control Lubrol concentration. Addition of further detergent inactivated the enzyme. We were thus able to confirm the clinical diagnoses in all seven patients and also demonstrated increased 'sensitivity' of the enzyme to detergent in the two type II cases.

All of the microassays described so far were performed using 3 mmol/L (final concentration) UDPGA as described by Black and colleagues (1969). The HPLC traces in Figure 3 were obtained during bilirubin UDPGT assay of liver from case 4 (SI) and a control. The effect of increasing the final concentration of UDPGA to

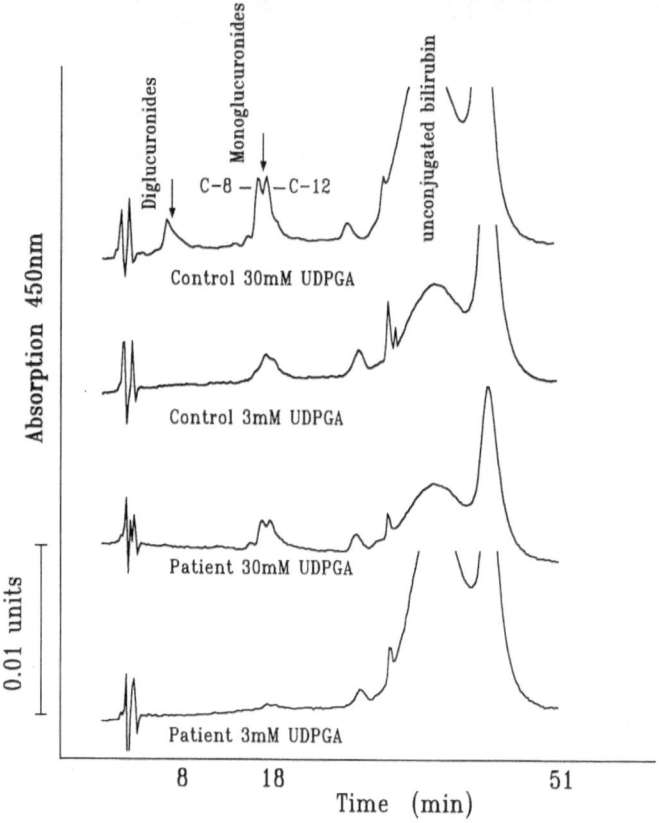

Figure 3 Bilirubin glucuronide production by Crigler–Najjar type II liver homogenate: the effect of UDPGA concentration. HPLC chromatograms obtained after incubation of human liver homogenates with bilirubin and 3 mmol/L or 30 mmol/L UDPGA. Top two traces: adult control liver. Bottom two traces: Crigler–Najjar type II liver. Separation was performed on a μBondapak (Waters) C18 reversed phase column using the gradient system of Odell and colleagues (1990)

30 mmol/L was demonstrated. The patient's measured bilirubin UDPGT activity rose 7.7-fold compared to a 3.3-fold rise in control activity, although the significance of this result is difficult to interpret. When the higher concentration of UDPGA was used, diglucuronides were detected in the control, whereas only monoglucuronides were produced by the Crigler–Najjar type II tissue. This data is in agreement with the *in vivo* evidence that Crigler–Najjar type II patients' bile contains only monoconjugates of bilirubin. The retention time of the diglucuronides was 8 min and of the monoglucuronides 17.5 min (C-8 monoglucuronides) and 18.5 min (C-12 monoglucuronides).

Immunoblot analysis of UDP-glucuronosyltransferases in human liver microsomes from Crigler–Najjar patients

The clinical features of Crigler–Najjar syndrome type II are known to be markedly decreased bilirubin UDPGT activity, but it is not known whether this is due to a reduction in enzyme protein levels or to inadequate catalytic activity of the enzyme. Immunoblot analysis was performed on liver homogenates from Crigler–Najjar patients (three type I and one type II samples) and from 'normal' human controls. The results using three different antibodies are shown in Figure 4. The antibody used in panel A recognized at least four major immunoreactive proteins ranging from 52 to 56.5 kDa in seven control liver microsomes and a similar pattern was observed in two of the type I liver microsomes. Examination of the type I and type II microsomes in lanes 8 and 9 respectively shows that three of these UDPGT proteins were not detected using this antibody. This apparent loss of transferase proteins is not due to the age of the Crigler–Najjar type II patient as control liver from humans of a similar age shows a normal spectrum of immunodetectable bands. One of the proteins not detected in lanes 8 and 9 would appear to be a human phenol UDPGT whose molecular weight and mobility are demonstrated by the cloned/expressed enzyme in lane P. Similar results were observed in panel B where the antibody specially raised against rat bilirubin/phenol GT recognized up to three major polypeptides. The more specific detection of the 52 kDa protein recognized by anti-testosterone UDPGT antibody is demonstrated in all samples in panel C (Figure 4), indicating that levels of this transferase are unaffected in Crigler–Najjar syndromes. A surprising feature of the immunostaining pattern of the Crigler–Najjar liver microsomes was the considerable increase in immunostaining of the 52 kDa polypeptide (lanes 8 and 9, Figure 4C). This UDPGT protein induction may well be related to the measured increase in the microsomal testosterone UDPGT activity (Burchell *et al.*, 1987). The Crigler–Najjar infants were treated with barbiturates, which may explain the results obtained (the testosterone UDPGT isoenzyme is induced by phenobarbitone in rat liver).

The apparent loss of transferase proteins in two cases of Crigler–Najjar syndrome may not be due to lack of synthesis of proteins, but may be due to alteration of the protein structure such that epitopes normally recognized by these antibody preparations are no longer 'visible'. Nonetheless, this analysis has demonstrated the heterogeneity of the molecular basis of this disorder within the patient population.

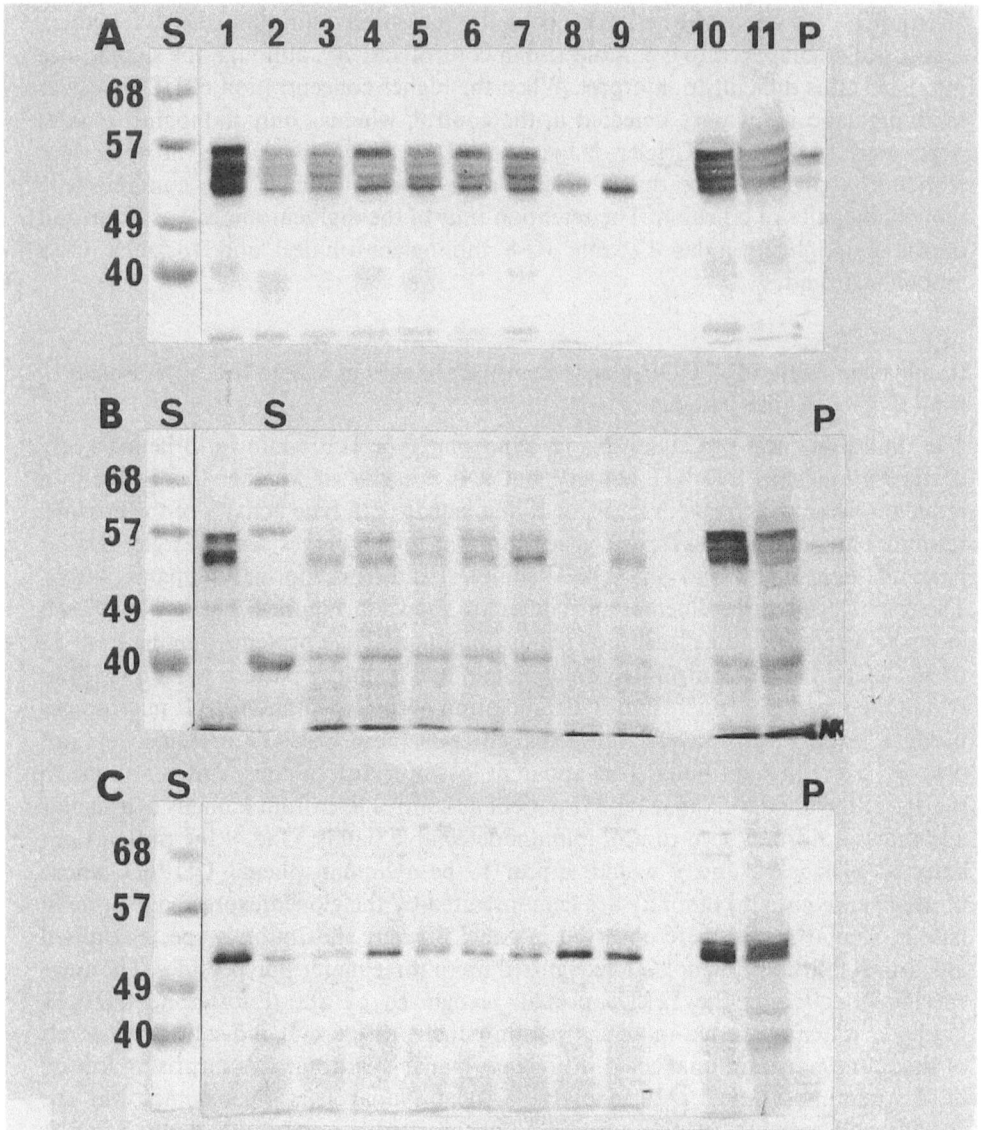

Figure 4 Immunoblot analysis of UDP-glucuronosyltransferases in liver homogenates from patients with Crigler–Najjar syndrome. Immunoblot analysis was performed as described in the experimental section. The primary antibodies are: panel A, anti-rat liver UDPGTs; panel B, anti-rat kidney UDPGT; panel C, anti-rat liver testosterone UDPGT. Liver homogenates (approximately 20 μg of protein) were loaded in each lane as follows; lanes 1–5, five different samples of adult human liver homogenate; lane 6, patient liver B1 (type I); lane 7, patient liver MS (type I); lane 8, patient liver B2 (type I); lane 9, patient liver EM (type II); lanes 10 and 11, liver homogenate from 73- and 71-year-old males. Lane P, cloned human phenol UDPGT in NIH3T3 cell homogenate (10 μg protein). Lanes S indicate protein molecular weight standards; albumin, 68 kDa; pyruvate kinase, 57 kDa; fumarase, 49 kDa; aldolase, 40 kDa (5 μg protein)

DISCUSSION

Biochemical assay of UDPGTs in Crigler–Najjar syndrome

Persistent, congenital defects of bilirubin metabolism are rare, with the exception of Gilbert syndrome (Owens and Evans, 1975). Nevertheless, an understanding of their pathogenesis is likely to provide valuable insight into the normal mechanisms of intracellular biotransformation and bilirubin excretion.

UDPGT activities measured in liver microsomes from Crigler–Najjar patients were determined for four aglycone substrates, after optimal activation with detergent. These enzyme activities were also determined in 'normal' *post mortem* liver samples from infants of the same age. Bilirubin UDPGT activity was determined by micro-HPLC analysis of the glucuronides formed. In the work reported here, no UDPGT activity towards bilirubin was detectable in liver homogenates from Crigler–Najjar type I patients, whereas activity towards 1-naphthol as substrate was determined to be the same value as the control. Our studies of Crigler–Najjar type II showed the synthesis of low levels of bilirubin monoconjugates only catalysed by liver homogenates, and again levels of 1-naphthol UDPGT activity were the same as controls.

Some of the variation in the results previously reported may be due to (a) lack of optimal activation of the UDPGTs during enzyme assay, (b) poor liver sample storage and preparation and (c) treatment with barbiturates as demonstrated in this paper. Measurement of menthol glucuronidation has also been proposed to be diagnostic for Crigler–Najjar syndrome (Szabo and Ebry, 1963), although some instances of normal menthol glucuronidation have been detected in these patients (Arias *et al.*, 1969; Bloomer *et al.*, 1971; G. B. Odell, personal communication). Our *in vitro* analyses show that menthol is a poor competitive inhibitor of bilirubin glucuronidation and that menthol glucuronidation was normal in the absence of bilirubin glucuronidation measured in liver from one patient. Our preliminary studies on purification of menthol UDPGT from rat liver show that this transferase activity was separated from bilirubin UDPGT by ion exchange chromatography (unpublished work). Furthermore, Odell (personal communication) has determined defective menthol glucuronidation after oral administration (1 g) to a 'normal' non-icteric individual, confirming the proposal that defects in menthol glucuronidation and bilirubin glucuronidation can occur independently in the population by molecular lesions affecting different UDPGT isoenzymes (Burchell and Coughtrie, 1990).

We also considered the possibility that the defect in Crigler–Najjar syndrome type II may be in the integrity of the UDPGA transporter which facilitates the passage of the co-substrate across the microsomal/endoplasmic reticulum membrane (Burchell and Coughtrie, 1989). The transverse topology of bilirubin UDPGT in the membrane has been described such that only a small portion of the enzyme is cytoplasmic and that the active site is intraluminal (Vanstapel and Blanckaert, 1988; Shepherd *et al.*, 1989). All the UDPGT isoenzymes require UDPGA as a co-substrate and little is known about the mechanism of transport of UDPGA, or of the primary substrates, across the membrane of the endoplasmic reticulum. It is reasonable to assume that one UDPGA transporter may serve all of the UDPGT isoenzymes. We have demonstrated that activation of 1-naphthol UDPGT is similar in control livers and

Crigler–Najjar II patient livers and therefore a defect in UDPGA transport does not explain the severely reduced levels of the bilirubin glucuronidation in these patients. The inactivation of the enzyme by the Lubrol concentrations required for maximal activation of control tissues suggests enzyme instability. Also, the 7.7-fold rise in bilirubin UDPGT activity when tissue from case SI was incubated with $10\times$ UDPGA contrasts with the 3.3-fold increase when control tissue was similarly treated (Table 1). There is therefore a possibility that at least some patients with Crigler–Najjar type II bilirubin UDPGT may have a reduced affinity for UDPGA.

Immunoblot analysis of UDPGT proteins in liver samples from Crigler–Najjar patients

The existence of several distinct UDPGTs in man is now well known (Coughtrie and Burchell, 1989) and these different transferases can be detected using specific antibodies. Immunoblot analyses of liver microsomes from Crigler–Najjar patients revealed that in certain cases the slightly larger UDPGTs such as a phenol UDPGT were not detectable with two different antibodies, whereas in other cases a 'normal' spectrum of proteins was observed. These results indicated a heterogeneity of the genetic lesion affecting this gene family with the patient population in agreement with a recently reported similar study (Van Es *et al.*, 1990).

UDPGT genes and genetic variation in Crigler–Najjar syndrome

Recent molecular genetic examination of UDPGT genes in rats and man has provided a possible explanation for the variability in expression of bilirubin UDPGT and other UDPGT isoenzymes. Studies of the genetic deficiency in Gunn rats has indicated an absence of phenol and bilirubin UDPGT activity and proteins, and a reduced level of specific mRNAs (Burchell and Coughtrie, 1989).

Recently a point mutation in phenol UDPGT cDNA from Gunn rat livers was identified which would result in the synthesis of a truncated or very unstable protein (Iyanagi *et al.*, 1989). A truncated protein has recently been identified (El Awady *et al.*, 1990). The cloning of rat liver bilirubin UDPGT has shown that the C-terminal halves of the bilirubin and phenol UDPGT proteins are identical, suggesting that the two proteins are synthesized from the same gene by differential splicing of messenger RNA (Sato *et al.*, 1990). A single point mutation in the exon encoding the C-terminal portion of the two proteins would therefore cause a simultaneous loss of bilirubin and phenol glucuronidation, resulting in hyperbilirubinaemia in Gunn rats. The N-terminal of UDPGTs is believed to bind the variable substrate, whereas the common substrate UDP glucuronic acid would bind more in the C-terminal region (see introduction). Point mutations in regions of the genes responsible for encoding these different substrate binding sites could affect a single transferase activity or multiple enzymes synthesized within this gene subfamily. The gene subfamily responsible for synthesizing steroid glucuronidating enzymes does not appear to function in this manner since a defect in androsterone glucuronidation in LA rats caused by a large gene deletion (Burchell and Coughtrie, 1989) does not affect testosterone glucuronidation although the two protein sequences show 85% identity.

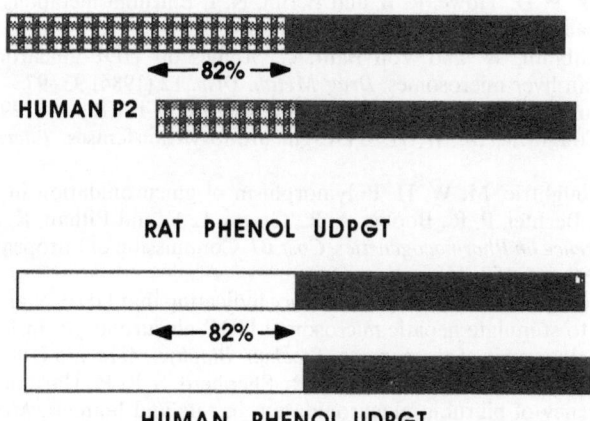

Figure 5 Comparison of human and rat liver UDPGT cDNA sequences. This schematic diagram shows that rat and human liver phenol UDPGT cDNAs show considerable sequence similarity (76% overall identity). Likewise, rat and human liver bilirubin UDPGTs(?) show considerable sequence identity in the 5' portion sequenced. The human phenol and bilirubin(?) UDPGT show complete sequence identity within the C-terminal halves of the proteins

Our studies of UDPGT genes in man have suggested that a human gene may be responsible for synthesis of a phenol UDPGT and a bilirubin UDPGT similar to the rat gene (Figure 5). A full-length cDNA clone encoding HP2 (bilirubin UDPGT?) is currently being isolated. This cDNA will then provide the basis for further study of the human gene and the genetic deficiency in Crigler–Najjar syndrome. Furthermore, a molecular genetic diagnosis of this disorder should soon be available.

ACKNOWLEDGEMENTS

We thank Dr B. Kristiansen (Gottenburg, Sweden), Dr E. Sokal (Louvain, Belgium), Dr A. Boobis (Royal Postgraduate Medical School, London), Drs M. Tarlow and D. Kelly (Children's Hospital, Birmingham), Dr A. Mowat (King's College Hospital, London) and Professor B. Billing (Royal Free Hospital, London) for providing liver samples, etc. We also thank Professor G.B. Odell, Madison, Wisconsin for many stimulating discussions. Funding for this work was awarded by the Scottish Home and Health Department, the MRC, The Wellcome Trust, The Cunningham Trust and Tenovus, Scotland.

REFERENCES

Arias, I. M., Gartner, L. M., Cohen, M., Ezzer, J. B. and Levi, A. J. Chronic non-hemolytic hyperbilirubinemia with glucuronyl transferase deficiency. *Am. J. Med.* 47 (1969) 395–409

Black, M., Billing, B. H. and Heirwegh, K. P. M. Determination of bilirubin UDP-glucuronyl transferase activity in needle biopsy specimens of human liver. *Clin. Chim. Acta* 29 (1970) 27–35

Blanckaert, N. Analysis of bilirubin and bilirubin mono- and di-conjugates. *Biochem. J.* 185 (1980) 115–128

Bloomer, J. R., Berk, P. D., Howe, R. B. and Berlin, N. I. Bilirubin metabolism in congenital non-haemolytic jaundice. *Pediatr. Res.* 5 (1971) 256–264

Bock, K. W., Lilienblum, W. and Von Bahr, C. Studies on UDP-glucuronosyltransferase activities in human liver microsomes. *Drug Metab. Disp.* 12 (1984) 93–97

Burchell, A. Molecular pathology of glucose-6-phosphatase. *FASEB J.* 4 (1990) 2978–2988

Burchell, B. and Coughtrie, M. W. H. UDP-glucuronosyltransferases. *Pharmacol. Ther.* 43 (1989) 261–289

Burchell, B. and Coughtrie, M. W. H. Polymorphism of glucuronidation in man. In Alvan, G., Balant, L. P., Bechtel, P. R., Boobis, A. R., Grann, L. F. and Pithan, K. (eds.), *European Consensus Conference on Pharmacogenetics, Cost B1*, Commission of European Communities, Luxembourg, 1990, pp. 153–160

Burchell, B., Weatherill, P. J. and Berry, C. Evidence indicating that UDP-N-acetylglucosamine does not appear to stimulate hepatic microsomal UDP-glucuronosyltransferase by interaction with the catalytic unit of the enzyme. *Biochim. Biophys. Acta* 735 (1983) 309–313

Burchell, B., Coughtrie, M. W. H., Jackson, M. R., Shepherd, S. R. P., Harding, D. and Hume, R. Genetic deficiency of bilirubin glucuronidation in rats and humans. *Mol. Aspects Med.* 9 (1987) 429–455

Coughtrie, M. W. H., Burchell, B., Leaky, J. E. A. and Hume, R. The inadequacy of perinatal glucuronidation: Immunoblot analysis of the developmental expression of individual UDP-glucuronosyltransferase isoenzymes in rat and human liver microsomes. *Mol. Pharmacol.* 34 (1988) 729–735

Coughtrie, M. W. H., Ask, B., Rane, A., Burchell, B. and Hume, R. The enantioselective glucuronidation of morphine in rats and humans. *Biochem. Pharmacol.* 38 (1989) 3273–3280

Crigler, J. F. and Najjar, V. A. Congenital familial non-hemolytic jaundice with kernicterus. *Pediatrics* 10 (1952) 169–179

El Awady, M., Roy Chowdhury, J., Kesari, K., van Es, H., Jansen, P. L. M., Lederstein, M., Arias, I. M. and Roy Chowdhury, N. Mechanism of the lack of induction of UDP-glucuronosyltransferase activity in Gunn rats by 3-methylcholanthrene. *J. Biol. Chem.* 265 (1990) 10752–10758

Gollan, J. L., Huang, S. N., Billing, B. and Sherlock, S. Prolonged survival in three brothers with severe type 2 Crigler–Najjar syndrome. Ultrastructural and metabolic studies. *Gastroenterology* 68 (1975) 1543–1555

Iyanagi, T., Watanabe, T. and Uchiyama, Y. The 3-methylcholanthrene-inducible UDP-glucuronosyltransferase deficiency in the hyperbilirubinaemic rat (Gunn rat) is caused by a -1 frameshift mutation. *J. Biol. Chem.* 264 (1989) 21302–21307

Jackson, M. R., McCarthy, L. R., Hardy, D., Wilson, S., Coughtrie, M. W. H. and Burchell, B. Cloning of a human liver UDP-glucuronosyltransferase cDNA. *Biochem. J.* 242 (1987) 581–588

Labrune, P., Myara, A., Hennion, C., Gout, J. P., Trivin, F. and Odievre, M. Crigler–Najjar type II disease inheritance: a family study. *J. Inher. Metab. Dis.* 12 (1989) 302–306

Laemmli, U. K. Cleavage of structural proteins during the assembly of the head of bacteriophage T. *Nature* 227 (1970) 680–685

Lowry, O. H., Rosebrough, N. J., Farr, A. L. and Randall, R. J. Protein measurement with the Folin phenol reagent. *J. Biol. Chem.* 193 (1951) 265–275

Muraca, M. and Blanckaert, N. Liquid chromatographic assay and identification of mono- and diester conjugates of bilirubin in normal serum. *Clin. Chem.* 29 (1983) 1767–1771

Odell, G. B., Mogilevsky, W. S. and Gourley, G. R. High performance liquid chromatographic analysis of bile pigments as their native tetrapyrroles and as their dipyrrolic azosulfanilate derivatives. *J. Chromatog.* 529 (1990) 287–298

Onishi, S., Itoh, S., Kawade, N., Isobe, K. and Sugiyama, S. An accurate and sensitive analysis by high pressure liquid chromatography of conjugated and unconjugated bilirubin IX in various biological fluids. *Biochem. J.* 185 (1980) 281–284

Otani, G., Abou-el-Makarem, M. M. and Bock, K. W. UDP-Glucuronosyltransferase in perfused rat liver and in microsomes. III – Effects of galactosamine and carbon tetrachloride on the glucuronidation of 1-naphthol and bilirubin. *Biochem. Pharmacol.* 25 (1976) 1293–1297

Owens, D. and Evans, J. Population studies on Gilbert's syndrome. *J. Med. Genet.* 12 (1975) 152–156

Puig, J. F. and Tephly, T. R. Isolation and purification of rat liver morphine UDP-glucuronosyltransferase. *Mol. Pharmacol.* 30 (1986) 558–565

Sato, H., Koiwai, O., Tanabe, K. and Kashiwamota, S. Isolation and sequencing of rat liver bilirubin UDP-glucuronosyltransferase cDNA: Possible alternative splicing of a common primary transcript. *Biochem. Biophys. Res. Commun.* 169 (1990) 260–264

Schmid, R. and McDonagh, A. F. Hyperbilirubinemia. In: Stanbury, J. B., Wyngaarden, J. B. and Fredrickson, D. S. (eds.), *The Metabolic Basis of Inherited Disease*, 4th edn., McGraw-Hill, New York, 1978, pp. 1221–57

Shepherd, S. R. P., Baird, S. J., Hallinan, T. and Burchell, B. An investigation of the transverse topology of bilirubin UDP-glucuronosyltransferase in rat hepatic endoplasmic reticulum. *Biochem. J.* 259 (1989) 617–620

Strebel, L. and Odell, G. B. Bilirubin uridine diphospho-glucuronosyltransferase in rat liver microsomes: Genetic variation and maturation. *Pediatr. Res.* 5 (1971) 548–59

Svensson, J-O., Rane, A., Sawe, J. and Sjoqvist, F. Determination of morphine, morphine-3-glucuronide and (tentatively) morphine-6-glucuronide in plasma and urine using ion-pair, high performance liquid chromatography. *J. Chromatog.* 230 (1982) 427–432

Szabo, L. and Ebrey, P. B. Studies on the inheritance of Crigler–Najjar syndrome by the menthol test. *Acta Paediatr. Hung.* 4 (1963) 153–158

Towbin, H., Staehelin, T. and Gordon, J. Electrophoretic transfer of proteins from polyacrylamide gels to nitrocellulose sheets: procedures and some applications. *Proc. Natl. Acad. Sci. USA* 76 (1979) 4350–4354

Van Es, H., Goldhoorn, B., Paul-Abrahamse, M., Oude-Elferink, R. P. J. and Jansen, P. L. M. Immunochemical analysis of UDP-glucuronosyltransferase in four patients with Crigler–Najjar type I syndrome. *J. Clin. Invest.* 85 (1990) 1199–1205

Van Roy, P. and Heirwegh, K. P. M. Determination of bilirubin glucuronide and assay of glucuronosyltransferase with bilirubin as acceptor. *Biochem. J.* 107 (1968) 507–518

Vanstapel, F. and Blanckaert, N. Topology and regulation of bilirubin UDP-glucuronosyltransferase in sealed native microsomes from rat liver. *Arch. Biochem. Biophys.* 263 (1988) 216–225

Wolkoff, A. W., Roy Chowdhury, J. and Arias, I. M. Hereditary jaundice and disorders of bilirubin metabolism. In: Stanbury, J.B., Wyngaarden, J. B. and Fredrickson, D. S. (eds.), *The Metabolic Basis of Inherited Disease*, 5th edn., McGraw-Hill, New York, 1983, pp. 1385–1420

J. Inher. Metab. Dis. 14 (1991) 580–595
© SSIEM and Kluwer Academic Publishers.

Niemann–Pick Disease Type C: An Update

M.T. Vanier[1,2], P. Pentchev[3], C. Rodriguez-Lafrasse[1] and R. Rousson[1]

[1]*Department of Biochemistry, INSERM U 189, Faculté de Médecine Lyon-Sud, BP 12 , F-69921 Oullins Cedex, France;* [2]*Fondation Gillet-Mérieux, Centre Hospitalier Lyon-Sud, F-69310 Pierre-Bénite, France;* [3]*Developmental and Metabolic Neurology Branch, National Institute of Neurological Disorders and Stroke, National Institutes of Health, Bethesda, MD 20892, USA*

Summary: The concept of Niemann–Pick disease type C as a secondary sphingomyelin storage disorder (in contrast to the sphingomyelinase-deficient types A and B) has become more and more prevalent, in view of the complex lipid storage pattern and variable sphingomyelinase activities. Although the primary lesion is still unknown, studies conducted over the past six years have led to a breakthrough by showing that this disorder is characterized by unique abnormalities of intracellular translocation of exogenous cholesterol. In cultured fibroblasts of patients, this block leads to a delayed induction of the homeostatic responses to exogenous cholesterol, in particular cholesteryl ester formation, and to the accumulation of unesterified cholesterol in a vesicular, essentially lysosomal, compartment. The transport of endogenous cholesterol is apparently unaffected. The spectrum of phenotypic heterogeneity in relation to abnormal LDL-processing has been defined in a large patient population. Clinical presentation of the disease is also reviewed and biochemical correlations are discussed. This discovery has had immediate medical applications, by providing the first strategy for reliable prenatal diagnosis of the disorder and easy diagnosis of patients. To date, the exact implication of the cholesterol transport defect in the pathogenesis of Niemann–Pick type C is not known; recent observations have opened up new possible approaches for the understanding of this lesion. Although final classification of Niemann–Pick disease type C must await elucidation of the primary defect(s), present knowledge already establishes that the disease is a nosological entity distinct from Niemann–Pick disease type A and B, and suggests that it might be the model for a new molecular concept of neurolipidosis — and even of inherited metabolic disease.

Niemann–Pick disease constitutes a clinically and biochemically heterogeneous group of recessively inherited disorders sharing accumulation of variable amounts of sphingomyelin in liver and spleen, historically divided in four main subtypes, A to D (Crocker, 1961; Fredrickson and Sloan, 1972). In type C, the substantially smaller increase in tissue sphingomyelin content compared to that in type A and B was already emphasized by Crocker (1961). Subsequent biochemical characterization of

Niemann–Pick disease established a primary sphingomyelinase (EC 3.1.4.12) deficiency in types A and B, while the concept of Niemann–Pick type C as a secondary sphingomyelin storage disease increased in strength in view of the complex lipid storage pattern and the lack of consistent defects in sphingomyelinase observed in this disorder (Brady, 1983; Vanier *et al.*, 1986; Spence and Callahan, 1989). At a meeting held in Prague in 1983, a consensus was reached to separate the 'sphingomyelinase-deficient' forms, designated as Niemann–Pick disease group I (including types A and B), from the other forms, or Niemann–Pick disease group II (including types C and D) (Elleder and Jirasek, 1983), a distinction that has since gained general acceptance (Spence and Callahan, 1989).

A new approach to characterizing the latter group, which changed from the study of sphingomyelin catabolism to focus on intracellular cholesterol processing, soon led to a breakthrough in the understanding of the underlying biochemical lesion in Niemann–Pick disease type C. Studies conducted over the past six years, which will be reviewed below, have shown that this disorder is characterized by unique abnormalities of intracellular translocation of exogenous cholesterol. This discovery has had immediate medical implications by providing the first strategy for reliable prenatal diagnosis of the disorder (Vanier *et al.*, 1989) and facilitated the diagnosis of patients. Subsequent and current studies have aimed at unravelling the causal mechanism. To date, the exact relationship between the cholesterol transport defect and the primary molecular lesion(s?) is still unknown. Although final classification of Niemann–Pick disease type C must await elucidation of the primary defect(s), present knowledge already establishes that the disease is a nosological entity distinct from Niemann–Pick disease types A and B, and suggests it might be the model for a new molecular concept of neurolipidosis, and even of inherited metabolic disease.

SPECTRUM OF CLINICAL PHENOTYPES

The variability of clinical phenotypes encountered in Niemann–Pick type C has been discussed in several recent articles or reviews (Vanier *et al.*, 1988a; Fink *et al.*, 1989; Spence and Callahan, 1989). The following review is largely based upon our experience of 125 clinically and biochemically defined patients studied in the laboratory.

Although neurological deterioration is a central characteristic of the disease, severe liver involvement may occur in the first months of life, before the onset of any neurological symptom, and even prenatal manifestations (fetal ascites) have been reported (Manocochie *et al.*, 1989, and unpublished personal observations). Prolonged neonatal icterus with predominantly conjugated hyperbilirubinaemia and progressive hepatosplenomegaly has been observed in nearly half of the patients for whom information regarding this period of life was obtained. In most cases, the jaundice spontaneously regressed between the second and the fourth months of life, but a rapid worsening of the condition leading to liver failure and death before the end of the first half-year could occur (Guibaud *et al.*, 1979; Jaeken *et al.*, 1980). This *severe neonatal cholestatic rapidly fatal form*, which constituted 12% of our cases, has often been misdiagnosed ('neonatal hepatitis') in the past. Classification of the other patients is best achieved from the analysis of the neurological symptomatology, more especially the age of onset and type of first symptom. Figure 1 gives an outline of the age of neurological onset in our patient population, and illustrates the wide heterogeneity observed.

In the *severe infantile form*, hypotonia and delay of developmental motor milestones were the first symptoms and became evident around the age of 1–1.5 years. The subsequent clinical course included a loss of acquired motor skills, mental regression being proportionally less marked and, finally, spasticity with pyramidal tract involvement. Intention tremor was often noted, but supranuclear paresis of the vertical gaze was usually absent, and these children seldom developed epilepsy. Hepatosplenomegaly (mild to severe) was present. Many of these patients died between the ages of 3 and 5 years. This form was observed in 30% of our patients.

Cerebellar involvement is one of the prominent features of the *late infantile form* and the *juvenile form*, the most common clinical subtypes (respectively 23% and 30% in our series). The first evident manifestation in children with a neurological onset by the age of 3–5 years was most often an ataxic gait. In those aged 6–12 years, poor school performance due to a combination of mental regression and coordination problems, especially of fine hand movements, was in many cases the first symptom. Later symptoms included ataxia, dysarthria, cataplectic attacks, epileptic manifestations, in some cases prominent dystonic features. Finally, in these patients, vertical supranuclear ophthalmoplegia was almost invariable from the age of 6–7 years. Progressive mental regression was a general observation, although the timing and the severity of the downward course varied considerably. Severe visceromegaly was rarely observed; a moderate, sometimes transient (hepato)splenomegaly was the most common finding; however, repeated absence of clinically detectable hepatosplenomegaly was found in approximately 10% of the cases. Many of these patients died in

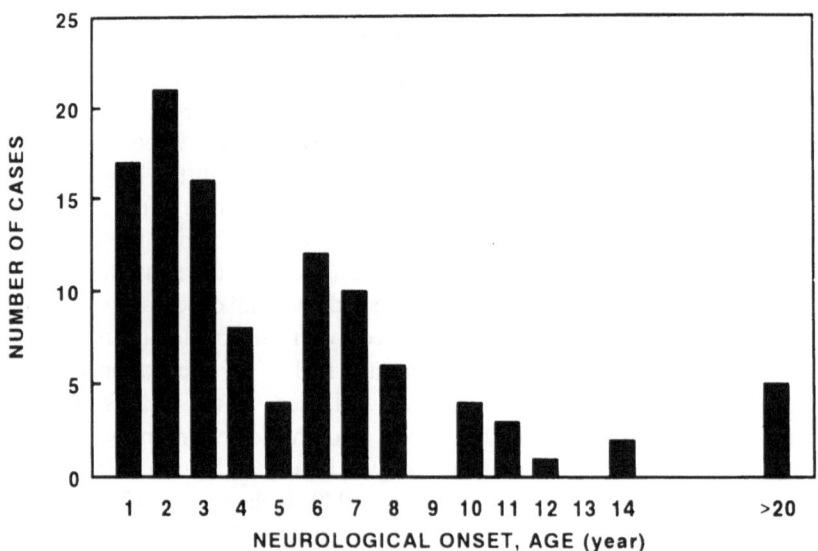

Figure 1 Age at onset of neurological symptoms in a population of 125 patients with Niemann–Pick disease type C

their second decade, with a trend for patients with a late infantile onset to die earliest. However, several of them are still alive in their twenties.

Very few Niemann–Pick type C cases with an *adult onset* (Longstreth *et al.*, 1982) have so far been reported, but their number might have been underestimated owing to the previous difficulty of biochemical confirmation. In our series, this form, which presented with the symptomatology of an attenuated juvenile form or with prominent psychiatric involvement, constituted 5% of the cases.

Patients with Niemann–Pick type C have been described under many different names, such as juvenile dystonic lipidosis, DAF syndrome and neurovisceral storage disorder with vertical supranuclear ophthalmoplegia (see Spence and Callahan, 1989, for review). Biochemical studies also permitted definitive reassessment of the one described case of lactosylceramidosis (Dawson *et al.*, 1971) as infantile Niemann–Pick type C (Vanier *et al.*, 1988a).

MAIN CHARACTERISTICS OF THE LIPID STORAGE PATTERN

Liver and spleen

In contrast with Niemann–Pick disease types A and B, in which a massive (20–50 times normal value) sphingomyelin accumulation is largely predominant over other ancillary lipid changes, the lipid storage pattern observed in type C is that of a complex lipidosis, with a moderate increase of sphingomyelin, but also of bis(monoacylglycero)phosphate, of glucosylceramide and of unesterified cholesterol (for review, see Brady, 1983; Spence and Callahan, 1989). In our experience, the changes were always more pronounced in spleen (5 times the normal concentration for sphingomyelin, 2–3 times for unesterified cholesterol, 20–30 times for glucosylceramide) than in liver, although of a similar type in both tissues (Vanier, 1983). Finally, the lipid storage was almost as pronounced in fetal tissues as in the final stage of the disease (Vanier *et al.*, 1988b); this is a unique situation compared to any of the sphingolipidoses, suggesting a distinct accumulation mechanism.

Brain

We have been able to study (Vanier *et al.*, 1988b) the brain tissue of 7 cases (age at death ranging from 3 months up to 19 years), covering the spectrum of clinical phenotypes to the exception of the adult form. In accordance with previous studies (Spence and Callahan, 1989), no abnormal increase of sphingomyelin or of unesterified cholesterol was found in cerebral cortex. In white matter, the concentration of these lipids was decreased in relation to the degree of demyelination, which ranged from nil (cholestatic rapidly fatal form) or mild (older cases) to severe (neurological infantile form). But significant alterations of the glycolipids were observed in cerebral cortex from all the patients. The ganglioside profiles were modified, with a uniform 5–10-fold elevation of the GM3 and GM2 species, and a compensatory slight diminution of GD1a and GD1b. Glucosylceramide showed the most striking (20–50-fold) increase. Abnormal levels of lactosylceramide and gangliotriaosylceramide were also found. These data emphasize that in Niemann–Pick type C brain abnormalities are primarily located in the grey matter, confirm the glycolipid nature of the neuronal storage (Elleder *et al.*, 1985), and establish that a similar type of changes occurs in the different clinical forms of the disease.

SPHINGOMYELINASE ACTIVITY

Sphingomyelinase activity (reviewed by Brady, 1983, and by Spence and Callahan, 1989) has shown normal or elevated levels in leukocytes, liver, spleen or brain tissue, while a partial deficiency has been reported in cultured skin fibroblasts of a majority (60–70%) of patients, using the conventional *in vitro* assay or measuring the degradation of radiolabelled sphingomyelin added to the culture medium of living fibroblasts. In cultured cells, a modulation of sphingomyelinase activity in relation to the presence or absence of lipoproteins in the culture medium, with an adverse effect of LDL, has recently been reported (Thomas *et al.*, 1989; Vanier *et al.*, 1991).

ABNORMAL INTRACELLULAR CHOLESTEROL METABOLISM IN CULTURED SKIN FIBROBLASTS

These investigations were initiated by the discovery of a mutant mouse with a neurovisceral disease associated with a lipid storage pattern very similar to that in Niemann–Pick type C (Pentchev *et al.*, 1980), in which intracellular cholesterol storage was shown to be associated with a deficiency in the esterification of exogenously derived cholesterol in cultured skin fibroblasts (Pentchev *et al.*, 1984). These studies soon led to the key findings that Niemann–Pick type C fibroblasts were uniquely and severely deficient in their ability to esterify exogenously derived cholesterol, despite apparently normal acyl-CoA:cholesterol acyltransferase (EC 2.3.1.26) activity (Pentchev *et al.*, 1985, 1986), and stored abnormal amounts of unesterified cholesterol in an intracellular vesicular compartment when cultured in a cholesterol-containing medium (Pentchev *et al.*, 1985; Kruth *et al.*, 1986). Fully normal results were observed in Niemann–Pick type A and type B fibroblasts, providing an ultimate argument to dissociate type C from the sphingomyelinase-deficient types of Niemann–Pick disease.

Regulatory responses to LDL-derived cholesterol show a delayed induction

Further characterization of cholesterol metabolism in mutant Niemann–Pick type C cell lines demonstrated that low-density lipoproteins (LDL) were internalized and transported to the lysosome, in which both their protein and their lipid moieties were normally hydrolysed. However, as illustrated in Figure 2, all three major control mechanisms associated with intracellular cholesterol homeostasis, namely (1) up-regulation of acyl-CoA:cholesterol acyltransferase, the key enzyme in the regulation of intracellular cholesterol esterification, (2) down-regulation of 3-hydroxy-3-methyl-glutaryl CoA reductase (EC 1.1.1.34), the rate-limiting enzyme in *de novo* synthesis of cholesterol, (3) down-regulation of the LDL-receptors mediating LDL internalization, showed a considerably delayed induction (Pentchev *et al.*, 1986, 1987; Liscum and Faust, 1987). In parallel, the unesterified cholesterol content of Niemann–Pick type

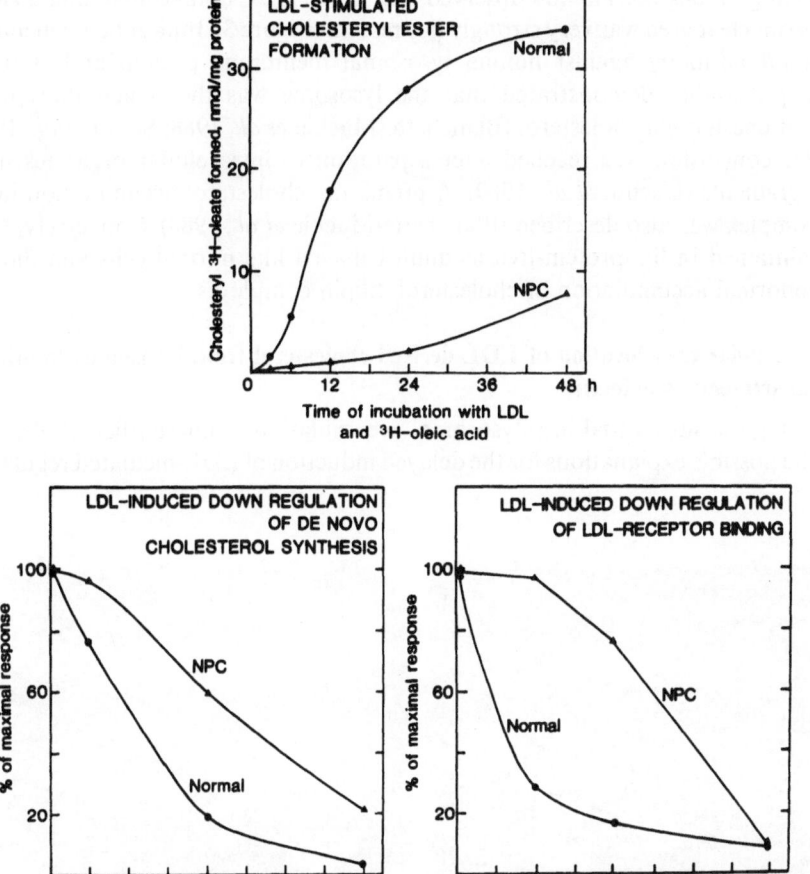

Figure 2 Regulatory responses to LDL-derived cholesterol in skin fibroblast cultures. Delayed induction in Niemann–Pick disease type C. (Adapted from Pentchev *et al.*, 1987)

C cells, which was essentially identical to that of normal cells after 3 days of culture in lipoprotein-deficient medium, increased continuously during the first 48 h of LDL uptake, as the result of impaired regulatory responses (Pentchev *et al.*, 1986, 1987). All three responses could, however, be normally mediated by mevalonate (Liscum and Faust, 1987), suggesting a normal endogenous pathway, and by 25-hydroxycholesterol (a soluble derivative that bypasses the lysosome), providing a confirmation of the functional integrity of acyl-CoA : cholesterol acyltransferase and emphasizing the role of the lysosome in the intracellular cholesterol dysregulation.

The lysosome is the preferential site of storage of unesterified cholesterol

Filipin, a fluorescent histochemical probe specific for unesterified cholesterol, proved an invaluable tool in the study of the intracellular cholesterol storage. In Niemann–Pick type C cells cultured in presence of LDL, an abnormally high level of intracellular fluorescent granules was already observed after 2 h of LDL uptake, and after 24 h the entire perinuclear area was very strongly fluorescent (Figure 3). Immunocytochemistry using a rat antibody against human lysosomal membrane protein and electron-microscopic studies demonstrated that the lysosome was the preferential site of storage of unesterified cholesterol (Blanchette-Mackie *et al.*, 1988; Sokol *et al.*, 1988). A similar conclusion was reached after separation of intracellular organites using Percoll gradients (Liscum *et al.*, 1989). A premature cholesterol accumulation in the Golgi complex was also described (Blanchette-Mackie *et al.*, 1988). Conversely, NPC cells maintained in lipoprotein-free medium behaved like normal cells and did not show abnormal accumulation of cholesterol–filipin complexes.

The intracellular translocation of LDL-derived cholesterol from lysosomes to other cell compartments is defective

Considering the substantial intralysosomal accumulation of unesterified cholesterol, one of the possible explanations for the delayed induction of LDL-mediated regulatory

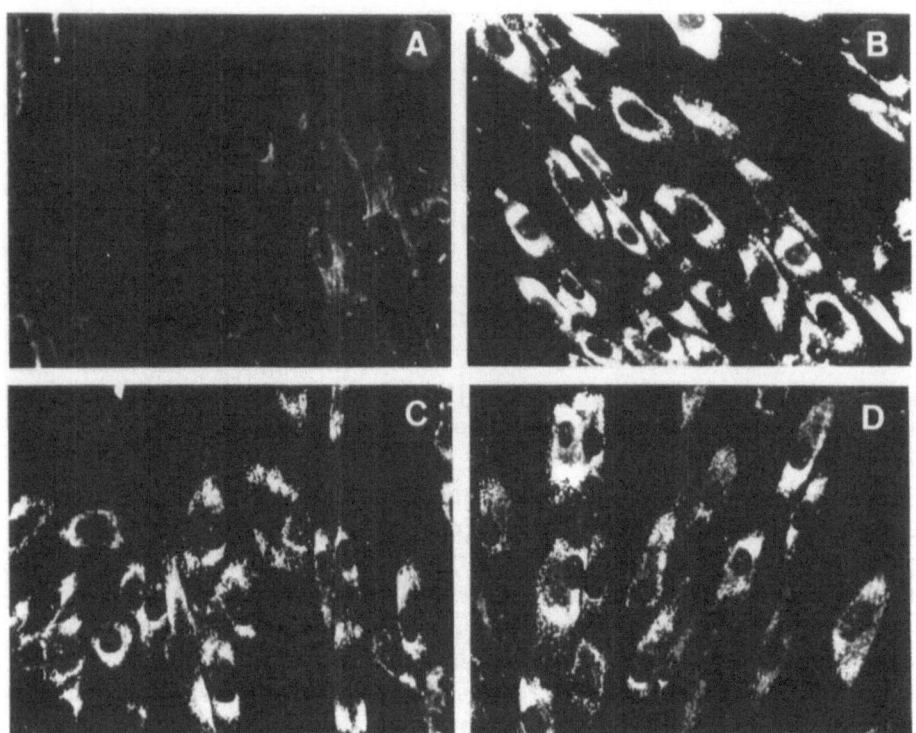

Figure 3   Localization of unesterified cholesterol by filipin staining in cultured skin fibroblasts grown in presence of LDL. Abnormal vesicular accumulation in Niemann–Pick disease type C. A, Normal subject. B, Classical Niemann–Pick type C. C, Intermediate Niemann–Pick type C homozygote. D, Variant Niemann–Pick type C homozygote. (Adapted from Vanier *et al.*, 1991)

responses could be a defective translocation of cholesterol from lysosomes to the site(s) of regulation (Liscum *et al.*, 1987; Mazière *et al.*, 1987; Pentchev *et al.*, 1987). The finding that *in vitro* esterification of cellular cholesterol was defective in cell homogenates with intact organelles but not in disrupted homogenates (Sokol *et al.*, 1988) supported the hypothesis of an abnormal sequestration of LDL-derived cholesterol in a metabolically latent pool. Further, a decreased rate of transport of cholesterol from the lysosome to the plasma membrane, studied by feeding the cells with LDL labelled with [^{3}H]cholesteryl linoleate and measuring the rate of appearance of labelled cholesterol in the medium (Liscum *et al.*, 1989) or at the plasma membrane (Argoff *et al.*, 1991), has been documented. Transport of endocytosed [^{3}H]cholesterol to the endoplasmic reticulum also appears to be impaired (Argoff *et al.*, 1991). On the contrary, the transport of endogenously synthesized cholesterol to the plasma membrane (Liscum *et al.*, 1989), and of cholesterol inserted in the plasma membrane to the endoplasmic reticulum (Slotte *et al.*, 1989) seems to occur at a normal rate. Available data thus lead to the conclusion that there is defective intracellular translocation of LDL-derived (and more generally, of exogenous) cholesterol in Niemann–Pick type C.

SPECIFICITY OF CHOLESTEROL METABOLISM ALTERATIONS

Cell lines from a large number of lysosomal and/or neurological diseases other than Niemann–Pick type C and from disorders affecting cholesterol metabolism have been studied to assess the specificity of the abnormalities in intracellular cholesterol processing described above (Pentchev *et al.*, 1985; Inui *et al.*, 1989; Omura *et al.*, 1989;Vanier *et al.*, 1991). LDL-mediated regulatory responses were affected in disorders with impaired LDL internalization (familial hypercholesterolaemia) or lysosomal hydrolysis (acid lipase deficiencies), but without abnormal intracellular accumulation of unesterified cholesterol assessed by histochemical filipin staining. Zellweger syndrome, in which alterations of sterol-carrier-protein 2 have been reported, showed no abnormality. Only I-cell disease displayed both deficient regulatory responses and an abnormal storage of unesterified cholesterol evaluated by filipin staining, which could at least in part be explained by the documented impaired lysosomal hydrolysis of the LDL. All other pathological states investigated gave normal results.

Our experience to date is that the best biochemical markers for diagnosis of patients are the study in cultured cells of the early phase (first 4–6 hours) of LDL-induced cholesteryl ester formation, combined with the histochemical evaluation (filipin staining after 24 h of LDL uptake) of the LDL-induced intracellular accumulation of unesterified cholesterol. These tests have been described in detail and are applicable to cultured skin fibroblasts (Vanier *et al.*, 1988a, 1991), cultured lymphocytes (Argoff *et al.*, 1990) and cultured chorionic villus cells or amniotic fluid cells (Vanier *et al.*, 1989). Cholesteryl ester formation studied with a non-lipoprotein [^{3}H]cholesterol source, the method initially proposed as a diagnostic test, has been shown not to permit identification of all patients (Vanier *et al.*, 1988a, b), as discussed below.

SPECTRUM OF BIOCHEMICAL ABNORMALITIES OF CHOLESTEROL METABOLISM: CORRELATION WITH CLINICAL PHENOTYPES

The above strategy, applied to fibroblast cultures from 125 Niemann–Pick type C patients (Vanier *et al.*, 1991) established that abnormalities of intracellular cholesterol metabolism are a constant feature of the disease, but also disclosed a variable phenotypic expression. Profound alterations (esterification rates less than 10% of normal with numerous intensely fluorescent cholesterol–filipin granules) were demonstrated in 86% of cases, depicting the '*classical*' *Niemann–Pick type C phenotype*. In these cases, esterification studied with a non-lipoprotein cholesterol source (Pentchev *et al.*, 1985; Vanier *et al.*, 1988a,b; Fink *et al.*, 1989; Inui *et al.*, 1989; Omura *et al.*, 1989) was also profoundly deficient. The remaining cell lines showed a graded, less severe impairment (Figure 4) and more transient delay in the induction of LDL-mediated cholesteryl esterification, along with an attenuated accumulation of

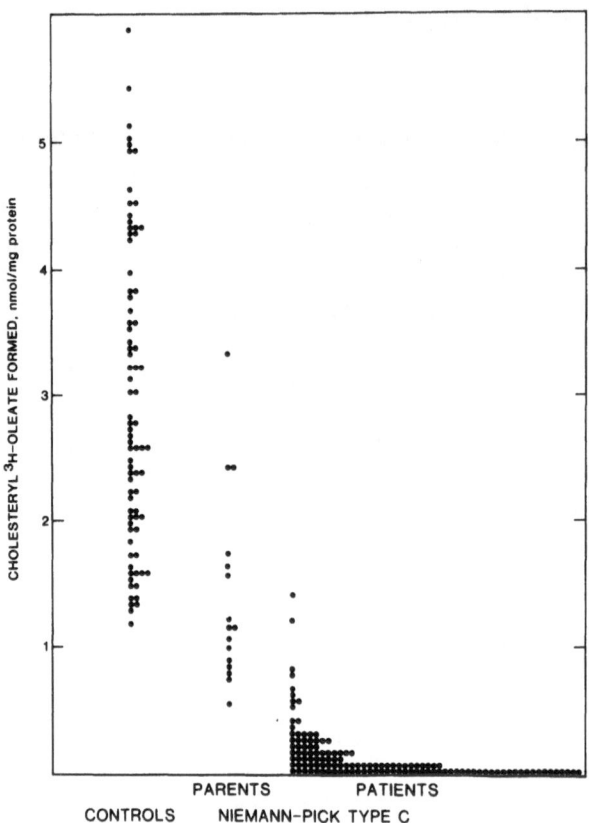

Figure 4 Cumulative rates of cholesteryl ester synthesis after 4.5 h of LDL uptake in cultured skin fibroblasts from control subjects, patients with Niemann–Pick disease type C and obligate heterozygotes. Rates are expressed as the difference between the levels of cholesteryl [³H]oleate formed in the presence and in the absence of lipoproteins. (Adapted from Vanier *et al.*, 1991)

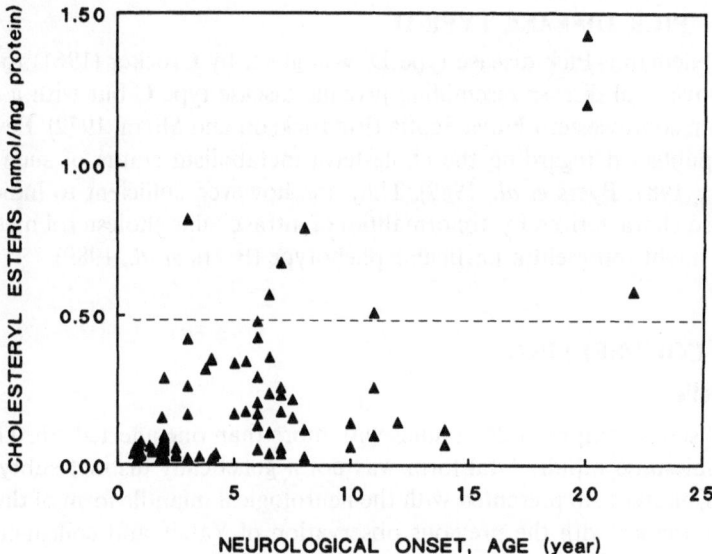

Figure 5 Coorrelation between the clinical subtype (evaluated from the age at onset of neurological symptoms) of Niemann–Pick disease type C patients and the rate of LDL-induced cholesteryl ester formation in their skin fibroblast cultures. The dotted line distinguishes the 'variant' biochemical phenotype (cholesteryl ester formation > 0.5 nmol/mg protein) from the classical and intermediate groups

unesterified cholesterol (Figure 5). In particular, cells from a small group of patients showed only slight alterations of esterification, restricted to the early phase of LDL uptake (Vanier *et al.*, 1991; Argoff *et al.*, 1991) and the diagnosis was reached by demonstration of an abnormal cholesterol–filipin fluorescence, which, although moderate, was evident (Figure 3) provided pure LDL were used and rigorous experimental conditions were followed. This group, comprising 7% of the cases, has been referred to as the '*variant*' *phenotype*. A third, less clearly individualized group (7%) of patients, differing from the classical phenotype mostly by higher rates of cholesteryl ester formation (10–15% of the mean normal value using a lipoprotein cholesterol source but up to 60% using a non-lipoprotein source), has been designated as the '*intermediate phenotype*' to encompass a more difficult diagnosis of such patients and its bearing in terms of genetic counselling (see below). The significance of this phenotypic variation in terms of genetic heterogeneity has still to be demonstrated.

The correlation between the severity of alteration in intracellular cholesterol homeostasis and the clinical phenotype has been studied by us in 80 cases, and the results are outlined in Figure 5. Patients with the cholestatic rapidly fatal form (not included in the figure) and the severe infantile form (24 cases) invariably belonged to the 'classical' biochemical phenotype. Conversely, the 3 cases with an adult onset were included in the 'variant' group. However, cases with a late-infantile or juvenile form had an unpredictable biochemical behaviour.

NIEMANN–PICK DISEASE TYPE D

The name 'Niemann–Pick disease type D' was given by Crocker (1961) to patients with a neurovisceral disease resembling juvenile disease type C but with a common ancestry from southwestern Nova Scotia (Fredrickson and Sloan, 1972). Few studies have been published regarding the cholesterol metabolism status of such patients (Butler *et al.*, 1987; Byers *et al.*, 1989). They are, however, sufficient to indicate that type D is also characterized by abnormalities of intracellular cholesterol metabolism, although it might represent a particular phenotype (Byers *et al.*, 1989).

GENETIC COUNSELLING

Familial studies

Our clinical series comprised 24 families with more than one affected sib. The severe neonatal cholestatic rapidly fatal form was not a genetically distinct subtype, since in 5 families, another sib presented with the neurological infantile form of the disease, in good accordance with the previous observation of Yatziv and colleagues (1983). Otherwise, a similar clinical subtype and rather comparable course of the disease was the usual rule in siblings.

In our laboratory, cholesterol homeostasis could be studied in skin fibroblasts of 14 pairs of siblings. The results were consistent with a given biochemical phenotype within a family, an important observation with regard to prenatal diagnosis.

Prenatal diagnosis

Definition of the biochemical phenotype of the index case appeared an absolute prerequisite to adequate genetic counselling in a given family. Prenatal diagnosis has now proved a safe procedure in families with the classical biochemical phenotype, from our experience of 27 pregnancies at risk monitored to-date, mostly using cultured chorionic villus cells (Vanier *et al.*, 1989, and unpublished results). Other laboratories have reached the same conclusion (D. Wenger, Philadelphia; M. Zeigler, Jerusalem, personal communications). However, prenatal diagnosis is clearly not feasible at present in the 'variant' families and, in our opinion, not totally reliable in families with an 'intermediate' phenotype.

CELLULAR LEVEL OF THE CHOLESTEROL METABOLISM DEFECT: WORKING HYPOTHESES

Although progress has been made in delineating the mechanism of cholesterol movement from its site of synthesis in the endoplasmic reticulum to the plasma membrane, the mechanism(s) of intracellular transport of LDL-derived cholesterol from the lysosome to other cellular sites is essentially unknown. Type C Niemann–Pick disease might prove to be a very useful model leading to a better understanding of the latter pathway. A first question, yet unanswered, is to define whether the lysosomal sequestration of unesterified cholesterol observed in Niemann–Pick type C is due to a defect directly affecting the lysosomal egress of the compound, or to a more distal block, the lysosome then playing the role of a reservoir.

One or several of four sequential steps could in theory be altered: (1) delivery of newly released cholesterol to the lysosomal membrane; (2) active passage or flip-flop through the lysosomal membrane; (3) transport by acceptor particles/sterol-carrier protein(s); (4) activation of the regulatory responses.

Experimental data are scarce. It has been shown that acyl-CoA:cholesterol acyltransferase, hydroxymethylglutaryl CoA reductase and LDL-receptor synthesis can be regulated normally in Niemann–Pick type C cells by the endogenous pathway or by 25-hydroxycholesterol (Liscum and Faust, 1987). There is no support for a topologically misplaced acyl-CoA:cholesterol acyltransferase (Sokol *et al.*, 1988). Although a block in the formation of a putative regulatory metabolite cannot be ruled out, such a metabolite has not been demonstrated in normal cells. In Niemann–Pick type C cells, it has, however, been suggested that decreased cholesterol substrate availability is only partly responsible for the observed esterification defect (Byers *et al.*, 1989). To date, there is no published study of sterol-carrier proteins in Niemann–Pick type C tissues, nor of cholesterol egress from type C lysosomes, and none of the above hypotheses can really be favoured. Another important observation to be kept in mind is that transport of LDL-derived cholesterol is not blocked, but rather retarded. From available experimental data, it cannot be ruled out that a concomitant impairment of several of the above steps could be under the dependence of a common factor, possibly related to a more general membrane disturbance.

RELATIONSHIP BETWEEN ALTERATIONS OF CHOLESTEROL PROCESSING AND THE PRIMARY LESION

Can the observed alterations in cholesterol processing explain most of the biochemical features of the disease?

The finding of variable but statistically significant alterations of LDL-induced cholesterol homeostasis in skin fibroblast cultures from Niemann–Pick type C obligate heterozygotes (Kruth *et al.*, 1986; Vanier *et al.*, 1988a, 1991; and Figure 4) suggests that these modifications are in close relationship to the primary lesion. Recent studies (Thomas *et al.*, 1989; Vanier *et al.*, 1991) also indicate that in Niemann–Pick type C patients impaired sphingomyelin catabolism might be under the influence of cholesterol metabolism abnormalities. But there is yet no such evidence to explain the pronounced glycolipid abnormalities, and even less to explain the morphological and lipid changes in brain tissue.

Several cationic amphiphilic agents can mimic the Niemann–Pick type C phenotype in normal cultured cells

We have underlined previously (Vanier *et al.*, 1986) the similarities between the lipid storage pattern observed in Niemann–Pick type C and that in lipidoses induced *in vivo* or in cell cultures by a large number of drugs with a common cationic amphiphilic structure. Of interest is also the marked reduction of sphingomyelinase activity induced in cell culture by many of these agents. More recently, it has been shown that a number of such compounds, in particular imipramine (Rodriguez-Lafrasse *et al.*, 1990), but also propranolol, chlorpromazine, W7, AY9944 (Mason *et al.*, 1990; Rodriquez-Lafrasse *et al.*, 1990; Yoshikawa and Sakuragawa, 1990), added to fibroblast cultures to a concentration that did not affect lysosomal hydrolysis of low-density lipoproteins, induced an intracellular accumulation of unesterified cholesterol and a delay in LDL-mediated regulatory responses, due to impaired mobilization of LDL-derived cholesterol. Similar results have been obtained with the cholesterol synthesis inhibitor U18666A (Liscum and Faust, 1989; Liscum, 1990), which appears also to be a hydrophobic weak base amine, and more recently, with stearylamine and sphinganine (Roff *et al.*, 1990).

Elucidation of the mechanism by which these agents act upon intracellular transport of exogenously derived cholesterol, which is under current investigation, may cast a new light on the pathogenesis of Niemann–Pick type C (abnormal production of a 'toxic' metabolite?). In particular, the hypothesis of a possible involvement of sphingoid bases, with their assumed regulatory functions, opens up an exciting new aspect of research.

CONCLUSION

Available data have convincingly demonstrated that in Niemann–Pick type C, defective intracellular transport of exogenously derived cholesterol is a pathognomonic abnormality closely (but not necessarily immediately) related to the primary defect. Although this defect is still elusive, Niemann–Pick type C already qualifies as an original model among inherited metabolic disorders.

ACKNOWLEDGEMENTS

We are greatly indebted to all paediatricians and other colleagues who kindly provided us with detailed clinical data from their patients.

REFERENCES

Argoff, C. E., Kaneski, C. R., Blanchette-Mackie, E. J., Comly, M., Dwyer, N. K., Brown, A., Brady, R. O. and Pentchev, P. G. Type C Niemann–Pick disease: documentation of abnormal LDL processing in lymphocytes. *Biochem. Biophys. Res. Commun.* 171 (1990) 38–45

Argoff, C. E., Comly, M. E., Blanchette-Mackie, J., Kruth, H. S., Pye, H. T., Goldin, E., Kaneski, C., Vanier, M. T., Brady, R. O. and Pentchev, P. Type C Niemann–Pick disease: Cellular uncoupling of cholesterol homeostasis is linked to the severity of disruption in the intracellular transport of exogenously derived cholesterol. *Biochim. Biophys. Acta* 1906 (1991) (in press)

Blanchette-Mackie, E. J., Dwyer, N. K., Amende, L. M., Kruth, H. S., Butler, J. D., Sokol, J., Comly, M. E., Vanier, M. T., August, J. T., Brady, R. O. and Pentchev, P. G. Type C Niemann–Pick disease: low-density lipoprotein uptake is associated with premature cholesterol accumulation in the Golgi complex and excessive cholesterol storage in lysosomes. *Proc. Natl. Acad. Sci. USA* 85 (1988) 8022–8026

Brady, R. O., Sphingomyelin lipidosis: Niemann–Pick disease. In: Stanbury, J. B., Wyngaarden, J. B., Fredrickson, D. S., Goldstein, J. L. and Brown, M. S. (eds.) *The Metabolic Basis of Inherited Disease.* McGraw-Hill, New York, 1983, pp. 834–841

Butler, J. D., Comly, M. E., Kruth, H. S., Vanier, M. T., Filling Katz, M., Fink, J., Barton, N., Weintroub, H., Quirk, J., Tokoro, T., Marshall, D. C., Brady, R. O. and Pentchev, P. Niemann–Pick variant disorders: comparison of errors of cellular cholesterol homeostasis in group D and group C fibroblasts. *Proc. Natl. Acad. Sci. USA* 84 (1987) 556–560

Byers, D. M., Rastogi, S. R., Cook, H. W., Palmer, F. B. and Spence, M. W. Defective activity of acyl-CoA: cholesterol O-acetyltransferase in Niemann–Pick type C and type D fibroblasts. *Biochem. J.* 262 (1989) 713–719

Crocker, A. C. The cerebral defect in Tay–Sachs disease and Niemann–Pick disease. *J. Neurochem.* 7 (1961) 68–80

Dawson, G., Matalon, R. and Stein, A. O. Lactosylceramidosis: lactosylceramide galactosyl hydrolase deficiency and accumulation of lactosylceramide in cultured skin fibroblasts. *J. Pediatr.* 79 (1971) 423–429

Elleder, M. and Jirasek, A. International symposium on Niemann–Pick disease. *Eur. J. Pediatr.* 140 (1983) 90–91

Elleder, M., Jirasek, A., Smid, F., Ledvinova, J. and Besley, J. T. N. Niemann–Pick disease type C. Study on the nature of the cerebral storage process. *Acta Neuropathol.* 66 (1985) 325–336

Fink, J. K., Filling-Katz, M. R., Sokol, J., Cogan, D. G., Pikus, A., Sonies, B., Soong, B., Pentchev, P. G., Comly, M. E., Brady, R. O. and Barton, N. W. Clinical spectrum of Niemann–Pick disease type C. *Neurology* 39 (1989) 1040–1049

Fredrickson, D. S. and Sloan, H. R. Sphingomyelin lipidosis: Niemann–Pick disease. In: Stanbury, J. B., Wyngaarden, J. B. and Fredrickson, D. S. (eds.) *The Metabolic Basis of Inherited Disease.* McGraw-Hill, New York, 1972, pp. 783–807

Guibaud, P., Vanier, M. T., Malpuech, G., Gaulme, J., Houllemare, R., Goddon, R. and Rousson, R. Forme infantile précoce, cholestatique, rapidement mortelle de la sphingomyelinose de type C. A propos de deux observations. *Pediatrie* 43 (1979) 103–114

Inui, K., Nishimoto, J., Okada, S. and Yabuuchi, H. Impaired cholesterol esterification in cultured skin fibroblasts from patients with I-cell disease and pseudo-Hurler polydystrophy. *Biochem. Int.* 18 (1989) 1129–1135

Jaeken, J., Proesmans, W., Eggermont, E., Van Hoof, F., Den Tandt, W., Standaert, L., Van Herck, G. and Corbeel, L. Niemann–Pick type C disease and early cholestasis in three brothers. *Acta Paediatr. Belg.* 33 (1980) 43–46

Kruth, H. S., Comly, M. E., Butler, J. D., Vanier, M. T., Fink, J. K., Wenger, D. A., Patel, S. and Pentchev, P. G. Type C Niemann–Pick disease. Abnormal metabolism of low-density lipoprotein in homozygous and heterozygous fibroblasts. *J. Biol. Chem.* 261 (1986) 16769–16774

Liscum, L. Pharmacological inhibition of the intracellular transport of low-density lipoprotein-derived cholesterol in Chinese hamster ovary cells. *Biochim. Biophys. Acta* 1045 (1990) 40–48

Liscum, L. and Faust, J. R. Low-density lipoprotein (LDL)-mediated suppression of cholesterol synthesis and LDL uptake is defective in Niemann–Pick type C fibroblasts. *J. Biol. Chem.* 262 (1987) 17002–17008

Liscum, L. and Faust, J. R. The intracellular transport of low density lipoprotein-derived cholesterol is inhibited in chinese hamster ovary cells cultured with 3-β-[2-(diethylamino)-ethoxy]androst-5-en-17-one. *J. Biol. Chem.* 264 (1989) 11796–11806

Liscum, L., Ruggiero, R. M. and Faust, J. R. The intracellular transport of low-density lipoprotein-derived cholesterol is defective in Niemann–Pick disease type C fibroblasts. *J. Cell. Biol.* 108 (1989) 1625–1636

Longstreth, W. T., Daven, J. R., Farell, D. F., Bolen, J. W. and Bird, T. D. Adult dystonic lipidosis: clinical, histologic and biochemical findings of a neurovisceral disease. *Neurology* 32 (1982) 1295–1299

Manocochie, I. K., Chong, S., Mieli-Vergani, G., Lake, B. D. and Mowat, A. P. Fetal ascites: an unusual presentation of Niemann–Pick disease type C. *Arch. Dis. Child.* 64 (1989) 1391–1393

Masson, M., Turpin, J. C., Spezzati, B. and Baumann, N. Defect of exogenous cholesterol ester biosynthesis in cultured fibroblasts in genetic and drug-induced neurolipidoses. *Congrès GERLI*, Nice (1990) Abstr. P48

Mazière, C., Mazière, J. C., Mora, L., Lageron, A., Polonovski, C. and Polonovski, J. Alterations in cholesterol metabolism in cultured fibroblasts from patients with Niemann–Pick disease type C. *J. Inher. Metab. Dis.* 10 (1987) 339–346

Omura, K., Suzuki, Y., Norose, N., Sato, M., Maruyama, K. and Koeda, T. Type C Niemann–Pick disease: clinical and biochemical studies on 6 cases. *Brain Dev.* 11 (1989) 57–61

Pentchev, P. G., Gal, A. E., Booth, A. D., Omodeo-Sale, F., Fouks, J., Neumeyer, B. A., Quirk, J. M., Dawson, G. and Brady, R. O. A lysosomal storage disorder in mice characterized by a dual deficiency of sphingomyelinase and glucocerebrosidase. *Biochim. Biophys. Acta* 619 (1980) 669–679

Pentchev, P. G., Boothe, A. D., Kruth, H. S., Weintroub, H., Stivers, J. and Brady, R. O. A genetic storage disorder in Balb/c mice with a metabolic block in esterification of exogenous cholesterol. *J. Biol. Chem.* 259 (1984) 5784–5791

Pentchev, P. G., Comly, M. E., Kruth, H. S., Vanier, M. T., Wenger, D., Patel, S. and Brady, R. O. A defect in cholesterol esterification in Niemann–Pick disease type C patients. *Proc. Natl. Acad. Sci. USA* 82 (1985) 8247–8251

Pentchev, P. G., Kruth, H. S., Comly, M. E., Butler, J. D., Vanier, M. T., Wenger, D. A. and Patel, S. Type C Niemann–Pick disease. A parallel loss of regulatory responses in both the uptake and esterification of low density lipoprotein-derived cholesterol in cultured fibroblasts. *J. Biol. Chem.* 251 (1986) 16775–16780

Pentchev, P. G., Comly, M. E., Kruth, H. S., Tokoro, T., Butler, J., Sokol, J., Filling-Katz, M., Quirk, J. M., Marshall, D. C., Patel, S., Vanier, M. T. and Brady, R. O. Group C Niemann–Pick disease: faulty regulation of low-density lipoprotein uptake and cholesterol storage in cultured fibroblasts. *Faseb J.* 1 (1987) 40–47

Rodriguez-Lafrasse, C., Rousson, R., Bonnet, J., Pentchev, P., Louisot, P. and Vanier, M. T. Abnormal cholesterol metabolism in imipramine-treated fibroblast cultures. Similarities with Niemann–Pick type C disease. *Biochim. Biophys. Acta* 1043 (1990) 123–128

Roff, C. F., Goldin, E., Comly, M. E., Cooney, A., Brown, A., Vanier, M. T., Miller, S. P. F., Brady, R. O. and Pentchev, P. G. Type C Niemann–Pick disease: use of hydrophobic amines to study defective cholesterol transport. *Devel. Neurosci.* (1991) (in press)

Slotte, J. P., Hedström, G. and Bierman, E. L. Intracellular transport of cholesterol in type C Niemann–Pick fibroblasts. *Biochim. Biophys. Acta* 1005 (1989) 303–309

Sokol, J., Blanchette-Mackie, E. J., Kruth, H. S., Dwyer, N. K., Amende, L. M., Butler, J. D., Robinson, E., Patel, S., Brady, R. O., Comly, M. E., Vanier, M. T. and Pentchev, P. G. Type C Niemann–Pick disease: lysosomal accumulation and defective intracellular mobilization of LDL-cholesterol. *J. Biol. Chem.* 263 (1988) 3411–3417

Spence, M. W. and Callahan, J. W. Sphingomyelin-cholesterol lipidoses: the Niemann–Pick group of diseases. In: Scriver, C. R., Beaudet, A. L., Sly, V. S. and Valle, D. (eds.) *The Metabolic Basis of Inherited Disease*. McGraw-Hill, New York, 1989, pp. 1655–1676

Thomas, G. H., Tuck-Muller, C. M., Miller, C. S. and Reynolds, L. W. Correction of sphingomyelinase deficiency in Niemann–Pick type C fibroblasts by removal of lipoprotein fraction from culture media. *J. Inher. Metab. Dis.* 12 (1989) 139–151

Vanier, M. T. Biochemical studies in Niemann–Pick disease. I — Major sphingolipids of liver and spleen. *Biochim. Biophys. Acta* 750 (1983) 178–184

Vanier, M. T., Rousson, R., Zeitouni, R., Pentchev, P. G. and Louisot, P. Sphingomyelinase and Niemann–Pick disease. In: Freysz, L., Dreyfus, H., Massarelli, R. and Gatt, S. (eds.) *Enzymes of Lipid Metabolism II*. Plenum Press, New York, 1986, pp. 791–802

Vanier, M. T., Wenger, D. A., Comly, M. E., Rousson, R., Brady, R. O. and Pentchev, P. G. Niemann–Pick disease group C: clinical variability and diagnosis based on defective cholesterol esterification. A collaborative study on 70 patients. *Clin. Genet.* 33 (1988a) 331–348

Vanier, M. T., Pentchev, P. G. and Rousson, R. Pathophysiological approach of Niemann–

Pick disease type C; definition of a biochemical heterogeneity and reevaluation of the lipid storage process. In: Salvayre, R., Douste-Blazy, L. and Gatt, S. (eds.) *Lipid Storage Disorders: Biological and Medical Aspects*. Plenum Press, New York, 1988b, pp. 175–185

Vanier, M. T., Rousson, R. M., Mandon, G., Choiset, A., Lake, B. and Pentchev, P. G. Niemann–Pick disease: prenatal diagnosis on cultured chorionic villus cells. *Lancet* 1 (1989) 1014–1015

Vanier, M. T., Rodriguez-Lafrasse, C., Rousson, R., Gazzah, N., Juge, M. C., Pentchev, P., Revol, A. and Louisot, P. Type C Niemann–Pick disease: spectrum of phenotypic variation in disruption of intracellular LDL-derived cholesterol processing. *Biochim. Biophys. Acta* 1096 (1991) (in press)

Yatziv, S., Leibovitz ben Gershon, Z., Ornoy, A. and Bach, G. Clinical heterogeneity in a sibship with Niemann–Pick disease type C. *Clin. Genet.* 23 (1983) 125–131

Yoshikawa, H. and Sakuragawa, N. Reduction of cholesterol esterification in human fibroblasts induced by AY-9944. *5th International Congress of Inborn Errors of Metabolism*, Asilomar (1990) Abstr. P84

J. Inher. Metab. Dis. 14 (1991) 596–603

Paediatric Liver Transplantation: Review of Current Experience

J.A.C. BUCKELS

Liver Unit, Queen Elizabeth Hospital, Birmingham, B15 2TH, UK

Summary: During the 1980s the results of liver replacement in children improved dramatically, with 12-month survival rates rising from around 20% to over 85% at the most experienced centres. This improvement has been due to several factors, including better patient selection and timing of transplantation, advances in immunosuppressive therapy, and developments in liver preservation. Moreover, the learning curve effect has contributed with advances both in surgical technique and in the rapid diagnosis and treatment of complications, including the need to retransplant patients in whom the first graft has been irreversibly damaged. One major development is the refinement of the anatomically reduced grafts where a larger, usually adult, graft is cut down to fit a child. This has allowed a greater number of children to be grafted, including emergency cases such as fulminant hepatic failure in whom there is insufficient time to wait for a size-matched donor.

INTRODUCTION

The first attempt at liver transplantation was performed by Thomas Starzl in 1963. The patient did not survive the early postoperative period nor did several others grafted over the next few years. The first successful transplant was again performed by Starzl in 1967, with the patient surviving for over 12 months only to die from recurrence of the liver tumour that had been the original indication for grafting. Throughout the next 15 years only a small number of liver transplants were performed at a limited number of centres, with survival rates of only 20–30%. Nevertheless, the quality of life in these surviving patients was so good as to encourage these pioneers to persist in their efforts and to continue to refine and improve techniques and postoperative care.

In the early 1980s the introduction of a new and more effective immunosuppressive agent, cyclosporin, coincided with a marked improvement in survival. This led to a National Consensus Conference on Liver Transplantation held in the USA in 1983 that became a milestone in the history of liver transplantation. The conference concluded that liver grafting had evolved from an experimental stage to that of a procedure with a wide application for patients dying of liver failure. Since then there has been a marked increase in the number of transplants performed both in the USA and elsewhere that continues to date as an increasing number of indications for liver replacement are identified. This paper will describe the current indications for liver transplantation in the paediatric population, recent developments in operative techniques and immunosuppression, and discuss the common complications. Finally the current results will be presented together with a view of possible future developments.

PATIENT SELECTION

The indications for liver replacement in children match those for adults, being chronic liver failure, acute fulminant liver failure, primary liver tumours that are untreatable by conventional liver surgery, and inborn errors of metabolism. Liver transplantation for inborn errors of metabolism is the subject of another paper from this symposium and will not be discussed further (Burdelski, 1990). A breakdown of paediatric liver transplants in Europe up to the end of 1989 relating to underlying disease is shown in Table 1.

Chronic liver failure is by far the largest group, with extrahepatic biliary atresia being the commonest indication. If diagnosed within 6 weeks of birth and treated surgically by portoenterostomy (Kasai operation) a majority of these patients will become jaundice free, with a proportion of long-term survivors. Unfortunately, only a minority are so treated and currently only around 25% overall are cured by the Kasai procedure (McClement *et al.*, 1985). The remainder either remain jaundiced and progress to end-stage liver disease within the first year of life, or clear the jaundice but progress to cirrhosis with failure to thrive and end-stage disease within 2–3 years. Thus currently there is an ongoing need to transplant the majority of biliary atresia patients. Other forms of chronic liver failure treatable by liver replacement in children include chronic active hepatitis, cryptogenic cirrhosis and neonatal hepatitis.

Timing of liver replacement in these patients is an imprecise science that is governed by two main factors: (1) unpredictability of complications, leading to rapid decompensation and death; (2) a possibly lengthy search for a donor liver. Because of these factors we would aim to place non-urgent patients on the transplant waiting list at an early stage, given that a donor liver for such cases may take up to 6 months to find. It is imperative not to delay the decision to transplant as operations performed late are far less likely to be successful due to complications relating to muscle wasting, renal impairment, severe portal hypertension and infection.

Malignant liver tumours are rare in children and this has been an infrequent

Table 1 Indications for transplantation in 733 paediatric patients[a]

Biliary atresia	379
Metabolic disease	119
Acute hepatic failure	59
Cirrhosis	48
Hepatic malignancy	29
Other diagnoses	99

[a]Data from the European Liver Transplant Registry (December 1989)

indication for liver grafting. Obviously, lesions that can be treated by conventional resection are not transplant candidates. Long-term results of grafting are limited by a high recurrence rate, indicating that preoperative tests to diagnose micrometastases outside the liver are imprecise. Nevertheless, around 30% will survive long term and thus all such patients should be considered for liver replacement.

Acute fulminant liver failure is an excellent indication for liver replacement in children as long as this is performed before brain damage has developed. The commonest causes in children are virus hepatitis and drugs. Unfortunately, the period available to find and implant a new liver is limited to days or even hours in some patients. Earliest referral is thus important, together with an ability to cooperate with other transplant centres, including those overseas, in order to find a donor. In Europe anatomical reduction of an adult liver to enable this to fit into a child has been employed in almost half of the children transplanted for fulminant hepatic failure.

OPERATIVE TECHNIQUES

In practice the transplant operation commences in the donor hospital. Donor livers for specific recipients are chosen on the basis of blood group, urgency for transplantation and size. The ongoing shortfall in paediatric donors has led to the development of anatomical reduction referred to earlier with a larger child's or even an adult liver cut down to fit into the paediatric recipient (de Hemptinne *et al.*, 1987). In this way donor-to-recipient weight ratios of up to 10:1 have been successfully implemented. Donor liver removal is usually part of a multiorgan removal with the abdominal organs perfused *in situ* with preservation fluid. Until recently this allowed safe storage of the liver for up to 6 hours, which meant that the majority of transplants were performed at night. A newly developed preservation fluid, University of Wisconsin Solution, allows safe storage of livers for up to 24 hours, permitting daytime grafting, which allows for a better utilization of donors and hospital resources (Todo *et al.*, 1989).

The transplant operation comprises two procedures: removal of the diseased liver, followed by implantation of the new liver. The recipient hepatectomy is a potentially dangerous undertaking owing to a combination of portal hypertension, defective coagulation and the presence of adhesions in patients who have had previous surgery. After securing haemostasis, the new liver is inserted by performing the caval then the portal vein anastomosis. At this stage the new liver is reperfused and following this the hepatic artery and biliary anastomoses are performed (Figure 1). In patients with biliary atresia and in small infants the bile duct is drained via a Roux jejunal loop. In larger children with a normal biliary tree a bile duct-to-duct anastomosis is possible, which is usually stented with a t-tube. During the anhepatic phase the patient develops a metabolic acidosis but this is rapidly reversed as the new liver starts to function. Expert anaesthetic and laboratory support is needed with frequent estimations of acid–base balance, electrolytes, ionized calcium, blood count and coagulation parameters.

In patients receiving anatomically reduced grafts the surgery is modified. The donor liver is first cut down on the back table, removing the unwanted segments but

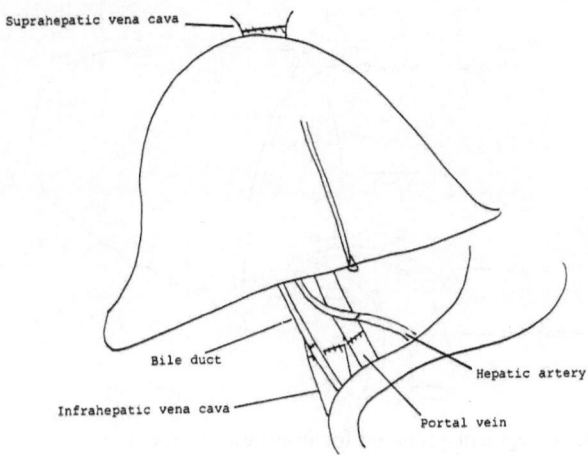

Figure 1 Whole liver graft after insertion

carefully preserving the attached vessels and bile duct for the anastomoses. The cut-down is performed with the liver immersed in slushed Ringer's solution to prevent warming that would damage the graft. Vessels on the cut surface are carefully ligated and the raw area is then treated with fibrin glue to aid haemostasis. If the donor-to-recipient weight ratio is less than 4:1, the vena cava is retained with the portion of liver (usually the left lobe or left lateral segments) and implanted as for a whole graft (Figure 2). If the donor-to-recipient weight ratio exceeds 4:1 the left lateral segment alone is usually used, with the vena cava removed and the left hepatic vein prepared for anastomosis to the recipient vena cava, which is preserved (Figure 3). In this way the major discrepancies in caval size are overcome. The portal, hepatic artery and biliary anastomoses are then performed as for a whole graft.

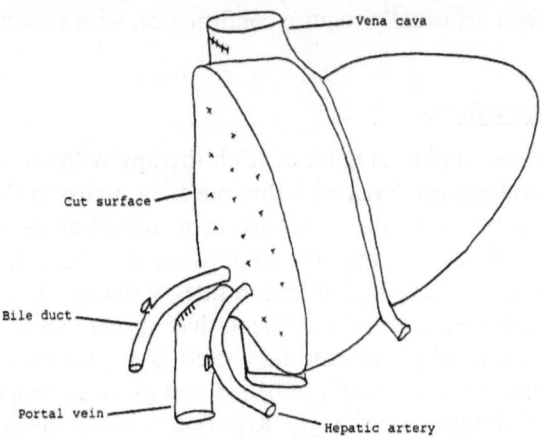

Figure 2 Left lobe prepared for insertion

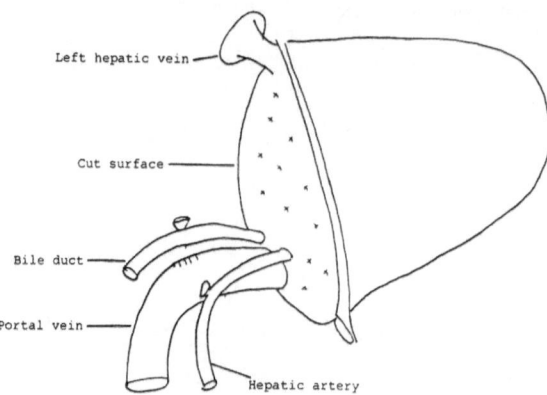

Figure 3   Left lateral segment prepared for insertion

POSTOPERATIVE CARE

Postoperatively the patient is usually ventilated in intensive care for 24–48 hours. Ongoing assessment of graft function includes coagulation studies, blood sugar and acid–base balance. Liver function tests usually show initially high transaminase levels that progressively fall during the first few postoperative days. Excretion of bile with a rapid reduction of jaundice is an indication of a well-functioning graft. Abnormal liver function tests require a specific protocol of investigations to determine the cause. In patients with a t-tube, a cholangiogram will demonstrate patency of the biliary tree. In patients without a t-tube, an ultrasound of the liver can exclude biliary obstruction and demonstrate patency of the portal vein and hepatic artery. If thrombosis is suspected this can be confirmed by angiography. Needle biopsy is carried out next and is the gold standard for diagnosing rejection. Other diagnoses such as preservation injury or viral hepatitis in the graft can also be diagnosed. However, viral infections usually require confirmation with specific antibody tests.

IMMUNOSUPPRESSION

The majority of centres employ a regime of 'triple therapy' with low-dose prednisolone, azathioprine and cyclosporin. Even with this, rejection occurs in the majority of liver transplant recipients but is usually controlled by increased doses of steroid. Regimes using higher doses of baseline immunosuppression may have lower incidences of rejection but are likely to have high infection rates with considerable morbidity and even morality. Moreover, each of the agents has specific toxic effects. The most troublesome are found with cyclosporin, which is nephrotoxic and also causes neurological complications. Toxicity can be reduced by measuring cyclosporin blood levels and adjusting dosages accordingly. Rejection is less frequent after the first few weeks, such that immunosuppression doses at 3 months are quite modest with minimal infection risks to the patients.

New immunosuppressive agents are being developed and two of these deserve mention. A monoclonal antibody to T3 lymphocytes, OKT3, has been shown to be useful in reversing steroid-resistant rejection (rescue therapy). Some units have used OKT3 in the immediate postoperative period in an attempt to prevent any early rejection damage followed by conventional immunosuppression with triple therapy (so-called sequential therapy). As yet there is no documented evidence that this is more effective in terms of graft survival than when it is used for rescue therapy. Moreover, most units using OKT3 have a particularly high incidence of severe viral infections, especially with cytomegalovirus (CMV). Finally, one further agent being assessed is FK-506, a fungal-related compound from Japan. Early studies indicate that it is an extremely powerful immunosuppresssant but that it also shares many of the toxic side-effects of cyclosporin, including nephrotoxicity and neurotoxicity.

COMPLICATIONS

The more frequent complications are listed in Table 2. Peroperative haemorrhage in children is usually less of a problem than in adults, even though the majority of the children will have had previous surgery on the liver. This is most likely due to the fact that portal hypertension as measured by portal vein pressure is less severe in the child than in the adult, possibly a result of more effective collateral vessel formation.

Hepatic artery thrombosis is a major problem in paediatric liver transplantation. Rates vary between units from 10% to 25%. When this occurs in the early postoperative period the resulting ischaemia produces either acute graft failure or biliary tree infarction with bile leakage and intra- or extrahepatic abscess formation. The only treatment is urgent regrafting. Late arterial thrombosis is uncommon and produces less damage to the graft, possibly owing to the development of collaterals, and does not require retransplantation unless major biliary complications ensue.

Acute rejection occurs in the majority of recipients as discussed above but is usually reversible with increased steroid therapy. Chronic rejection is manifested by destruction of small bile ducts shown on biopsy. This form of rejection is not reversible by high-dose immunosuppression. This diagnosis should not be accepted until it has been shown on repeated histology. The only treatment is retransplantation.

Table 2   Complications of liver transplantation

Haemorrhage
Primary non-function
Hepatic artery thrombosis
Acute rejection
Chronic rejection
Infection
Bacterial
Opportunistic – viral (e.g. CMV)
– fungal
– pneumocystis

Infection is a significant risk in all immunosuppressed patients. As mentioned above, infection rates are highest if large doses of immunosuppression are used. As well as common bacterial infections, usually in the respiratory and biliary tracts, opportunistic infections are a potential problem. The commonest of these are cytomegalovirus (CMV) and fungal infections. CMV infections can be minimized by matching CMV status between donor and recipient of both graft and blood and blood products. In the event of a CMV-positive graft being implanted in a CMV-negative recipient, prophylaxis with acyclovir has been shown to be effective in minimizing the severity of any resulting CMV infection. Fungal infections are common in liver transplant recipients as most patients with chronic liver disease are heavily colonized with candida. Oral prophylaxis and the restricted use of broad-spectrum antibiotics may lessen the incidence and severity of fungal sepsis. Pneumocystis is a further risk in these patients and any such infections carry a high mortality. Fortunately, prophylaxis with oral cotrimoxazole is nearly always effective.

RESULTS

The results of liver grafting are closely related to the severity of illness in the recipient prior to transplantation. Thus patients in the terminal phase of chronic liver failure, with advanced muscle wasting, renal impairment, encephalopathy and recurrent variceal bleeding, are less likely to survive compared to patients transplanted at an earlier stage. The long wait associated with finding a paediatric donor can lead to many recipients being grafted too late or even to their dying on the waiting list. The development of the anatomical reduction techniques has allowed an increased rate of paediatric liver replacement with improving results. One further aspect that has improved results has been an active policy of retransplantation for patients with failing first grafts. Regraft rates in children run at 15–25%, roughly double the rate for adults, which relates to the higher incidence of hepatic artery thrombosis in children.

It is important to specify the original indication when analysing results of liver grafting. The biggest group by far is biliary atresia and overall actuarial survival in Europe at 12 and 36 months is 70% (Figure 4). However, these results cover the past 10 years and recent series from the more experienced units have survival rates of over 85% (Otte *et al.*, 1988). Results for patients with metabolic disease are of the same order. Patients transplanted for tumours have a high incidence of recurrent disease with long-term survival rates around 30%. Cerebral injury has been the commonest cause of death in children grafted for fulminant hepatic failure. This is evidence of the donor shortage in that grafts are performed after irreversible brain damage has occurred. Current 12-month survival rates for this group remain poor at 48%. Apart from the tumour cases, the survival curves are flat and these patients can be expected to survive long term, probably into adulthood and beyond. Current data do not show an ongoing failure rate after liver grafting, as is seen with heart and kidney transplants.

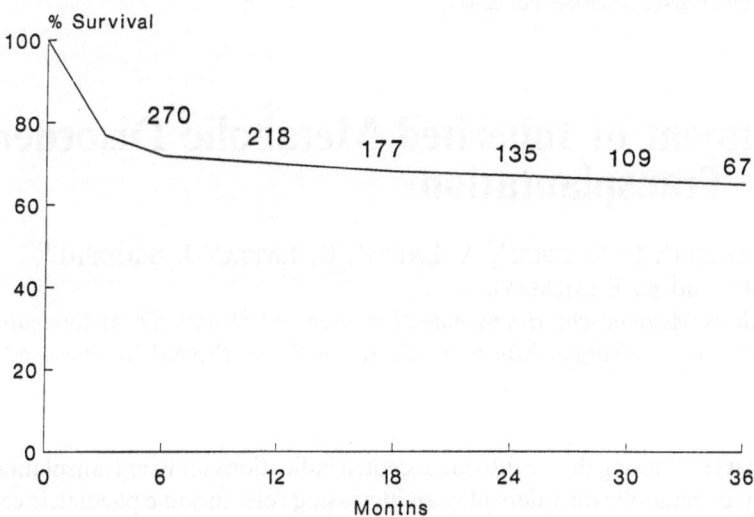

Figure 4 Actuarial survival after liver transplantation for biliary atresia in Europe. Data from the European Liver Transplant Registry

THE FUTURE

Possible developments in the long term include 'dialysis' for chronic liver failure and the use of hepatocyte grafts for both chronic and acute liver failure. Neither of these goals is close to fruition, although hepatocyte grafts are being tried in patients with metabolic disorders who are deficient in a specific enzyme and do not have cirrhosis. Living related donors is another approach currently being explored at a limited number of centres. However, it seems inappropriate to risk the life of the donor (a parent) when currently the majority of both adult and paediatric donor liver offers in the United Kingdom are not being taken because of limited resources (usually a lack of intensive care beds) in the recipient hospitals. More immediate developments to improve the results of paediatric liver transplantation must surely be both an earlier referral of potential recipients and better utilization of current resources.

REFERENCES

Burdelski, M., Rodeck, B., Latta, A., Latta, K., Brodehl, J., Ringe, B. and Pichlmayr, R. Treatment of inherited metabolic disorders by liver transplantation. *J. Inher. Metab. Dis.* 14 (1991) 604–618

de Hemptinne, B., de Ville de Goyet, J., Kestens, P. J. and Otte, J. B. Volume reduction of the liver graft before orthotopic transplantation: Report of a clinical experience in 11 cases. *Transplant. Proc.* 14 (1987) 3317–3322

McClement, J. W., Howard, E. R. and Mowat, A. P. Results of surgical treatment of extrahepatic biliary atresia in United Kingdom, 1980–82. *Br. Med. J.* 290 (1985) 345–347

Otte, J. B., Yandza, T., de Ville de Goyet, J., Tan, K. C., Salizzoni, M. and de Hemptinne, B. Paediatric liver transplantation: Report on 52 patients with a 2-year survival of 86%. *J. Paediatr. Surg.* 23 (1988) 250–253

Todo, S., Nery, J., Yanaga, K., Podesta, L., Gordon, R. D. and Starzl, T. E. Extended preservation of human liver grafts with UW solution. *J. Am. Med. Assoc.* 261 (1989) 711–714

J. Inher. Metab. Dis. 14 (1991) 604–618

Treatment of Inherited Metabolic Disorders by Liver Transplantation

M. Burdelski[1], B. Rodeck[1], A. Latta[1], K. Latta[1], J. Brodehl[1], B. Ringe[2] and R. Pichlmayr[2]
[1]*Kinderklinik Medizinische Hochschule Hannover and* [2]*Klinik für Abdominal- und Transplantations-Chirurgie, Konstanty Gutschow Str. 8, D-3000 Hannover 61, Germany*

Summary: Among the worldwide accepted indications for liver transplantation, inherited metabolic disorders play an increasing role. In some paediatric centres this indication runs second after extrahepatic biliary atresia.

The aim of liver transplantation in inherited metabolic disorders is twofold: the first is to save a patient's life, the second is to accomplish phenotypic and functional cure of his disease. These aims may be achieved in disorders presenting with cirrhosis, hepatoma, life-threatening progression or failure of other organs with preserved liver function. The timing of liver transplantation has become easier with development of surgical techniques of reduced-size donor livers. These techniques enable the performance of liver transplantation with ABO blood group compatible organs of almost any size if indicated either by deterioration of liver function or impending complications such as hepatoma or life-threatening progression. In comparison with other indications such as extrahepatic biliary atresia, postnecrotic liver cirrhosis or acute liver failure, the results of transplantation in patients with inherited metabolic disorders seem to be better, reaching up to 78–95% actuarial 1-year survival rates. However, lifelong immunosuppressive therapy is necessary. This seems to be acceptable even in disorders with only partial liver function defects.

Liver transplantation in inherited disorders of metabolism has a twofold aim. The first is to save the patient's life since the disorder may cause either acute or chronic liver failure, hepatoma or failure of other organs. The second aim is to cure the underlying metabolic defect. This aim may be achieved by phenotypic and functional cure; a genetic cure, however, is not possible (Esquivel *et al.*, 1988). Nevertheless, phenotypic and functional cure enable a normal life style in children who otherwise would have died. In addition, from a scientific point of view, liver transplantation represents a new concept in clarifying the pathogenesis in hepatic-based metabolic disorders (Starzl, 1988a).

When compared to conventional indications for liver transplantation, such as extrahepatic biliary atresia or postnecrotic cirrhosis, there are both similarities and major differences that can be recognized. As in extrahepatic biliary atresia, the most frequent indication for liver transplantation in paediatric patients (Calne *et al.*, 1986; Burdelski *et al.*, 1987; Schade, 1987; Mowat, 1987; Shaw *et al.*, 1988; Bismuth, 1989; Starzl *et al.*, 1989a; Starzl, 1989), liver transplantation may cure the disease in inherited metabolic disorders. This only can happen if the defect is restricted to the liver itself. On the other hand, in some diseases involving not only the liver but also other organs, e.g. the kidneys in tyrosinosis or the heart in glycogen storage disease type IV (Burdelski *et al.*, 1987; Starzl *et al.*, 1989a), the risk of progress of the metabolic disorder in these organs seems to be lower than the risk of recurrence of hepatitis B infection in patients with hepatitis B-induced liver cirrhosis (Starzl *et al.*, 1989b). In generalized metabolic disorders such as Niemann–Pick disease (Daloze *et al.*, 1977; Starzl *et al.*, 1989a) and other storage diseases the metabolic defect will affect the transplanted liver within a short period of time without any real phenotypic or functional cure since the reticular endothelial system of the donor will be replaced by that of the recipient within a few months.

The purpose of this review is to elaborate the role of liver transplantation in inherited metabolic disorders on the basis of published, communicated or personally gathered experience.

Metabolic disorders with liver cirrhosis such as α_1-antitrypsin deficiency have been classical indications for liver transplantation from the very beginning (Starzl *et al.*, 1989a). Many of these diseases such as Byler disease or fumaryl hydrolase deficiency type 1a are mainly of paediatric concern, since the natural course of the diseases causes death during infancy or childhood. Other diseases such as Wilson disease are found in both adult and paediatric series (Groth *et al.*, 1973; Sternlieb, 1984, 1988; Sokol *et al.*, 1985; Esquivel *et al.*, 1988; Gottrand *et al.*, 1988; Ringe *et al.*, 1988). The remarkable advances of liver transplantation during the last ten years (Keating *et al.*, 1985; Gordon *et al.*, 1986; Burdelski *et al.*, 1987; Martinez *et al.*, 1987; Shade, 1987; Shaw *et al.*, 1988; Bismuth, 1989; Starzl, 1989b) have been the extension of the indications for liver replacement to metabolic disorders with only partial defects of liver function. Nevertheless, it must be stressed that, in many of the metabolic disorders accepted for transplantation today, the results need further evaluation because the follow-up period is not long enough or the experience is based on case reports only.

FREQUENCY AND VARIETY OF DISORDERS FOR TRANSPLANTATION

The frequency with which liver transplantation is used for inherited metabolic disorders varies between 10.8% in the Pittsburgh series (Starzl *et al.*, 1989a) and 4.9% reported in the European Liver Transplantation Registry (Bismuth, 1989). In reports of individual European centres, however, the percentage of inherited metabolic disorders ranges between 12% and 35% (Figure 1). The spectrum of metabolic disorders treated with liver transplantation also varies from centre to centre. In Europe, Byler disease is the most frequent indication, at least in Paris and Hanover, whereas in the USA α_1-antitrypsin deficiency seems to be the most important disease (Esquivel *et al.*, 1988; Starzl *et al.*, 1989a). However, due to a lack of a clear definition

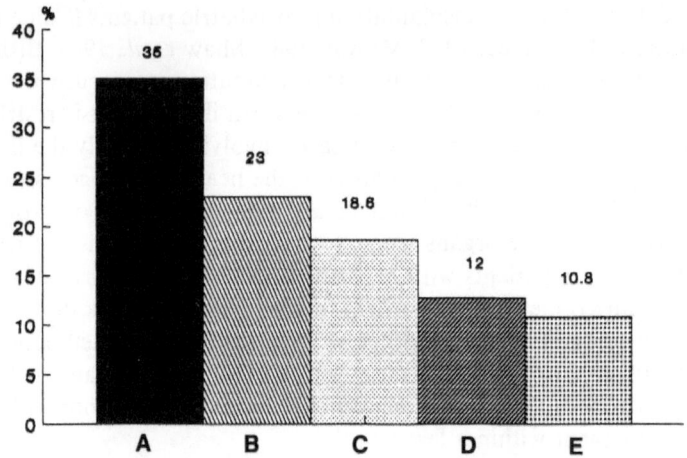

Figure 1 Frequency of liver transplantation in hepatic metabolic disorders in different transplantation centres: A: Paris (Alagille, personal communication); B: London (Cohen *et al.*, 1991); C: Hanover, authors' data; D: Brussels (Otte, personal communication); E: Pittsburg (Starzl, 1989a).

of Byler disease, some of these patients may be hidden in the group of 'cholestatic syndromes'.

A classification of the indications for liver transplantation in metabolic disorders according to the mode of clinical presentation is shown in Figure 2. The most frequent indication is liver failure, in either acute or chronic clinical course, followed by

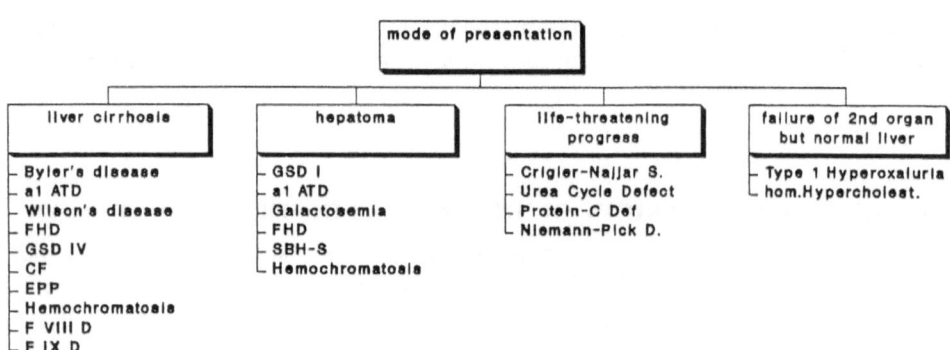

Figure 2 Classification of inherited metabolic disorders according to clinical modes of presentation. Abbreviations: α_1ATD = α_1-antitrypsin deficiency; FHD = fumaryl hydrolase deficiency; GSD IV = glycogen storage disease type IV; CF = cystic fibrosis; EPP = erythropoietic protoporphyria; F VIII D = haemophilia A; F IX D = haemophilia B; GSD I = glycogen storage disease type I; SBH-S = seablue histiocyte syndrome

hepatoma in normal or cirrhotic liver, life-threatening progression of the disease without liver failure, and finally failure of a second organ induced by isolated hepatic metabolic defects.

The results of liver transplantation in metabolic disorders will be reviewed on the basis of this classification. Special emphasis is laid on the phenotypic and functional cure achieved and on specific complications observed in these disorders.

RESULTS

Inherited metabolic disorders with cirrhosis (Table 1)

Cirrhosis of the liver may be the result of the metabolic defect or secondary due to hepatitis acquired in replacement therapy, as in factor VIII or IX deficiency. Phenotypic cure after transplantation is observed in all these disorders. Even in cystic fibrosis improvement of pulmonary function has been observed, the mechanism, however, being unclear (Mieles *et al.*, 1989).

As far as functional cure is concerned, complete normalization of metabolism is accomplished in Byler disease (apo-A1 metabolism: Sturm *et al.*, 1990), α_1-antitrypsin deficiency (α_1-antitrypsin, PI type ZZ Esquivel: *et al.*, 1988; Hood *et al.*, 1980; Pichlmayr *et al.*, 1987), Wilson disease (copper metabolism: Groth *et al.*, 1973; Groth and Ringden, 1984; Polson *et al.*, 1987; Gottrand *et al.*, 1988; Kreuzpaintner *et al.*, 1988; Starzl *et al.*, 1989a; Cohen *et al.*, 1991), erythropoietic protoporphyria (protoporphyrin metabolism: Polson *et al.*, 1988; Samuel *et al.*, 1988; Bloomer *et al.*, 1989; Johnson and Fusaro, 1989), haemochromatosis (iron metabolism: Esquivel *et al.*, 1988; Starzl *et al.*, 1989a) and in factor VIII (Lewis *et al.*, 1985) and factor IX (Merion *et al.*, 1988) deficiency. The significance of ongoing urinary succinylacetone

Table 1 Liver transplantation and phenotypic and functional cure in metabolic disorders with cirrhosis

Disease	*Cure*		*Complications*
	Phenotypic	*Functional*	
Byler disease	+	+ (apo A1?)	
α_1-Antitrypsin deficiency	+	+(α_1-AT, Pi type)	Aneurysm Pulmonary AV shunts
Wilson's disease	+	+ (Cu metabolism)	
Tyrosinaemia	+	(+) (Succinylacetonuria)	
Glycogen storage disease IV)	+	(+) (Cardial amylopectin)	Cardiomyopathy
Cystic fibrosis	±	±	Progress?
E. protoporphyria	+	+ (Protoporphyrin metabolism)	
Haemochromatosis	+	+ (Iron metabolism)	Cardiac arrhythmia
Factor VIII deficiency[a]	+	+ (Factor VIII)	Hepatitis
Factor IX deficiency[a]	+	+ (Factor IX)	Hepatitis

[a]Secondary cirrhosis due to hepatitis after replacement therapy
+ = complete, (+) = incomplete; − = no cure.

excretion in tyrosinaemia (Starzl et al., 1985; Kvittingen, 1986; Kvittingen et al., 1986; van Thiel et al., 1986; Tuchman et al., 1987) is not known yet. As far as glycogen storage disease IV is concerned, there is evidence of cardial deposits of amylopectin after transplantation (Starzl et al., 1989a).

Specific complications are reported in α_1-antitrypsin deficiency where pulmonary arteriovenous shunts may be the reason for postoperative severe hypoxaemia. In two of our patients suffering from this disorder arterial aneurysms have occurred after transplantation. In haemochromatosis severe cardiac arrhythmia has been observed after revascularization of the transplanted liver, which seemed to be caused by the cardiac involvement in haemochromatosis (Esquivel et al., 1988). Recurrence of hepatitis is a major concern in patients with factor VIII or IX deficiency (Starzl et al., 1989b). Septicaemia originating from pulmonary Pseudomonas infection in cystic fibrosis has been observed less frequently than one might have expected (Mieles et al., 1989).

Inherited disorders with hepatoma (Table 2)

Hepatoma may occur in cirrhotic and non-cirrhotic livers. In glycogen storage disease I those adenomata that are not influenced by appropriate dietary therapy (Malatack et al., 1983; Howell, 1984; Coire et al., 1987) and optimized metabolic correction seem to predispose to carcinoma. Except in patients with seablue histiocyte syndrome (Gartner et al., 1986), phenotypic and functional cure is observed in all these disorders after transplantation (Groth and Ringden, 1984; Starzl et al., 1985; Kvittingen, 1986; van Thiel et al., 1986; Burdelski et al., 1987; Esquivel et al., 1988, 1989; Dehner et al., 1989; Otto et al., 1989). The biology of these tumours seems to be different from that of primary hepatocellular carcinoma (Esquivel et al., 1989; Starzl et al., 1989b) since only a few tumour recurrences have been reported in these metabolically induced malignancies (Esquivel et al., 1988). The chance of tumour-free survival thus

Table 2 Liver transplantation and phenotypic and functional cure in metabolic disorders with hepatoma

Disease	Cure		Complications
	Phenotypic	Functional	
Glycogen storage disease I	+	+ (CH-metabolism)	Tumour recurrence
Galactosaemia	+	+ (Galactose metabolism)	Tumour recurrence
Tyrosinaemia	+	(+) (Succinylacetonuria)	Tumour recurrence
α_1-Antitrypsin deficiency	+	+ (α_1AT, Pi type)	Tumour recurrence
Haemochromatosis	+	+ (Fe metabolism)	Tumour recurrence
Seablue histiocyte syndrome	−	−	Disease progress

+ = complete; (+) = incomplete; − = no cure

is much higher in metabolic disorders with malignant lesions than in primary malignancies.

Inherited metabolic disorders with partial liver function defects characterized by life-threatening progression (Table 3)

In these disorders there is no hepatocellular injury leading to cirrhosis (Daloze *et al.*, 1977; Kauffman *et al.*, 1986; Pett and Mowat, 1987; Pichlmayr *et al.*, 1987; Shevell *et al.*, 1987; Casella *et al.*, 1988; Tuchman, 1989). The defect may lead to the production of a metabolite that is non-toxic to the liver but toxic to other organs. In protein-C deficiency the metabolic defect causes a disequilibrium of clotting factors leading to thrombosis. The natural course of all these disorders is characterized by a life-threatening progress. This progression may occur in early life as in protein-C deficiency and urea-cycle defects or in the second decade as in Crigler–Najjar syndrome. Phenotypic and functional cure is achieved in Crigler–Najjar syndrome and in protein-C deficiency (Starzl *et al.*, 1989a). In urea-cycle defects there is a phenotypic cure, but acitrullinaemia after transplantation requiring citrullin supplementation may be observed (Tuchman, 1989).

In Niemann–Pick disease, recurrence of sphingomyelin storage in hepatocytes and Kupffer cells of the transplanted liver and further progress of the disease in other organ systems has been seen (Daloze *et al.*, 1977; Starzl *et al.*, 1989a).

Inherited hepatic metabolic disorders leading to failure of a second organ (Table 4)

In this category, hyperoxaluria type 1 (Watts *et al.*, 1985, 1987; Cochat *et al.*, 1989; Danpure, 1989; McDonald *et al.*, 1989; Morgan and Watts, 1989; Latta and Brodehl, 1990) and homozygous hypercholesterolaemia type IIa (Bilheimer *et al.*, 1986; Starzl *et al.*, 1984; East *et al.*, 1986; Figuera *et al.*, 1986; Starzl *et al.*, 1989a) are to be found. Detoxification, synthesis, excretion and metabolic capacities of the diseased livers are normal except for alanine : glyoxalate aminotransferase in the case of primary hyperoxaluria type I and low-density lipoprotein production and receptors in homozygous hypercholesterolaemia type IIa. Transplantation of the liver enables phenotypic and functional cure of the diseases. As far as alanine : glyoxalate amino-transferase deficiency is concerned, hyperoxaluria will continue due to accumulated

Table 3 Liver transplantation and phenotypic and functional cure in metabolic disorders with life-threatening progression

Disease	Cure		Complications
	Phenotypic	*Functional*	
Crigler–Najjar syndrome	+	+ (Glucuronyltransferase)	
Urea-cycle defect	+	(+) (Acitrullinaemia)	
Protein-C deficiency	+	+ (Protein-C)	
Niemann–Pick disease type A	–	–	Disease progress

+ = complete; (+) = incomplete; – = no cure

Table 4 Liver transplantation and phenotypic and functional cure in metabolic disorders with failure of a second organ

Disease	Cure		Complications
	Phenotypic	*Functional*	
Hyperoxaluria type 1	+	(+) (Oxaluria)	Bone disease LTX/KTX
Homozygous hypercholesterolaemia	+	+ (Cholesterol metabolism, hep.LDL receptors	LTX/HTX

LTX = liver transplantation; KTX = kidney transplantation; HTX = hearttransplantation; LDL = low-density lipoproteins; + = complete; (+) = incomplete cure

oxalate (Latta and Brodehl, 1990). In contrast to the other groups of indications, transplantation of a second organ such as kidney in hyperoxaluria and heart in hypercholesterolaemia is necessary in most of the patients since these organs represent the targets for the metabolic defect.

Timing of transplantation (Table 5)

Timing of transplantation in hepatic-based metabolic disorders is very complex and depends especially on the donor situation of the individual centre. In disorders with liver cirrhosis, deterioration of liver function as indicated by scores (Malatack *et al.*, 1987) or dynamic liver function tests (Düwel *et al.*, 1989; Oellerich *et al.*, 1989a,b,c, 1990; Burdelski *et al.*, 1990) are essential for timing of transplantation. However, clinical experience with regard to the natural course of the disease will help to define the optimum timing of transplantation. Disorders that are at risk of developing liver carcinoma require transplantation before this is likely to occur. This means that most of these disorders should be transplanted before the age of 2 years (Dehner *et al.*, 1989). This recommendation can only be accomplished if adult donor organs are utilized using the surgical technique of reducing the liver to either the left lateral segment or the left or right liver lobe (Bismuth and Houssain, 1984; de Hemptinne *et al.*, 1987; Brölsch *et al.*, 1988; Ringe *et al.*, 1988).

Table 5 Proposal for timing of liver transplantation in hepatic metabolic disorders

Disease/Mode of presentation	Indicators
Cirrhosis	Liver function, dynamic liver function tests
Tumour	Natural course
Life-threatening progression	Nature course
Failure of second organ	Hyperoxaluria: GFR > 50 ml/min: LTX GFR < 20 ml/min: LTX/KTX Hypercholesterolaemia Cardiac infarction: LTX/HTX

GFR = glomerular filtration rate; LTX = liver transplantation; KTX = kidney transplantation; HTX = heart transplantation

Immunosuppression after liver transplantation

Immunosuppression after liver transplantation is the price patients with metabolic disorders have to pay for phenotypic and functional cure. In most centres the immunosuppressive regimen is performed on the basis of cyclosporin A plus prednisolone (Calne *et al.*, 1986; Burdelski *et al.*, 1987; Gordon *et al.*, 1986; Marsh *et al.*, 1987; Schade, 1987; Shaw *et al.*, 1988; Starzl *et al.*, 1989b; Starzl, 1989). Patients with impairment of renal function profit from additional azathioprine, which allows the reduction of the cyclosporin concentration. Thus cyclosporin-induced nephrotoxicity may be avoided (Burdelski *et al.*, 1987). Future immunosuppressive therapy may include new drugs like FK 506, which is being used in clinical studies at the present (Fung *et al.*, 1990).

Clinical results of liver transplantation

Patients with inborn errors of metabolism tend to have better results from liver transplantation than those with all other conventional indications (Table 6) (Starzl, 1989a). In our own experience, the 4-year survival of patients with metabolic disorders is 88%. The results in patients with postnecrotic cirrhosis (72%), biliary atresia (47%) and tumour (30%) range far behind (Figure 3). In centres reporting the actuarial 1-year survival after liver transplantation in patiénts with hepatic-based metabolic diseases, the results range between 75% and 95% (Figure 4). Quality of life improves to the same extent. Strict dietary regimens and complex metabolic controls become redundant. On the other hand, new diseases such as viral infections in the immunocompromised patient may have deleterious effects on the results of liver transplantation (Burdelski *et al.*, 1987; Starzl *et al.*, 1989b).

DISCUSSION

According to these results, liver tansplantation in hepatic metabolic disorders is acceptable if phenotypic and functional cure is achieved (Tables 1–4). With the exception of cystic fibrosis, seablue histiocyte syndrome and Niemann–Pick disease, the aim of phenotypic and functional correction of the metabolic defect has become possible by means of the surgical procedure of liver transplantation. The future role of liver transplantation in cystic fibrosis cannot be predicted at the moment. Since it

Table 6   One-year survival probabilities with different indications (according to Bismuth, 1989; Burdelski *et al.*, 1987; East *et al.*, 1986)

Disease	Probability of 1-year survival (%)
Fulminant liver failure	57
Budd–Chiari syndrome	57
Postnecrotic cirrhosis	65
Biliary atresia	70
Metabolic disorders	78–95

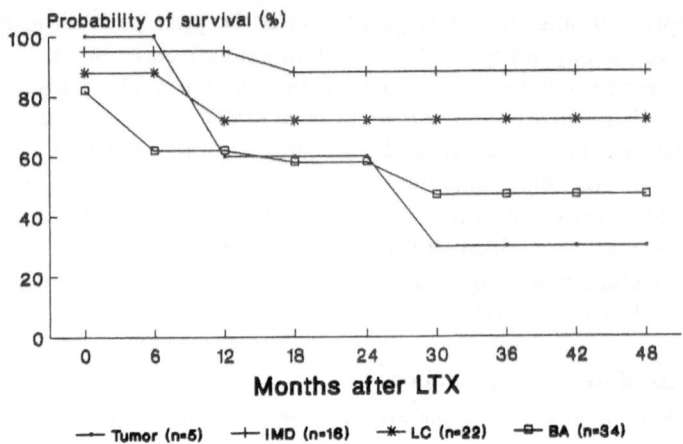

Figure 3 Comparison of results in liver transplantation with different indications in Hanover. Abbreviations: IMD = inborn metabolic disorders; LC = postnecrotic liver cirrhosis; BA = biliary atresia

is a systemic disease of all exocrine glands, progression of the disease in other affected organs will occur. This means that pulmonary disease and diabetes and diseases related to these complications are likely to contribute to post-transplant morbidity and mortality. In generalized metabolic disorders such as Niemann–Pick disease, combined bone-marrow and liver transplantation may be considered on an experimental basis.

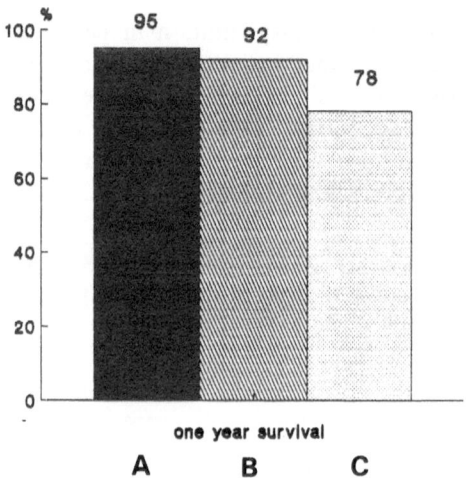

Figure 4 Comparison of actuarial 1-year survival in liver transplantation of metabolic disorders in different centres. A: Hanover (authors[1] data); B: Paris (Alagille, personal communication); C: Pittsburg (Starzl, 1989a, b).

There are residual functional impairments, however, in tyrosinaemia, glycogen storage disease IV, urea-cycle defects and type 1 hyperoxaluria (Tables 1–4). The implications of these functional impairments remain to be elucidated since numbers and follow-up periods are too small to permit definite conclusions. Severe clinical complications have been reported in glycogen storage disease type IV (Starzl *et al.*, 1989a). In patients with liver cirrhosis due to hepatitis B in factor VIII or IX deficiency the risk of hepatitis B recurrence is as high as 80–90% (Starzl, 1989b). The role of either ortho- or heterotopic auxiliary transplantation of liver segments, leaving parts or the whole original liver, in metabolic disorders with only partial defects is a subject of future investigation. Concerning haemophilia this concept would mean the resection of the left lateral segment and its replacement by a transplanted liver segment before infection of the native liver has taken place or factor VIII inhibitors develop. In metabolic disorders producing toxic metabolic compounds, e.g. hyperoxaluria type 1, this concept would not work, since the production of this compound in the remaining liver would overcome the benefit from the correct metabolic processing in the transplanted segment.

The surgical technique of segmental transplantation to replace the whole liver has enabled transplantation in small infants with body weight below 6 kg. This has made transplantation possible in tyrosinaemia type 1 and urea-cycle defects that would not be suitable for transplantation if only ABO blood group and body-weight-compatible organs were used. This early transplantation is of special interest in disorders at risk of developing carcinoma (Dehner *et al.*, 1989; Cohen *et al.*, 1991). Fifty per cent of the patients with tyrosinaemia transplanted in Pittsburgh had liver malignancy at time of operation (Esquivel *et al.*, 1988). Avoidance of this potential risk of tumour disease after transplantation will increase the chance of survival in these disorders. Patients with extrahepatic tumour manifestations should be excluded from transplantation.

In primary hyperoxaluria type 1 and in homozygous hypercholesterolaemia, functional impairment of other organs than the liver will determine the indication for transplantation. Since the results of kidney transplantation alone in hyperoxaluria have been disappointing, combined transplantation of both liver and kidney are proposed in patients with renal insufficiency (Watts *et al.*, 1987). In patients with glomerular filtration rate above 50 ml/min liver transplantation alone might be sufficient for phenotypic and functional cure. On the other hand, bone disease may be a long-standing problem after transplantation (Latta and Brodehl, 1990). Homozygous hypercholesterolaemia is not a primary indication for liver transplantation as long as coronary arteriosclerosis can be prevented by plasmapheresis. If coronary heart disease occurs despite this therapy, or if it is present at the time of diagnosis, combined heart and liver transplantation is needed.

The appropriate timing of liver transplantation in metabolic disorders leading to liver cirrhosis is very difficult. Our data on the prognostic use of dynamic liver function tests in prospective studies in both adult and paediatric patients with liver cirrhosis have shown that the indocyanine green test and monoethylglycinexylidide formation after intravenous lidocaine injection are superior to all clinical and biochemical parameters if the end-stage of the disease has been reached (Oellerich *et al.*, 1989a,b,c, 1990; Düwel *et al.*, 1989; Burdelski *et al.*, 1990). These tests will help to identify those patients with chronic end-stage liver disease who are at risk of expiring within the next 3- and 12-month periods and thus need the next available organ.

The reason for the better outcome after liver transplantation in hepatic metabolic disorders compared with biliary atresia is not yet clear. In our experience the comparatively good nutritional status of these patients and the lack of previous operations have the most important impact in this regard. These considerations are supported by the fact that there is an almost 15% difference (Figure 3) in early postoperative mortality between patients with inborn errors of metabolism and patients with biliary atresia. This finding is explained by the higher complication rate due to intestinal perforations in combination with bacterial infections in the group of patients with biliary atresia. In the later postoperative course, acquired viral infections and chronic rejection are the most important factors that will affect all different groups of indications almost to the same extent.

There are only two reports of accidental transplantation of inborn metabolic disorders to transplant recipients (Dzik *et al.*, 1987; Henne-Bruns and Kremer, 1988). The transplanted disorders were factor XI deficiency and Gilbert syndrome. In the case of factor XI deficiency the findings confirm the hypothesis that the liver is the site of production of this factor.

The decision to accept a patient suffering from an inborn metabolic disorder as a candidate for liver transplantation may be based on the results reported in this review. If the risk of not surviving the disease is greater than the risk of transplantation itself, and if the tansplantation will provide phenotypic and functional cure of the disease, this surgical approach to correcting the metabolic defect yields the best chance for the patient's survival.

REFERENCES

Bilheimer, D. W., Goldstein, J. L., Grundy, S. M., Starzl, T. E. and Brown, M. S. Liver transplantation to provide low-density lipoprotein receptors and lower hypercholesterolemia. *N. Engl. J. Med.* 311 (1984) 1658–1664

Bismuth, H. European liver transplantation registry 1989 (personal communication)

Bismuth, H. and Houssain, D. Reduced-size orthotopic liver graft in hepatic transplantation in children. *Surgery* 95 (1984) 367–370

Bloomer, J. R., Weimer, M. K., Bossenmaier, I. C., Snover, D. C., Payne, W. D. and Ascher, N. L. Liver transplantation in a patient with protoporphyria. *Gastroenterology* 97 (1989) 188–194

Brölsch, C. E., Emond, J. C., Thistlethwaite, J. R. *et al.* Liver transplantation with reduced-size donor organs. *Transplantation* 45 (1988) 519–523

Burdelski, M., Pichlmayr, R., Ringe, B., Rodeck, B. and Brodehl, J. Pediatric liver transplantation — Ten years' experience in Hanover. In: Terasaki, P. J. (ed.) *Clinical Transplants* UCLA Tissue Typing Laboratory, Los Angeles, 1987, pp. 55–62

Burdelski, M., Oellerich, M., Rodeck, B. and Düwel, J. Prognostic indicators in liver cirrhosis. *Pediatr. Res.* 27 (1990) 535

Calne, R. Y., Williams, R. and Rolles, K. Liver transplantation in the adult. *World J. Surg.* 10 (1986) 422–431

Casella, J. F., Lewis, J. H., Bontempo, F. A., Zitelli, B., Markel, H. and Starzl, T. E. Successful treatment of homozygous protein-C deficiency by hepatic transplantation. *Lancet* 1 (1988) 435–438

Cochat, P., Faure, J. L., Divry, P., Danpure, C. J., Descos, B., Wright, C., Takvorian, P. and Floret, D. Liver transplantation in primary hyperoxaluria type 1 (letter). *Lancet* 1 (1989) 1142–1143

Cohen, A. T., Mowat, A. P., Bhaduri, B. H., Noble-Jamieson, G., Williams, R., Barnes, N. and Calne, R. Y. Liver transplantation for inborn errors of metabolism and genetic disorders. In: Schaub, J., Van Hoof, F. and Vis, H. L. (eds.) *Inborn Errors of Metabolism.* Nestlé Nutrition Workshop Series, Vol. 24. Nestec Ltd., Vevey/Raven Press, New York, 1991, pp. 213–220

Coire, C. I., Qizilbash, A. H. and Castelli, M. F. Hepatic adenomata in type Ia glycogen storage disease. *Arch. Pathol. Lab. Med.* 111 (1987) 166–169

Daloze, P., Delvin, E. E., Glorieux, F. H., Corman, J. C., Bettez, P. and Toussi, T. Replacement therapy for inherited enzyme deficiency: liver orthotopic transplantation in Niemann–Pick disease type A. *Am. J. Med. Genet.* 1 (1977) 229–239

Danpure, C. J. Recent advances in the understanding, diagnosis and treatment of primary hyperoxaluria type 1. *J. Inher. Metab. Dis.* 12 (1989) 210–224

Dehner, L. P., Snover, D. C., Sharp, H. L., Ascher, N., Nakhleh, R. and Day, D. L. Hereditary tyrosinemia type I (chronic form): pathologic findings in the liver. *Hum. Pathol.* 20 (1989) 149–158

Düwel, J., Burdelski, M., Oellerich, M. and Rodeck, B. Evaluation of liver function tests as prognostic indicators in chronic pediatric liver disease. *Hepatology* 10 (1989) 660

Dzik, W. H., Arkin, C. F. and Jenkins, R. C. Transfer of congenital factor XI deficiency from a donor to a recipient by liver transplantation. *N. Engl. J. Med.* 316 (1987) 1217–1218

East, C., Grundy, S. M. and Bilheimer, D. W. Normal cholesterol levels with lovastatin (mevinolin) therapy in a child with homozygous familial hypercholesterolemia following liver transplantation. *J. Am. Med. Assoc.* 256 (1986) 2843–2848

Esquivel, C. O., Marino, I. R., Fioravanti, V. and van Thiel, D. H. Liver transplantation for metabolic disease of the liver. *Gastroenterol. Clin. N. Am.* 17 (1988) 167–175

Esquivel, C. O., Mieles, L., Todo, S., Makowka, L., Ambrosino, G., Nakazato, P. and Starzl, T. E. Liver transplantation for hereditary tyrosinemia in the presence of hepatocellular carcinoma. *Transplant. Proc.* 21 (1989) 2445–2446

Figuera, D., Ardaiz, J., Martin-Judez, V., Pulpon, L. A. *et al.* Combined transplantation of heart and liver from two different donors in a patient with familial type IIa hypercholesterolemia. *J. Heart Transplant.* 5 (1986) 327–329

Fung, I. J., Todo, S., Jaim, A., McCanley, J., Alessiani, M., Scotti, C. and Starzl, T. E. Conversion from cyclosporine to FK 506 in liver allograft recipients with cyclosporine-related complications. *Transplant. Proc.* 22 (1990) 6–12

Gartner, J. C., Bergman, I., Malatack, J. J., Zitelli, B. J. and Jaffe, R. Progression of neurovisceral storage disease with supranuclear ophthalmoplegia following orthotopic liver transplantation. *Pediatrics* 77 (1986) 104–106

Gordon, R. D., Shaw, B. W., Iwatsuki, S., Esquivel, C. O. and Starzl, T. E. Indications for liver transplantation in the cyclosporine era. *Surg. Clin. N. Am.* 66 (1986) 541–556

Gottrand, F., Razemon, M., Otte, J. B., Vigier, J. E. and Farriaux, J. P. Indications de la transplantation hepatique au cours d'une maladie de Wilson. *Arch. Fr. Pediatr.* 45 (1988) 187–188

Groth, C. G. and Ringden, O. Transplantation in relation to the treatment of inherited disease. *Transplantation* 38 (1984) 319–327

Groth, C. G., Dubois, R. S., Corman, J. *et al.* Metabolic effects of hepatic replacement in Wilson's disease. *Transplant. Proc.* 5 (1973) 829–833

de Hemptinne, B., de Ville de Goyet, J., Kestner, P. J., *et al.* Volume reduction of the liver graft before orthotopic transplantation: report of a clinical experience in 11 cases. *Transplant. Proc.* 19 (1987) 3317–3322

Henne-Bruns, D. and Kremer, B. Manifestation of Gilbert syndrome (Meulengracht disease) following orthotopic liver transplantation: a rare case of postoperative hyperbilirubinemia. *Klin. Wochenschr.* 66 (1988) 596–598

Hood, J. M., Koep, L. J., Peters, R. C. *et al.* Liver transplantation for advanced liver disease with α_1-antitrypsin deficiency. *N. Engl. J. Med.* 302 (1980) 272–275

Howell, R. R. Glycogen storage disease research and clinical problems: a reappraisal. *J. Pediatr. Gastroenterol. Nutr.* 3 (1984) 12–13

Johnson, J. A. and Fusaro, R. M. Prognosis of liver transplantation in patients with erythropoetic protoporphyria (letter). *Transplantation* 48 (1989) 175–176

Kauffman, S. S., Wood, R. P., Shaw, B. W., Jr., Markin, R. S., Rosenthal, P., Gridelli, B. and Vanderhoof, J. A. Orthotopic liver transplantation for type I Crigler–Najjar syndrome. *Hepatology* 6 (1986) 1259–1262

Keating, J. J., Johnson, R. D., Johnson, P. J. and Williams, R. Clinical course of cirrhosis in young adults and therapeutic potential of liver transplantation. *Gut* 26 (1985) 1359–1363

Kreuzpaintner, G., Lauchart, W., Frenzel, H., Stremmel, W., Berges, W., Pichlmayr, R. and Strohmeyer, G. Orthotopic liver transplantation in Wilson's disease and acute liver failure. *Dtsch. Med. Wochenschr.* 113 (1988) 1097–1100

Kvittingen, E. A. Hereditary tyrosinemia type I — an overview. *Scand. J. Clin. Lab. Invest. Suppl.* 1 184 (1986) 27–32

Kvittingen, E. A., Jellum, E., Stokke, O., Flatmark, A., Bergan, A., Sodal, G., Halvorsen, S., Schrumpf, E. and Gjone, E. Liver transplantation in a 23-year-old tyrosinemia patient: effects on the renal tubular dysfunction. *J. Inher. Metab. Dis.* 9 (1986) 216–224

Latta, K. and Brodehl, J. Primary hyperoxaluria type I. *Eur. J. Pediatr.* 149 (1990) 518–522

Lewis, J. H., Bontempo, F. A., Spiro, J. A., Ragni, M. V., Starzl, T. E. Liver transplantation in a hemophiliac. *N. Engl. J. Med.* 312 (1985) 1189–1190

Malatack, J. J., Finegold, D. N., Iwatsuki, S., Shaw, B. W., Jr, Gartner, J. C., Zitelli, B. J., Roe, T. and Starzl, T. E. Liver transplantation for type I glycogen storage disease. *Lancet* 1 (1983) 1073–1075

Malatack, J. J., Schaid, D. J., Urbach, A. H., Gartner, J. C., Zitelli, B. J., Rockette, H., Fischer, J., Starzl, T. E., Iwatsuki, S. and Shaw, B. W. Choosing a pediatric recipient for orthotopic liver transplantation. *J. Pediatr.* 111 (1987) 479–489

Marsh, J. W., Makowka, L., Todo, S., Gordon, R. D., Esquivel, C. O., Tzakis, A., Iwatsuki, S. and Starzl, T. E. Liver transplantation today. *Postgrad. Med.* 81 (1987) 13–16

Martinez-Ibanez, V., Margarit, C., Tormo, R., Infante, D. *et al.* Liver transplantation in metabolic diseases. Report of five pediatric cases. *Transplant. Proc.* 19 (1987) 3803–3804

McDonald, J. C., Landreneau, M. D., Rohr, M. S. and De Vault, G. A., Jr. Reversal by liver transplantation of the complications of primary hyperoxaluria as well as the metabolic effect. *N. Engl. J. Med.* 321 (1989) 1100–1103

Merion, R. M., Delius, R. E., Campbell, D. A., Jr. and Turcotte, J. G. Orthotopic liver transplantation totally corrects factor IX deficiency in hemophilia B. *Surgery* 104 (1988) 929–931

Mieles, L., Orenstein, D., Teperman, L., Podesta, L., Koneru, B. and Starzl, T. E. Liver transplantation in cystic fibrosis. *Lancet* 1 (1989) 1073

Morgan, S. H. and Watts, R. M. Perspectives in the assessment and management of patients with primary hyperoxaluria type 1. *Adv. Nephrol.* 18 (1989) 95–106

Mowat, A. P. Liver disorders in children: the indications for liver replacement in parenchymal and metabolic disorders. *Transplant. Proc.* 19 (1987) 3236–3241

Oellerich, M., Burdelski, M., Lautz, H. U., Rodeck, B. and Schmidt, F. W. Assessment of short-term prognosis in transplant candidates with cirrhosis. *J. Hepatol.* 9 (1989a) 67

Oellerich, M., Burdelski, M., Lautz, H. U., Rodeck, B. and Düwel, J. Prognostic value of the MEGX liver function test in transplant candidates. *Clin. Chem.* 35 (1989b) 1130

Oellerich, M., Burdelski, M., Lautz, H. U. Prognostic sensitivity and specificity of the monoethylglycinexylidide liver function test in transplant candidates. *J. Clin. Chem. Clin. Biochem.* 27 (1989c) 757

Oellerich, M., Burdelski, M., Lautz, H. U., Schulz, M., Schmidt, F. W. and Herrmann, H. Lidocaine metabolite formation as a measure of liver function in patients with cirrhosis. *Ther. Drug. Monit.* 12 (1990) 220–226

Otto, G., Herfarth, C., Senninger, N., Feist, G., Post, S. and Gmelin, K. Hepatic transplantation in galactosemia. *Transplantation* 47 (1989) 902–903

Pett, S. and Mowat, A. P. Crigler–Najjar syndrome types I and II. Clinical experience — King's College Hospital 1972–1978. Phenobarbitone, phototherapy and liver transplantation. *Mol. Aspects Med.* 9 (1987) 473–482

Pichlmayr, R., Ringe, B., Burdelski, M., Lauchart, W. and Schmidt, E. Liver transplantation in metabolic diseases. *Z. Gastroenterol. (Verh.)* 22 (1987) 57–60

Polson, R. J., Rolles, K., Calne, R. Y., Williams, R. and Marsden, D. Reversal of severe neurological manifestations of Wilson's disease following orthotopic liver transplantation. *Q. J. Med.* 64 (1987) 685–691

Polson, R. J., Lim, C. K., Rolles, K., Calne, R. Y. and Williams, R. The effect of liver transplantation in a 13-year-old boy with erythropoietic protoporphyria. *Transplantation* 46 (1988) 386–389

Ringe, B., Pichlmayr, R. and Burdelski, M. A new technique of hepatic vein reconstruction in partial liver transplantation. *Transplant. Int.* 1 (1988) 30–35

Samuel, D., Boboc, B., Bernuau, J., Bismuth, H. and Benhamou, J. P. Liver transplantation for protoporphyria. Evidence for the predominant role of the erythropoetic tissue in protoporphyrine overproduction. *Gastroenterology* 95 (1988) 816–819

Schade, R. R. The changing indications for liver transplantation. *Transplant. Proc.* 19 (1987) 2–6

Shaw, B. W., Jr, Wood, R. P., Kaufman, S. S., Williams, L., Antonson, D. L. and Vanderhoof, J. Liver transplantation therapy for children: Part 1. *J. Pediatr. Gastroenterol. Nutr.* 7 (1988) 157–166

Shevell, M. I., Bernard, B., Adelson, J. W., Doody, D. P., Laberge, J. M. and Guttman, F. M. Crigler–Najjar syndrome type 1: treatment by home phototherapy followed by orthotopic liver transplantation. *J. Pediatr.* 110 (1987) 429–431

Sokol, R. J., Francis, P. D., Gold, S. H., Ford, D. M., Lum, G. M. and Ambruso, D. R. Orthotopic liver transplantation for acute fulminant Wilson disease. *J. Pediatr.* 107 (1985) 549–552

Starzl, T. E. Surgery for metabolic liver disease. In: McDermott, W. V., Jr (ed.) *Surgery of the Liver.* Blackwell Scientific, Oxford, 1989a, pp. 127–136

Starzl, T. E. Transplantation. *J. Am. Med. Assoc.* 261 (1989b) 2894–2895

Starzl, T. E., Bilheimer, D. W., Bahnson, H. T., Shaw, B. W., Jr, Hardesty, R. L. *et al.*, Heart–liver transplantation in a patient with familial hypercholesterolemia. *Lancet* 1 (1984) 1382–1383

Starzl, T. E., Zitelli, B. J., Shaw, B. W., Jr *et al.* Changing concepts: liver replacement for hereditary tyrosinemia and hepatoma. *J. Pediatr.* 106 (1985) 604–606

Starzl, T. E., Demetris, A. J. and van Thiel, D. Liver transplantation (First of two parts). *N. Engl. J. Med.* 321 (1989a) 1014–1022

Starzl, T. E., Demetris, A. J. and van Thiel, D. Liver transplantation (Second of two parts). *N. Engl. J. Med.* 321 (1989b) 1092–1099

Sternlieb, I. Wilson's disease: indications for liver transplantation. *Hepatology* 4 (*Suppl.*) (1984) 15S–17S

Sternlieb, I. Wilson's disease: transplantation when all else has failed. *Hepatology* 8 (1988) 975–976

Sturm, E., Burdelski, M., Bojanowski, M., Hoeg, J. M., Tsokos, M., Schulz-Falten, J. and Bojanowski, D. Progressive intrahepatic cholestasis: a defect in apolipoprotein A-I synthesis? *Hepatology* 12 (2) (1990) 984

Tuchman, M., Freese, D. K., Sharp, H. L., Ramnaraine, M. L., Ascher, N. and Bloomer, J. R. Contribution of extrahepatic tissues to biochemical abnormalities in hereditary tyrosinemia type I: study of three patients after liver transplantation. *J. Pediatr.* 110 (1987) 399–403

Tuchman, M. Persistent acitrullinemia after liver transplantation for carbamylphosphate deficiency (letter). *N. Engl. J. Med.* 320 (1989) 1498–1499

van Thiel, D. H., Gartner, L. M., Thorp, F. K., Newman, S. L., Lindahl, J. A., Stoner, E., New M. I. and Starzl, T. E. Resolution of the clinical features of tyrosinemia following orthotopic liver transplantation for hepatoma. *J. Hepatol.* 3 (1986) 42–48

Watts, R. W., Calne, R. Y., Williams, R., Mansell, M. A., Veall, N. and Purkiss, P. Primary hyperoxaluria (type 1): attempted treatment by combined hepatic and renal transplantation. *Q. J. Med.* 57 (1985) 697–703

Watts, R. W., Calne, R. Y., Rolles, K., Danpure, C. J., Morgan, S. H., Mansell, M. A., Williams, R. and Purkiss, P. Successful treatment of primary hyperoxaluria type I by combined hepatic and renal transplantation. *Lancet* 2 (1987) 474–475

J. Inher. Metab. Dis. 14 (1991) 619–626
© SSIEM and Kluwer Academic Publishers.

The Place of Fetal Liver Transplantation in the Treatment of Inborn Errors of Metabolism

Reported by J.-L. TOURAINE
with the collaboration of S. LAPLACE, F. REZZOUG, K. SANHADJI,
P. VEYRON, C. ROYO, I. MAIRE, M. T. ZABOT, M. T. VANIER, M. O. ROLLAND,
E. GOILLOT, O. DE BOUTEILLER, J. L. GARNIER, C. POUTEIL-NOBLE,
P. RAFFAELE, J. M. LIVROZET and T. SAINT-MARC
Department of Transplantation and Clinical Immunology, Pavillon P, Hôpital E. Herriot, 69437 Lyon Cedex 03, France

Summary: Over the last 16 years, 202 fetal tissue transplants have been performed in our department to treat 29 patients with severe inborn errors of metabolism without immunodeficiency, 26 patients with congenital and severe immunodeficiency diseases, and 2 patients with severe aplastic anaemia. The actuarial survival curve of patients with inborn errors of metabolism treated with fetal liver transplantation shows a 12-year survival of 77%. The condition of many of these patients has been improved by the treatment, but transplantation has had to be repeated in order to maintain clinical amelioration. Enzyme levels were not significantly and durably increased in peripheral blood but the quantities of substrates detected in sera and urines were significantly reduced and tissue deposits were stabilized.

Bone marrow transplantation has been shown to be effective in correcting – or partially improving – a large variety of inborn errors of metabolism (Hobbs, 1981, 1989). To avoid the risk of complications associated with the pretransplant conditioning, the bone marrow aplasia and the allogeneic reactions (infections, haemorrhages, graft-versus-host disease), and to develop a treatment applicable also to patients lacking an HLA-identical donor, we have investigated an alternative form of therapy, fetal liver transplantation (FLT). Such transplants provide both the haematopoietic stem cells and the precursors of hepatocytes. They home preferentially in the liver, the spleen and the bone marrow. To reduce the risk of complications, we have not used pretransplant conditioning which would leave the patients in prolonged and severe aplasia since, using the current methods, FLT in man results in a progressive reconstitution of haematopoiesis over several months. In patients with severe combined immunodeficiency disease (SCID), FLT was found to reconstitute the immunological system and cure the underlying disease fully (Touraine, 1983; Touraine *et al.*, 1987); it was also very effective when undertaken on the sick fetus, *in utero*, immediately following prenatal diagnosis (Touraine, 1989; Touraine *et al.*, 1989). In patients with inborn errors of metabolism which did not involve any immunodeficiency, a prolonged and moderate immunosuppressive therapy was given to limit rejection of the transplanted cells; in these conditions, full chimerism and displacement of the patient's own stem cells were not obtained but the cell survival *in vivo* was sufficient to lead to some improvement (Touraine, 1982; Touraine and Marseglia, 1985).

These clinical studies were preceded and accompanied by *in vitro* tests on human cells (Veyron *et al.*, 1982) and *in vivo* experiments on animal models, especially on the LSD mice (Veyron and Touraine, 1990), which demonstrated the benefit procured by FLT in enzyme deficiencies. They were conducted in accordance with the rules defined by the French National Committee for Bioethics (Touraine, 1985).

PATIENTS, MATERIALS AND METHODS

In our institution, 202 fetal tissue transplants have been performed in 57 patients (Table 1). Some immunodeficiency diseases, e.g. the Di George syndrome (embryopathy of the third and fourth pharyngeal pouches), were treated with fetal thymus transplantation, others with both fetal liver and thymus transplantation. The inborn errors of metabolism due to enzyme defects which did not result in immunodeficiency are listed in Table 2; they were treated with FLT.

Livers and thymuses were obtained from dead fetuses aged 7–20 weeks. A cell suspension was prepared in culture medium and the transplant consisted of the

Table 1   202 fetal tissue transplants in 57 patients (October 1974 to June 1990)

No.	Condition
19	Severe combined immunodeficiency disease (FLTT)[a]
1	Bare lymphocyte syndrome (FTT)[b]
6	Di George syndrome (FTT)
2	Severe aplastic anaemia (FLT)[c]
29	Inborn errors of metabolism (FLT)

[a]FLTT: fetal liver and thymus transplantation
[b]FTT: fetal thymus transplantation
[c]FLT: fetal liver transplantation

Table 2   Fetal liver transplantation in inborn errors of metabolism

5 Fabry disease	2 Hurler disease
5 Gaucher disease	2 Metachromatic leukodystrophy
2 Fucosidosis	1 Adrenoleukodystrophy
1 Niemann–Pick A	1 Sanfilippo B
1 Niemann–Pick B	1 Familial amyloidosis
2 Niemann–Pick C	1 Hunter disease
1 Morquio B	1 Gangliosidosis (GM2)
2 Glycogenosis	1 β-Thalassaemia major

intraperitoneal injection or the intravenous infusion of the cell suspension. Special care was given to the prevention of the transmission of micro-organisms. Serological tests for HIV, HBV and CMV were routinely performed on the donor's maternal serum. Patients with normal immunity received steroids (2 mg/kg the first day, rapidly tapered) in addition to either azathioprine ($2\,mg\,kg^{-1}\,day^{-1}$) or cyclosporin ($6\,mg\,kg^{-1}\,day^{-1}$), then adjusted using trough levels.

RESULTS

Figure 1 and Table 3 report the results obtained in these various and severe diseases.

Of the 26 patients with immunodeficiency diseases, 14 are alive and well. Immunological reconstitution could develop without restriction despite HLA mismatch between donor and recipient (Touraine, 1983; Roncarolo *et al.*, 1986; Touraine *et al.*, 1987). Clinical and immunological data concerning these patients have previously been published and we shall not develop further the primary immunodeficiency cases here.

Of the 29 patients with inborn errors of metabolism and normal immunity, 24 are presently alive. By contrast with immunodeficiency disease patients, those with inborn errors were not cured of their underlying disease but their condition improved thanks

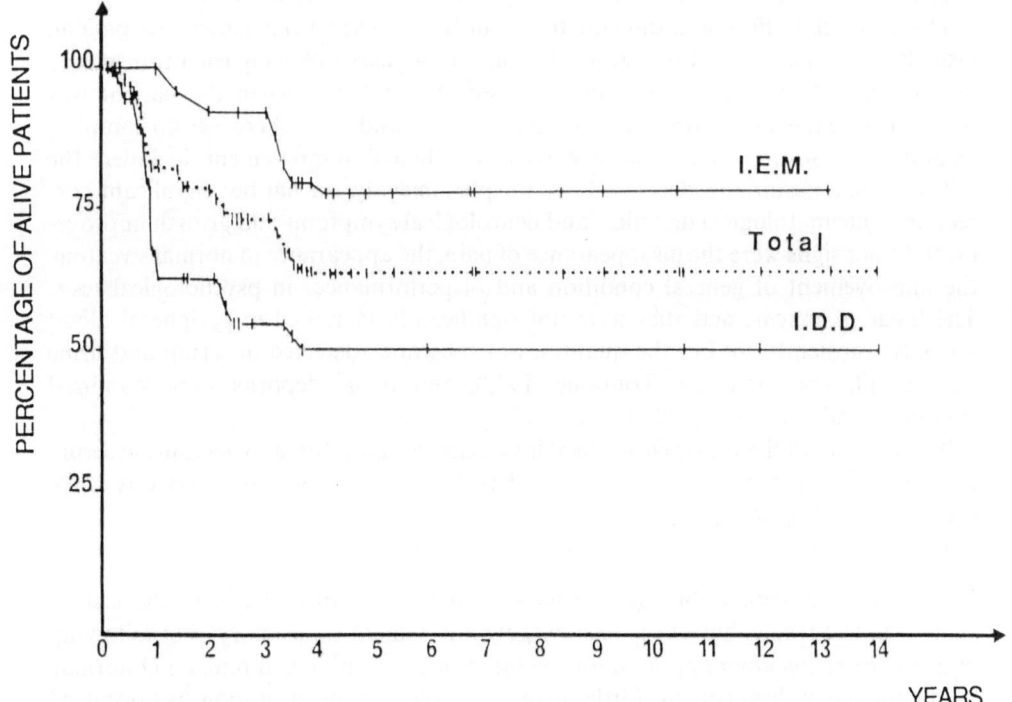

Figure 1 Survival of patients with severe immunodeficiency diseases or inborn errors of metabolism, treated in Lyon by fetal tissue transplantation, from 1974 to 1989

Table 3   Results of fetal tissue transplantation post- or prenatally in immunodeficiency diseases (IDD), inborn errors of metabolism (IEM) and severe aplastic anaemia (SAA)

No. of patients treated	Type of transplant	Alive and well	Success of transplant
26 IDD	FTT[a] (6 Di George,	5	4
	1 BLS[b])	0	0
	FLTT[c] [d] (19 SCID[e],	9	8
	including 3 BLS and 3		
	ADA[f] deficiency)		
29 IEM	FLT[g] [h]	24	24
2 SAA	FLT	0	0
Total 57		38	36

[a]FTT: Fetal thymus transplant
[b]BLS: Bare lymphocyte syndrome
[c]FLTT: Fetal liver and thymus transplant
[d]Two patients were transplanted *in utero* following prenatal diagnosis
[e]SCID: Severe combined immunodeficiency disease
[f]ADA: adenosine deaminase
[g]FLT: fetal liver transplant
[h]One patient was transplanted *in utero* following prenatal diagnosis

to the normal enzyme activity of the transplanted cells. In most patients, this improvement could be maintained only by using repeated transplants.

The beneficial effect was difficult to quantify; it varied from patient to patient. Usually it was partial and transitory (1 month to 4 years following each transplant). Generally, and as could be expected, the effect was better when the patient was treated before the most advanced stage of the disease and when there was no complete mental deterioration. The objective signs of clinical improvement included the following manifestations: decreased hepatosplenomegaly, partial but significant correction of haematological disorders and neurological symptoms and growth improvement. Other signs were the disappearance of pain, the appearance of normal sweating, the improvement of general condition and of performances in psychological tests. The levels of enzyme activities were not significantly increased in peripheral blood (or only transiently so) but the quantities of substrates detected in serum and urine were significantly reduced (Touraine, 1982), and tissue deposits were stabilized (Touraine and Marseglia, 1985).

The viability of the transplanted fetal liver cells was monitored by measuring serum levels of α-fetoprotein (AFP) which rose sharply, then decreased progressively while cells matured (Figure 2).

For the various diseases treated the results were as follows:

(i) Five patients with Fabry disease have been treated with FLT over the last 15 years. Clinical results have been encouraging and remain satisfactory after follow-up of 2–15 years. Sweating appeared for the first time, becoming and remaining normal; pain completely disappeared. Little further neurological deterioration has occurred since FLT. Renal involvement appeared to be stabilized, except in one patient who already had a partial renal failure at the time of FLT: the blood creatinine

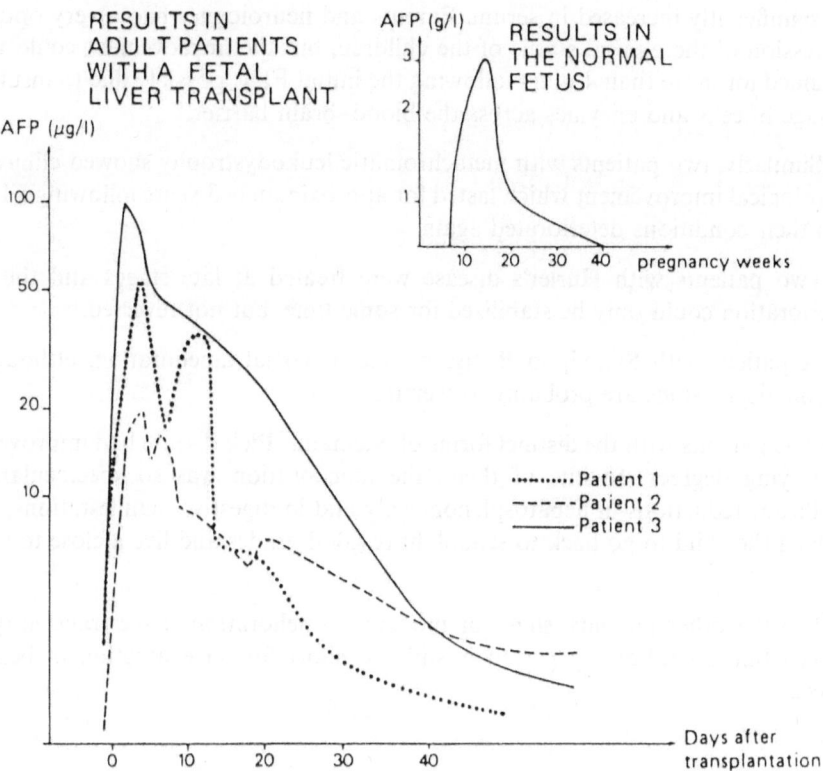

Figure 2 Variations in α-fetoprotein (AFP) levels in the serum of three patients with Fabry disease following fetal liver transplantation. Comparison with levels in the normal fetus

concentration was stabilized in this patient for a period of 4 years and then rose again with a slow progression. Cutaneous lesions seemed slightly decreased. The first patient apparently developed two rejection crises; the first one was successfully treated with an increased dosage of steroids. After the second rejection, pain reappeared but vanished again following a second FLT. The α-galactosidase A activity was not significantly increased in either leukocytes or sera. Trihexosylceramides were decreased in urine and in sera. The effect of FLT on Fabry disease itself in the very long term is still uncertain and no complete correction can be expected since glycosphingolipid deposits are not removed from a kidney even when transplanted into a non-Fabry recipient (Grunfeld *et al.*, 1975). The best results which can be hoped for from this form of therapy would not even attain the condition of heterozygote females who have a few clinical symptoms.

(ii) Five patients with Gaucher disease (one adult type and four severe forms in children) showed some improvement following FLT: amelioration of general condition, diminution of hepatosplenomegaly and slight reduction of thrombocytopenia.

(iii) Two patients received FLT for fucosidosis with neurological involvement. Their clinical condition improved for several years. The levels of α-fucosidase activity were not significantly increased in serum. Parents and neurologists had a very optimistic impression of the clinical status of the children, but the improvement could not be sustained for more than 4 years following the initial FLT, possibly due to insufficient passage of cells and enzymes across the blood–brain barrier.

(iv) Similarly, two patients with metachromatic leukodystrophy showed clinical and neurological improvement which lasted for approximately 3 years following FLT but then their conditions deteriorated again.

(v) Two patients with Hurler's disease were treated at late stages and the brain deterioration could only be stabilized for some time, but not reversed.

(vi) A patient with Sanfilippo B disease had a partial amelioration, although the neurological lesions are probably irreversible.

(vii) The patients with the distinct forms of Niemann–Pick disease had improvements to varying degrees. In one of them, the amelioration was so spectacular, with significant reductions in hepatosplenomegaly and in digestive manifestations, that it enabled the child to go back to school, have good grades and live a close to normal life.

(viii) In the other patients, slight or moderate ameliorations have transiently been noticed but the follow-up period is still too short for an evaluation of beneficial effects.

DISCUSSION

At the present time the methods for correction of enzyme deficiencies (Brady *et al.*, 1973) are only partially effective. Repeated enzyme infusions, blood product transfusions and fibroblast transplants have been relatively disappointing. In the future, the use of modified enzyme molecules or of gene therapy will offer possible treatments for some of the congenital errors of metabolism.

The current use of organ, bone marrow or fetal liver transplantation has given hope to patients with many of these diseases (Hobbs, 1989). The positive results obtained with organ transplants are described in other articles in this issue. As reported in another paper, bone marrow transplants lead to significant improvements in many inborn errors of metabolism: this procedure, however, is not without risk for the patient, especially when there is no HLA-identical sibling available. FLT in association with a moderate and prolonged immunosuppression represents a concrete possibility for partial amelioration in several inborn errors, provided that it is performed early enough in the course of the disease.

The mechanism of action may be interpreted in the light of *in vitro* results. In effect, when cells deficient in lysosomal enzymes were cocultured with normal cells, they were shown to incorporate some enzyme activity (Veyron *et al.*, 1982). We can therefore assume that the deficient cells from the patients could partially benefit from transplanted normal cells when the latter cells have migrated and come to rest in very close vicinity to the deficient cells. Such a phenomenon possibly occurs in the liver, the spleen, the bone marrow and, to a lesser degree, in other organs. The very clear efficacy of FLT in LSD mice (Veyron and Touraine, 1990) will offer an experimental model to test further this hypothesis for the mechanism of action *in vivo*.

To discriminate between the possible effects of steroids, azathioprine or cyclosporin and those of the transplanted fetal liver cells themselves, we have given this immunosuppressive therapy to some patients with Fabry disease for 2 months prior to FLT. No clinical improvement or laboratory alteration of ceramides was noticed during this pretreatment period, while modifications were observed from the very first weeks following FLT.

The ethical issues surrounding the treatment of children with very severe inborn errors of metabolism are numerous and incompletely solved. It is our belief that treating the very terminal patient – as we occasionally have done – may be disputable on the grounds that active prolongation of an almost agonic life is not a valid approach. Obviously all the above-described treatments were carried out with the informed consent of the parents, but this is certainly not sufficient to validate the procedure. At the present time, we tend to consider unethical the active treatments given without curative hope to prolong survival of patients with inborn errors of metabolism in the agonic phase, and we apply FLT in relatively less advanced stages.

REFERENCES

Brady, R. O., Tallman, J. F., Johnson, W. G., Gal, A. E., Leahy, W. R., Quirk, J. M., and Dekaban, A. S. Replacement therapy for inherited enzyme deficiency. Use of purified ceramidetrihexosidase in Fabry disease. *N. Engl. J. Med.* 289 (1973) 9

Grunfeld, J. P., Le Porrier, M., Droz, D., Bensaude, J., Hinglais, N. and Crosnier, J. La transplantation rénade chez les sujets atteints de maladie de Fabry. *Nouv. Presse Med.* 4 (1975) 2081

Hobbs, J. R. Bone marrow transplantation for inborn errors. *Lancet* 2 (1981) 735

Hobbs, J. R. *Correction of Certain Genetic Diseases by Transplantation*, 1 vol., Cogent, London, 1989

Roncarolo, M. G., Touraine, J. L. and Banchereau, J. Co-operation between major histocompatibility complex mismatched mononuclear cells from a human chimera in the production of antigen-specific antibody. *J. Clin. Invest.* 77 (1986) 673

Touraine, J. L. Fetal liver transplantation in congenital enzyme deficiencies in man. *Exp. Haematol.* 10 (suppl. 10) (1982) 46

Touraine, J. L., Bone marrow and liver transplantation in immunodeficiencies and inborn errors of metabolism: Lack of significant restriction of T-cell function in long-term chimeras despite HLA-mismatch. *Immunol. Rev.* 71 (1983) 103

Touraine, J. L. *Hors de la Bulle*, 1 vol., Flammarion, Paris, 1985

Touraine, J. L. New strategies in the treatment of immunological and other inherited diseases: allogeneic stem cells transplantation. *Bone Marrow Transplantation*, 4 (suppl. 4) (1989) 139

Touraine, J. L. and Marseglia, G. L. Fetal liver transplantation in congenital enzyme deficiency. *Perspect. Inher. Metab. Dis.* 6 (1985) 109

Touraine, J. L., Roncarolo, M. G. and Royo, C. Fetal tissue transplantation, bone marrow transplantation and prospective gene therapy in severe immunodeficiencies and enzyme deficiencies. *Thymus* 10 (1987) 75

Touraine, J. L., Raudrant, D., Royo, C., Rebaud, A., Roncarolo, M. G., Souillet, G., Philippe, N., Touraine, F. and Bétuel, H. *In utero* transplantation of stem cells in bare lymphocyte syndrome. *Lancet* 1 (1989) 1382

Veyron, P., Maire, I., Zabot, M. T., Mathieu, M., Bonneau, M. and Touraine, J. L. Fabry's disease: Attempted correction of α-galactosidase A deficiency in cell culture. In M. d'A. Crawfurd *et al.* (eds.) *Advances in the Treatment of Inborn Errors of Metabolism*, Wiley, Chichester, 1982, p. 333

Veyron, P. and Touraine, J. L. Survival of grafted BALB/c lysosomal storage disease mice. *Transplantation Proc.* 22 (1990) 2253

J. Inher. Metab. Dis. 14 (1991) 627–632
© SSIEM and Kluwer Academic Publishers.

Screening and Economics

J. A. STILWELL
Health Services Research Unit, Warwick Business School, University of Warwick, UK

Summary: Screening for disease involves expenditure now in order to reap benefits in the future. It is important to understand why future benefits should be *discounted* in the cost–benefit calculation. The reasons are derived from a societal preference for consumption now over consumption tomorrow, combined with the productivity of capital, which enables goods today to be transformed into more goods tomorrow.

It is also necessary to put costs and values on human lives. This is simplified at present in the UK because a highly restrictive immigration policy implies that the net value of the average additional citizen is zero (or even negative).

The cost–benefit calculations that are presented must be carried out highly systematically in order to avoid double counting or omission. A computerized spreadsheet is ideal for this purpose.

The special characteristics of a health screening programme are first that, initially (or for any one cohort), the costs occur earlier, and in some cases much earlier, than the benefits, and secondly that it is often possible to come to an unequivocal conclusion concerning the net value of a screening programme without recourse to any attempt to put a money value upon quality-of-life improvements.

By this I mean that a screening programme can in the first instance be seen as an investment that should pay for itself by reducing future health service costs by a greater present value than the costs incurred by the programme. Only if the programme cost is greater than the future cost savings is it necessary to appeal to the value of reduction in morbidity in order to justify the screening programme.

There are three issues, therefore, where economic theory makes a contribution to decision making in this area. After these issues have been tackled, the problem is reduced to a systematic enumeration of probable costs, where the information required comes from epidemiologists on the one hand and management accountants on the other. Later I give an example of a method by which a computer spreadsheet is used to display the information systematically and to make the necessary calculations.

The first issue is concerned with comparing present and future costs. How do we know whether a programme pays for itself or not? Double-glazing salesmen will claim that expenditure on new windows 'pays for itself in *x* years' But how big can *x* be? A payback period of 3 years is obviously better than a payback period of 5 years, but the householder still does not know whether or not to install the windows. A more sophisticated, and in private investment terms a satisfactory, decision rule is to ask whether such an investment would literally pay for itself. In other words, could the householder borrow the cost of the windows from the bank, and use the resulting energy savings to pay off the loan before the windows needed replacing again?

Obviously, in such a calculation, there are three crucial inputs; the initial costs, the flow of savings, and the rate of interest. The higher the rate of interest, the less likely it is that a given expected savings flow will be able to pay off the loan.

A private investor takes the rate of interest for granted; he may grumble at its high level, or take advantage if it is low, but to him the question whether or not the rate represents some real and genuine factor in the economy, or whether it is the result of nefarious manipulations of the international Aston-Martini set, is of no relevance.

However, when we consider a social cost–benefit analysis, where we want to answer the real and important question of whether or not it is to the benefit of society to embark upon a social investment, then we need to be able to understand and justify the rate of interest that will be used to discount the future benefit stream consequent upon, and to be compared with, a possible investment in a health screening programme.

Positive interest rates can be justified in terms of two factors — social time preference, and the productivity of capital. Social time preference is the community equivalent of personal time preference. In general, people prefer jam today rather than jam tomorrow, but after several pots of contemporary preserve, people are prepared to sacrifice an additional pot now for the sake of a pot tomorrow. To demonstrate this effect — which is an implication of the oldest and probably most powerful economic axiom concerning the behaviour of people, that of diminishing marginal utility — we must consider an *indifference curve*.

The indifference curve shown below is built up by linking all combinations of 'jam today' and 'jam tomorrow' that are considered by an individual, and by extension by society, to afford the same overall satisfaction (Figure 1). Consider the marked point on Figure 1 which represents an endowment of 16 pots today, and 20 pots tomorrow. The curve gives the information that this is equally as acceptable as 20 pots today and 16 pots tomorrow — a straight swap of four pots. But ask the person (society) to give up 4 pots today (leaving 12), and positive time preference will lead to a demand for 6 extra pots tomorrow. However, although present consumption is in general preferred to future consumption, as one progresses down the indifference curve diminishing marginal utility begins to outweigh this, and, for example, at a consumption today of 30 pots, 3 contemporary pots would be sacrificed in order to secure 2 pots tomorrow.

What is shown here is that an indifference curve is convex to the origin but is rotated slightly so that it approaches the horizontal axis faster than the vertical axis. Both these characteristics are important. An indifference curve is one line on an indifference map, which is a collection of indifference curves. The curves represent higher and higher levels of satisfaction the further they are from the origin of the diagram.

So far we have addressed the *demand* for jam. What about the supply side of the

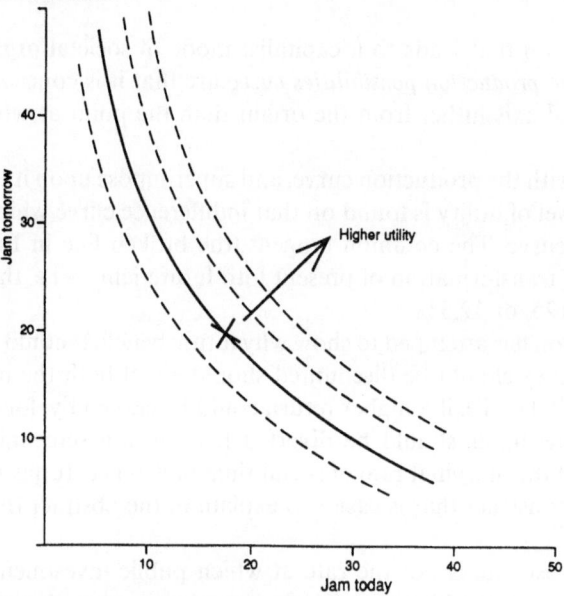

Figure 1 An indifference map showing the combinations of *jam today* and *jam tomorrow* that yield identical consumer satisfaction

equation? Jam today can be converted into jam tomorrow. We can abbreviate this demonstration; Figure 2 shows the different combinations of jam today and jam tomorrow that can be produced by a jam plant. In general, sacrificing today (investing) leads to greater production tomorrow. This is the quality of modern (i.e. post-industrial

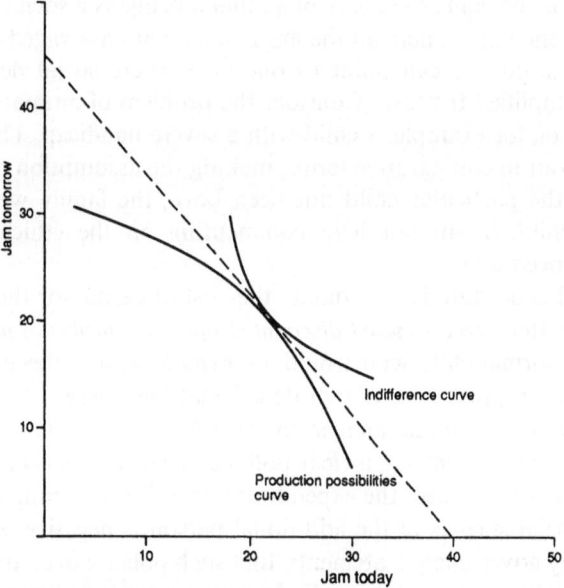

Figure 2 A production possibilities frontier superimposed on the indifference map showing how the highest point of social satisfaction can be attained when the curves are tangential, and that the common tangent is the *rate of interest*

revolution) production that leads to a capitalist mode of societal organization. The characteristics of the *production possibilities curve* are that it is concave to the origin and cuts the vertical axis futher from the origin than the point at which it cuts the horizontal.

Start, therefore, with the production curve, and superimpose upon it the indifference map; the highest level of utility is found on that indifference curve which is tangential to the production curve. The common tangent (the broken line in Figure 2) shows the solution rate of transformation of present into future jam — i.e. the interest rate. In this case it is 1.125, or 12.5%.

This demonstration has attemped to show why future benefits should be discounted. The rate at which they should be discounted should equal both the marginal social productivity of capital — i.e. if a higher return could be earned by, for example, road building, then public funds should be diverted from health screening to the road programme — and the marginal rate of social time preference. It has to be admitted that the latter is a construct that is easier to explain in the abstract than to quantify in practice.

The market interest rate is not the rate at which public investment programmes are discounted, because the Treasury is of course aware that there are influences upon interest rates that have nothing at all to do with underlying parameters of productivity. So from time to time the Treasury estimates the marginal social return to investment, and publishes a discount rate to be used in such exercises. This is a *real* rate — that is, inflation is removed from these calculations, usually by means of carrying them all out at constant prices (which is in any case the easiest way of doing them).

The second issue is the value *to society* of a human being as a social and economic animal. We cannot encompass here all the arguments that have raged over this issue in the past 25 years, but we can point to one area where social decision makers (politicians) have simplified the task. Consider the problem of estimating the *cost to society* of the birth of, for example, a child with a severe handicap. The calculations are usually carried out in comparative terms, making the assumption of *replacement*, meaning that had the particular child not been born, the family would have had another, normal, child. (I am not here commenting on the ethical or religious propriety of this procedure.)

The conventional procedure is to estimate the cost of caring for the handicapped child, and to add to that the *estimated discounted life-time surplus of production over consumption* of the normal child who would, *ex hypothese*, have been born had the handicapped child been prevented. Elaborate calculations ensue.

Luckily, now, for the economic analyst in the UK, although less luckily for the inhabitants of some other countries, a clear political decision has been made that no such social surplus exists. Indeed, the expenditure incurred on immigration controls suggests that the social surplus of the additional person is negative. And we know, of course, from many government statements, that such policies to control population growth are completely consistent over all classes or types of potential immigrant. But I do not think that this could easily or even logically be built into analyses of this type.

The ingredients of a screening cost-effectiveness analysis have been tabulated in a number of articles, of which the most influential over time has been Hagard and Carter's paper (1976) on the costs and benefits of Down syndrome screening, which, although subsequently subject to certain criticisms, is still a useful and readable model. Standard texts on health economics, such as Cullis and West (1979) or Drummond (1980) all describe the ingredients of such an analysis.

In brief, a screening programme is defined and a comparison table is drawn up. The first two elements given below are peculiar to the screening programme; the remaining need to be calculated for the situations with, and without, screening.

(1) The cost of screening
(2) The cost of unnecessary treatment due to the screening programme's less than 100% specificity
(3) Treating
(4) Public sector caring
(5) Private caring costs

These categories need to be disaggregated according to the specific programme. Clearly, the private costs of caring will be different in type between a screening programme for congenital abnormalities and one for breast cancer. For example, in the cited Down syndrome study, it was estimated (or assumed) that the participation in the labour force of young mothers of Down babies would be half the average (leading to a private sacrifice of income, mirroring a public sacrifice of production), but employment trends have changed so much over the intervening 15 years that we could not extrapolate the figures reached by this means to the present day.

Since all future costs need to be discounted, and since in this type of exercise clerical and arithmetical mistakes are frequently made in pre-publication drafts (always corrected, of course, by vigilant referees) I cannot stress too highly the advantages of computerized spreadsheets. What may seem extraordinarily unwieldly upon paper will fit into a minute part of the top left-hand corner of any reasonable commercial spreadsheet. Columns should represent types of costs, or benefits, and for all costs except the costs of finding and of iatrogenic morbidity there should be an identical column for the with-screening and without-screening situation. If the analysis is extended from a cost analysis to one that uses some concept of health measure such as an index designed specifically for the problem (in, perhaps, the case of mental impairment) or some more general measure such as the quality-adjusted life year, then each cost type can have its associated 'outcome' column.

Rows, of course, represent years, and it is a matter of simplicity to discount each row by the interest rate multiplied by (row-year minus base-year).

But perhaps the most compelling reason to use a spreadsheet for this purpose is to undertake *sensitivity analysis*. All estimates of costs (and outcomes) are subject to error, but some errors are more important than others. The arithmetical convenience of a spreadsheet means that the sensitivity of the 'figure in the bottom right hand corner' — the overall surplus of with-screening over without-screening costs — to a whole range of changes in assumptions or estimates, is made trivial, rather than, as was the case previously, so difficult as to be shelved by the exhausted, and perhaps, slightly disorganized?, researcher.

REFERENCES

Cullis, J. G. and West, P. A. *The Economics of Health, an Introduction*, Martin Robertson, Oxford, 1979

Drummond, M. F. *Principles of Economic Appraisal in Health Care*, Oxford University Press, Oxford, 1980

Hagard, S. and Carter, F. A. Preventing the birth of infants with Down's syndrome: a cost benefit analysis. *Br. Med. J.* 1(6012) (1976) 753–756

J. Inher. Metab. Dis. 14 (1991) 633–639

Economic Evaluation of Cost–Benefit Ratio of Neonatal Screening Procedure for Phenylketonuria and Hypothyroidism

J.-L. Dhondt[1]*, J.-P. Farriaux[1], J.-C. Sailly[2] and T. Lebrun[2]

[1]*Centre Régional de Dépistage des Maladies Métaboliques de l'Enfant, Faculté de Médecine, place de Verdun, 59000 Lille, France;* [2]*CRESGE, rue François Baës, 59046 Lille Cedex, France*

Summary: A comparison between the cost of identification and care of patients with phenylketonuria (PKU) and congenital hypothyroidism (CH) and the expenditure for the care of untreated retarded patients has been established on the basis of the activity of the Nord-Pas-de-Calais regional screening centre and of interviews with patients' families. The analysis yields a benefit–cost ratio of 6.6 for PKU and 13.8 for CH prophylaxis. However, cost–benefit varies depending on the economic partner, i.e. the patient's family, Social Security or Administration.

Neonatal screening programmes for phenylketonuria have been generally undertaken on the basis of purely medical considerations rather than for the serious estimation of cost–benefit advantages. In other words, programmes started with the presumption that screening activity was inherently 'good'. However, a lack of economic analysis can slow down future development and introduce a certain degree of apathy toward effecting changes or modifications. For example, after the publication in the USA of recommendations to improve neonatal screening programmes, reluctance to implement any changes was enhanced by budget problems faced by programmes in the different states (Hormuth, 1990). Adding new tests 'at a minimal cost' without any increase in the support of the non-laboratory components of the screening system also represents a major risk of alteration of an existing programme. Only frequent economic evaluation can prevent such problems.

This study reports on an approach to the cost–benefit analysis of the French neonatal screening programme. The study was carried out by a close collaboration of the Lille Regional Screening Centre and health economists, and aimed not only to prove an expected positive benefit–cost ratio, but mainly to serve as a model to develop an analytical framework which can be applied to new programmes.

---

*Correspondence: J.-L. Dhondt, Laboratoire de Biochimie, Hôpital Saint Philibert, 115 rue du Grand But, 59462 Lomme cedex, France

THE FRENCH PROGRAMME FOR NEONATAL SCREENING

The identification of the costs and benefits of screening depends on the organization of the public health services and of the screening programme. In France, neonatal screening is centralized under the auspices of the National Association founded in 1975 under a private statutory loan. In 1978 a convention was signed with the National Social Security (the funding agency) under an agreement with the Ministry of Public Health.

Up to the present the French programme has been voluntarily limited to the screening of phenylketonuria (PKU) and congenital hypothyroidism (CH). The programme (Dhondt and Farriaux, 1983; Frézal *et al.*, 1990) is characterized by an activity which is:

(i)   Systematic: almost all newborns (compliance rate over 99%) are subjected to the tests without existing legal obligation;

(ii)   Co-ordinated: the national organization is a federation of 21 Regional Associations. Each of them assumes the totality of the activities of screening and follow-up;

(iii) Controlled: the French association supervises the regional delegations and assumes responsibility towards the governmental agencies (national registry, interlaboratory quality assurance surveys);

(iv)   Egalitarian: all newborns benefit from the programme and all patients are taken care of free of charge (i.e., free delivery of dietary products for the treatment of PKU);

(v)   Financially balanced: the price of tests is periodically negotiated with the funding agency in regard to evolving aspects of the programme. For this reason the economic analysis of the programme is periodically updated; changes or implementation of new tests have to be first evaluated during pilot studies under the control of a technical committee. Such procedures are included in the contract between the French Association and Social Security.

COST–BENEFIT ANALYSIS

The aim of the study was to evaluate the cost–benefit ratio per detected case (Dhondt *et al.*, 1988). The evaluation was of an economic and monetary nature. It was realized globally and for each agent concerned with the procedure: the child and his family, Social Security and the community including state and local administrations.

The screening costs were calculated on the basis of the expenses of the Nord-Pas-de-Calais Regional Screening Centre which covers a tenth of the French population (80 000 newborns/year) with a single laboratory which has been managed by the same team for 20 years. Other economic data were obtained from the National Economic Statistical Agency (INSEE), from the analysis of 153 medical records (63 PKU, 90 CH) to establish medical costs and from interviews with 60 families (30 PKU, 30 CH) to evaluate additional costs.

A number of hypotheses have been adopted for the calculations:

(i)   The frequency of the diseases: PKU, 1/15937 and CH, 1/4041, with a coverage by the programme which is almost complete (99.8%), with all the identified cases effectively controlled and treated;

(ii) Life expectancy: (a) without early detection of the disease: PKU, 30 to 40 years, CH, 40 years when severely retarded (55% of the patients), 60 years when moderately or mildly retarded (25%) and 75 years in cases of normality; (b) after neonatal screening and proper treatment: normal life expectancy for PKU and CH.

(iii) Efficiency of the treatment (the child benefits from the treatment for its whole life for CH and for 8 years for PKU): the child detected and treated early is considered normal.

(iv) Duration of institutionalization (without detection): PKU, between 20 and 30 years, CH, variable according to the degree of the disease.

(v)   Monetary calculation: we used costs in 1985 French Francs with a discount rate of 4.5% (the computation has also been performed for the discount rates 7% and 10%).

In this evaluation we voluntarily omitted the costs connected with an increase in the incidence of PKU because of the treatment of detected patients, the incidence of false negatives (patients not detected by the screening test), and the follow-up of PKU mothers who have to return to the special diet during pregnancy (the problem of 'maternal PKU').

RESULTS AND COMMENTS

Tables 1 and 2 summarize the elements of the monetary analysis for each specific agent. Table 3 reports the cost–benefit ratio obtained for different discount rates. It is obvious that the monetary value of the global benefits due to the screening and treatment programme for CH (cost–benefit ratio = 13.8) is much higher than that obtained for the PKU programme (cost–benefit ratio = 6.6). This was to be expected because the incidence of CH is about five times higher and the cost of its treatment is much lower (7.6% of the medical costs vs 40% (Table 4)).

We have to be cautious with these first results. They are of a relative nature; indeed, it is difficult to provide a complete description and evaluation of all the benefits and costs of the programme. The major benefit usually argued is avoidance of the burden to society of the costs of caring for the mentally retarded child. However, the calculations for each specific agent demonstrate important variations in the cost–benefit ratio. As mentioned in previous reports (Dagenais *et al.*, 1985), some benefits can only be enumerated without being quantified (i.e., the increase in the well-being of parents and of affected children). The direct costs of the screening are easy to describe and quantify, although some of them are generally omitted (e.g. communication (Table 5)).

Table 1 Benefits and costs of neonatal screening procedure for PKU for each specific agent (in 1985 French Francs with a discount rate of 4.5%)

Benefits			Costs		
The child and family					
Gains of production		947 057	Taxes		291 657
Avoided costs of looking after the handicapped		34 784	Social contributions		35 771
			Allowances for a handicapped adult		34 784
			Part of medical expenses beyond age 30		1 733
	Total	981 841		Total	363 945
Social Security					
Social contributions		223 566	Cost of detection, confirmatory diagnosis, and regular follow-up		247 815
Avoided social placing					
For a child		1 479 789			
For an adult		660 883	Treatment		130 281
			Part of medical expenses beyond age 30		5 198
	Total	2 364 238		Total	383 294
State and other Administration					
Allowance for handicapped adult		34 784	Education		125 761
Taxes		291 657			
	Total	326 441		Total	125 761

More important is the possibility of progressive increases in costs due to 'minor' but additive changes in an ongoing programme. Improving the quality of therapeutic results is the goal of all metabolic units; this can be achieved at the screening or at the follow-up stage.

In PKU, the cost of dietary foods represents 1/10 (4.5 million FF) of the annual budget of the French Association. The mean annual cost per PKU infant for these diets is estimated at 15 000 FF with a wide range of variations depending on the substitute food product used (Figure 1). Since we are now aware of the risk of 'artificial' diets (vitamin and micronutrient supplements), improvement of the dietary foods may also imply the incurring of increasing costs. In addition, a longer period of dietary management is still under discussion.

In CH, improvement in the therapeutic results is believed to be obtained with a higher dosage of L-thyroxine for the early treatment and earlier follow-up of the patients. In fact, in our personal experience the mean age at diagnosis was 26 days (Dhondt et al., 1987). We can accelerate the screening logistics by taking blood earlier (day 3 vs day 5), by speeding up mail transport and by modifying the working schedule in the laboratory. With such changes it has been demonstrated that screening results can be obtained by day 12 of life in 96% of cases. However, the increased cost of the test is not negligible; the average cost of prestamped envelopes and special delivery was 1.6 FF per test (about 10% of the actual cost of the test).

Table 2 Benefits and costs of neonatal screening procedure for CH for each specific agent (in 1985 French Francs with a discount rate of 4.5%)

Benefits		Costs	
The child and family			
Gains of production	688 586	Taxes	205 899
Avoided costs of looking after		Social contributions	25 253
the handicapped	42 487	Allowances for a handicapped	
		adult	42 487
		Part of medical expenses	
		beyond age 30	629
Total	731 073	Total	274 268
Social Security			
Social contributions	157 831	Cost of detection, confirmatory	
Avoided institutionalization		diagnosis and regular follow-	
For a child	946 180	up	77 442
For an adult	623 108	Treatment	13 207
		Part of medical expenses	1 888
		beyond age 30	
Total	1 727 119	Total	92 537
State and other Administration			
Specialized education	89 975	Education	100 609
Allowance for handicapped			
adult	42 487		
Taxes	205 899		
Other institutions (psychiatric	127 263		
houses, etc.)			
Total	465 624	Total	100 609

Table 3 Cost–benefit ratio of PKU and CH screening

	PKU			Congenital hypothyroidism		
Discount rate	4.5%	7%	10%	4.5%	7%	10%
Global	6.6	4.7	3.3	13.8	9.7	6.9
Child–family	2.7	2.7	2.7	2.6	2.6	2.6
Social Security	6.2	4.6	3.3	18.7	12.9	8.8
State and other Administrations	2.6	1.7	1.1	4.6	3.2	2.4

Table 4 Costs of treatment of a PKU and a CH patient (in 1985 French Francs)

	PKU	CH
Hospitalization	23 673	3 157
Consultations	3 943	6 688
Drugs and diet	102 665	3 362
Total	130 281	13 207

Table 5   Definition of costs specific to a screening programme

1 – Organization/administration
2 – Sample collection
3 – Transmission of samples
4 – Laboratory procedure: equipment, salaries, reagents
5 – Programme evaluation
        Data collection
        Record keeping
        Procedure to recheck findings
        Epidemiology
        Quality assurance
6 – Confirmatory diagnostic procedure
7 – Interprogramme considerations
8 – Communication
        Documentation
        Public and parent education
        Training of health care personnel
        Staff training
9 – New areas of concern (other testing, newer techniques)

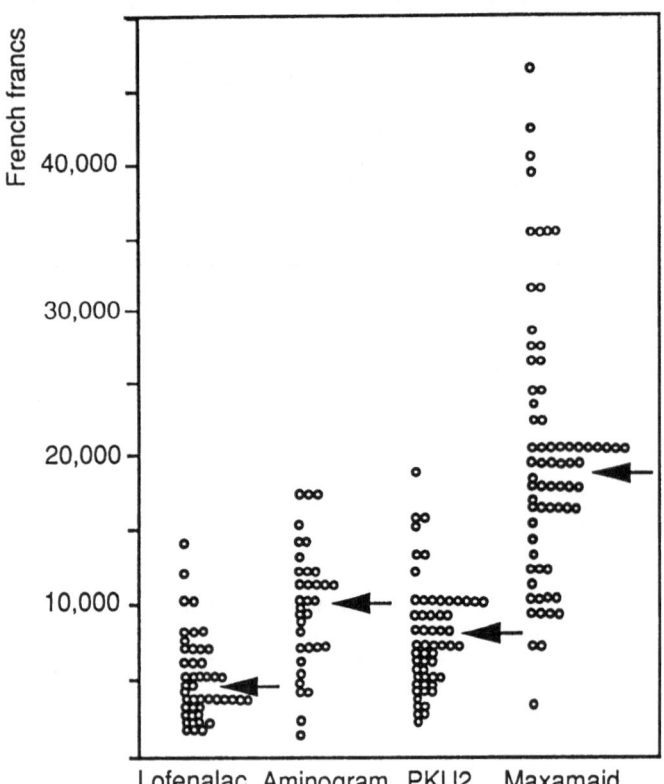

Figure 1   Annual cost of treating a PKU child with different dietary food products. The arrows indicate the mean for each group

These examples demonstrate that adaptations to new realities (further testing, newer techniques) have to be carefully evaluated and must be undertaken with prudence so as not to destabilize the ongoing programme. On behalf of the technical committee of the French Association, several prospective studies (pilot programmes) have been set up to evaluate the feasibility and utility of new screening procedures which may be included in the future in the actual programme.

CONCLUSION

Cost–benefit analysis constitutes an economic mechanism for collective and public decision making concerning the benefits and costs of handicap detection. The evaluation of the ongoing programme for PKU and CH screening was an opportunity to develop methodologies which can be applied to other detection or diagnostic procedures. The remaining problem is how to insert such analysis within a larger framework, taking into account the basic human and philosophical debates about life and handicap.

ACKNOWLEDGEMENT

This work was supported in part by grants from the Conseil Régional Nord-Pas-de-Calais and University of Lille II (B1*).

REFERENCES

Dagenais, D. L., Courville, L. and Dagenais, M. G. A cost-benefit analysis of the Quebec network of genetic medicine. *Soc. Sci. Med.* 20 (1985) 601–607

Dhondt, J. L. and Farriaux, J. P. Integration of neonatal screening procedure. The French experience. In Naruse, H. and Irie, M. (eds.) *Neonatal Screening*, Excerpta Medica, Amsterdam, 1983, pp. 438–443

Dhondt, J. L., Farriaux, J. P., Raux, M., Paux, E., Bouchery, A. M. and Debersée, J. Bilan du dépistage de la phénylcétonurie et de l'hypothyroïdie par le centre de Lille. *Arch. Fr. Pediatr.* 44 (1987) 787–790

Dhondt, J. L., Farriaux, J. P., Lebrun, T., Sailly, J. C. Etude coût/bénéfice du dépistage néonatal de la phénylcétonurie et de l'hypothyroïdie. *Pédiatrie* 43 (1988) 345–348

Frézal, J., Farriaux, J. P., Briard, M. L., Dhondt, J. L., Boschetti, R. and Travert, G. The French program of systematic neonatal screening. In Knoppers, B. M. and Laberge, C. (eds.) *Genetic Screening, From Newborns to DNA Typing*, Elsevier, Amsterdam, 1990, pp. 41–64

Hormuth, R. P. Update of the 1984 Chicago meeting on quality assurance in screening. In Knoppers, B. M. and Laberge, C. (eds.) *Genetic Screening. From Newborns to DNA Typing*, Elsevier, Amsterdam, 1990, pp. 3–10

J. Inher. Metab. Dis. 14 (1991) 640–651

Services for Thalassaemia as a Model for Cost–Benefit Analysis of Genetics Services

B. MODELL[1] and A. M. KULIEV[2]
[1]WHO Collaborating Centre for Community Control of Hereditary Diseases,
Department of Obstetrics and Gynaecology, UCMSM, University College, London,
UK; [2]WHO Collaborating Centre, National Medical Genetics Research Centre of
the Academy of Medical Sciences of the USSR, Moscow, USSR

Summary: Economic appraisal of genetics services is usually limited to consideration of financial costs and benefits, but this can generate misunderstandings about the aims of these services. We propose a general framework for economic analysis that includes non-financial costs and benefits, and the concept of genetic fitness.

The objective of genetics services is to help people with a genetic disadvantage to live and reproduce as normally as possible (*World Health Organization, 1985*).

According to Drummond (1980), a true cost–benefit analysis requires:

(1) A description of the service, including alternative *policies.*
(2) *Enumeration* of all identifiable financial and non-financial costs and benefits of these policies for the patient, the family and society.
(3) *Measurement* of these costs and benefits in any way that is possible and useful, and comparison of different policies.
(4) *Evaluation* of the costs and benefits of different policies, in equivalent units when possible.

Very few published cost–benefit analyses of individual genetics services, such as screening for Down syndrome (Hagard and Carter, 1976; Sadovnick and Baird, 1981), maternal serum AFP screening for neural tube defects (Chamberlain, 1978), or screening for thalassaemia (Attanasio *et al.*, 1980; Ostrowsky *et al.*, 1985; Old *et al.*, 1986) pretend to meet these rather demanding requirements. Most such analyses have been carried out to win financial support by demonstrating to health administrators that prenatal diagnosis saves money. Therefore money has been the main unit of measurement, and non-financial costs and benefits are excluded as 'intangibles' not susceptible to objective measurement. Most publications then attempt a 'cost-effectiveness' analysis, which means a comparison of the financial implications of alternative approaches to the same problem in order to identify the most efficient one. Patient treatment is viewed as an alternative to prevention by screening and prenatal diagnosis, and prevention is shown to be cheaper.

However, this type of analysis has the following serious disadvantages:

(1) It is hurtful to patients and families to hear themselves described as a financial burden rather than a benefit to society, especially when this is done by the medical profession.

(2) Treatment and prevention are complementary aspects of a single policy for a particular genetic disease. Separating them and treating them as alternatives frightens patients and the public.

(3) The implication seems to be that prevention is better because it is cheaper. In reality it is better if people want it.

(4) Cost is expressed in pounds per affected birth prevented, implying that the main objective in prenatal diagnosis is termination of affected pregnancies; but in reality it is the continuation of unaffected pregnancies. Henderson (1982) pointed out that the value of the healthy children born because of prenatal diagnosis is rarely considered. Only one analysis we know of (Gill *et al.*, 1986) takes account of the social and economic contribution of these healthy children. One analysis even argues that society obtains the best bargain when parents do not replace an aborted affected fetus with a healthy child, because the cost of schooling is saved!

(5) It is argued that the service should be funded at least to the point where financial cost equals financial savings. This has slipped into a tacit acceptance that it should be funded *only* to this point — effectively, that the service should pay for itself. This assumption, which is unique in medicine, does less than justice to genetics services.

(6) It is assumed that there is little indication to prevent conditions that lead to intrauterine death or death in early infancy and so do not cost the health service very much, despite the amount of distress involved.

From Drummond's viewpoint, all activities have costs and benefits. If the benefit of the above analyses has been funding for services, the cost has been confusion and misunderstanding because non-financial costs and benefits are excluded. When only money is considered, the aim of the service is inevitably presented as financial — namely, to save money. We need to develop a general approach for cost–benefit analysis of genetics services that is acceptable to the medical profession, patients and the public, and this will require improved dialogue between economists and clinicians.

Analysis of a medical service must be based on its objectives of ameliorating suffering and buying health, and requires valid non-financial units of measurement for costs and benefits. However, it can be difficult to assess even financial costs because of differences between patients, diseases and local standards of treatment, and differences in the distribution of costs between the health service, other social services and the family. Thalassaemia major is a particularly favourable condition for cost–benefit analysis, because it is a fairly uniform disorder, its natural history is known (Modell and Berdoukas, 1984), management is approximately standardized and reasonably successful (Modell and Petrou, 1983), and most of the financial costs of treatment fall on the hospital service. It can also be prevented in whole populations by a programme of community education, population screening, genetic counselling and the offer of prenatal diagnosis (Loukopoulos, 1988). Here we use the example of thalassaemia to demonstrate that many non-financial costs and benefits of genetics services can be measured objectively, and can and should be incorporated into their economic appraisal. We conclude that the concept of genetic fitness should be included in the description of services for genetic disease.

WHAT IS A POLICY?

A *policy* describes a comprehensive approach to a health problem. Treatment alone is not a policy and prevention alone is not a policy, because neither deals with the entire problem of a family at risk. Health policies for genetic disorders must include both patient care and prevention. The World Health Organization describes a 'control programme' for an inherited disease as 'an integrated approach combining the best possible patient care, with prevention* through community information, carrier screening and counselling, and the availability of prenatal diagnosis' (WHO, 1985).

In order to perform an analysis for thalassaemia that includes both treatment and prevention, it proved necessary to consider six 'policies', listed in Table 1. These policies really describe the successive stages in the evolution of treatment, carrier

Table 1 Explanation of 'policies'

Policy number	Treatment	Counselling		Prenatal diagnosis	
		Retrospective	Prospective	Late (> 18 wk)	Early (ca. 9 wk)
1	0	0	0	0	0
2	+	+	0	0	0
3	+	+	0	+	0
4	+	+	0	+	+
5	+	+	+	+	0
6	+	+	+	+	+

Examples

Policy 1: the situation for inherited diseases in most developing countries at present

Policy 2: the situation for inherited diseases where recurrence risk is known but laboratory diagnosis is not possible

Policy 3: e.g. only mid-trimester diagnosis is possible for immune-deficiency syndromes that must be diagnosed by fetal blood sampling after 20 weeks' gestation

Policy 4: first-trimester PND is available on a retrospective basis for many inherited conditions, e.g. cystic fibrosis in recent years

Policy 5: only mid-trimester diagnosis for thalassaemia (using fetal blood obtained at 18 weeks' gestation) is possible in areas such as Cyprus where DNA diagnosis is not yet available

Policy 6: community-based carrier screening and counselling, with first-trimester prenatal diagnosis, is being steadily developed throughout Greece and Italy.

---

*We use the term 'prevention' as a convenient shorthand for steps leading to identification and counselling of couples at risk, with or without the offer of prenatal diagnosis. The use of this term to describe screening and PND services is often criticized because the conception of affected fetuses is not prevented. However, the general aim is to prevent the distress associated with the unexpected or unwanted birth of a child affected by an avoidable disorder. PND is only one reason for the fall in the affected birthrate that often occurs after couples at risk are informed.

diagnosis and prenatal diagnosis for an inherited disease. In the past 25 years services for thalassaemia, for example, have evolved from a situation where very little could be done to effective management combined with community-based carrier screening and counselling and first-trimester prenatal diagnosis. Services for many other conditions are developing along the same lines, particularly rapidly in the case of cystic fibrosis.

As a starting point (*Policy 1*), it is conventional to define a baseline policy in which there is no treatment, genetic counselling or prenatal diagnosis, as in most developing countries today. Table 2, which summarizes costs and benefits to the patient,* the family and society in this situation, shows how terribly unequal the burden of ill-health can be. A principal aim of a National Health Service is to spread such burdens more equally.

Table 2   **Baseline situation: no NHS treatment or genetic counselling**

	Cost	Benefit	
Financial			
Community	Frequent visits to doctors, healers, priests		doctors
		Parents	other healers
		support	priests
			undertakers
Patient	Treated for wrong illness		
Family	Up to whole disposable income while child lives		
Siblings	Economic deprivation		
Health state			
Patient			
Survival	Death < 6 y	Up to 6 y of life	
Quality of life	Chronically sick		
Parents			
Health	Early bereavement	Loved child for 1–5 y	
	Knowledge that cannot afford treatment	Knowledge that doing best for child	
	Psychological disaster can disintegrate family		
Reproduction	25% recurrence risk	Ignorance of risk permits chance to have other, healthy children	
Siblings	Emotional deprivation	Sibling for 1–5 y	
	Poverty endangers health		
Productive output			
Community	Ignorance → prejudice and social isolation of family. This is ultimately a burden on society	No schooling for child	
Patient	No productive output		
Family	Loss of time, impoverishment, and poor morale → low output		

*A similar description, using the same headings, can be made for each of the six policies.

The introduction of effective treatment, and information on recurrence risk (*Policy 2*), resolves many severe problems and creates new ones. As patients live longer and there is more to be done for each one, the number of patients increases by the annual birth rate, and total NHS costs for treating the condition can increase quite rapidly. Genetic counselling provided after the birth of the first affected child ('retrospectively') has little effect on numbers. Even if all parents avoid a recurrence by having no more children, when final family size is 2 or 3 the affected birth rate will fall by only 12–18% (Fraser, 1972). The parents may be saved a recurrence, but are also deprived of the main compensation of ignorance (Table 2) — the chance of having at least one other, healthy child.

The introduction of retrospective prenatal diagnosis alleviates the latter problem. Its acceptability depends on the severity of the condition concerned, on social factors, and on timing of prenatal diagnosis, which is generally more acceptable in the first than in the second trimester of pregnancy. As acceptability affects the numbers of affected children born and the emotional costs to the parents, *Policy 3*, which includes prenatal diagnosis in the second trimester only, must be distinguished from *Policy 4*, in which prenatal diagnosis is available in the first trimester. The main benefit of retrospective prenatal diagnosis is that couples who want further, healthy children can complete their families. Statistically, since it is only possible to avoid recurrences, it has little more effect on the number of affected children born than does genetic counselling alone.

The introduction of 'prospective' carrier diagnosis (before the birth of an affected child) creates a fundamentally new situation, since all couples at risk can be identified and offered an informed choice about whether to undertake a pregnancy or to request prenatal diagnosis. Its effects depend on the adequacy of community information, laboratory diagnosis and counselling as well as on the prenatal diagnosis methods available. With *Policy 5*, prenatal diagnosis is available prospectively only in the second trimester, so carrier screening is often done in the antenatal clinic. In *Policy 6*, prenatal diagnosis is available prospectively in the first trimester of pregnancy. This, the most acceptable present approach, has important implications for service delivery, because to offer first-trimester prenatal diagnosis it is necessary to inform people before they become pregnant. That is, screening and counselling must be extended from the hospital setting into the community.

DESCRIBING TREATMENT

Management of thalassaemia major requires regular monthly blood transfusions, nightly subcutaneous infusion of the iron-chelating drug desferrioxamine (Desferal), and treatment of many possible complications. When the regimen is scrupulously followed the quality of life can be good — the burden of treatment is now one of the main problems of the disease. Patient survival is one key indicator of the effectiveness of treatment. Table 3 shows that the average financial cost per year of healthy life is of the order of £5370 per year per patient, about half for regular transfusions and investigations, and half for drugs. A *minimum* life-expectancy of 25 years (a realistic

Table 3 **Average annual costs of treating a patient with thalassaemia major in the UK. 1987 prices**

	Range (£)
Basic hospital care (12 transfusions, 12 OP visits, investigations	1624–2380
Drugs (mainly desferrioxamine + accessories)	2500–2875[a]
Annual investigations	616
Exceptional costs (averaged)	80
Total	4820–5950

[a]Add up to £1000/year if prescribed by GP
Calculations made with Dr B. Wonke

estimate now seems to be *at least* 35 years) gives a minimum (discounted) lifetime cost of £85 500 per patient.

DESCRIBING PREVENTION

Figure 1 is a flowchart describing a population screening and prenatal diagnosis service for thalassaemia that can also be used as a general framework for describing genetic prevention programmes (Royal College of Physicians, 1989). Non-financial costs are enclosed in broken boxes and benefits in full boxes. Estimated financial costs for each step (in 1987) are shown in the right-hand margin. Every step from community information to the birth of a baby has a corresponding benefit to set against financial cost.

The main benefit is seen to be informed choice on the part of couples at risk. Whatever their choice, as long as they are informed and offered counselling, the aim of the service has been achieved. Accepted affected children born because informed parents decided not to have prenatal diagnosis or not to terminate an affected pregnancy are counted as a benefit, not a cost. Termination of pregnancy is seen to be the main cost of the service, not its main benefit.

For three-quarters of couples at risk of thalassaemia, the price of a healthy child is one prenatal diagnosis, since they rarely complete a pregnancy in the absence of prenatal diagnosis (Modell *et al.*, 1980). For couples who find the pregnancy is affected, terminate and try again, the cost of replacing an affected fetus with a healthy one is two prenatal diagnoses. The financial cost of replacement (see Figure 1) is 30% of the annual cost, and 2% of the total (discounted) cost of treating a thalassaemic patient.

The flowchart is proposed only as an outline. To perform a full analysis, most aspects must be developed further, e.g. to include the numbers of the population at risk and carrier frequency, or to spell out the costs of misdiagnosis at any stage. The first half (population screening) would not apply in conditions where only retrospective carrier diagnosis and prenatal diagnosis were available, and only the part following on from pregnancy can be used to describe services for preventing conditions such

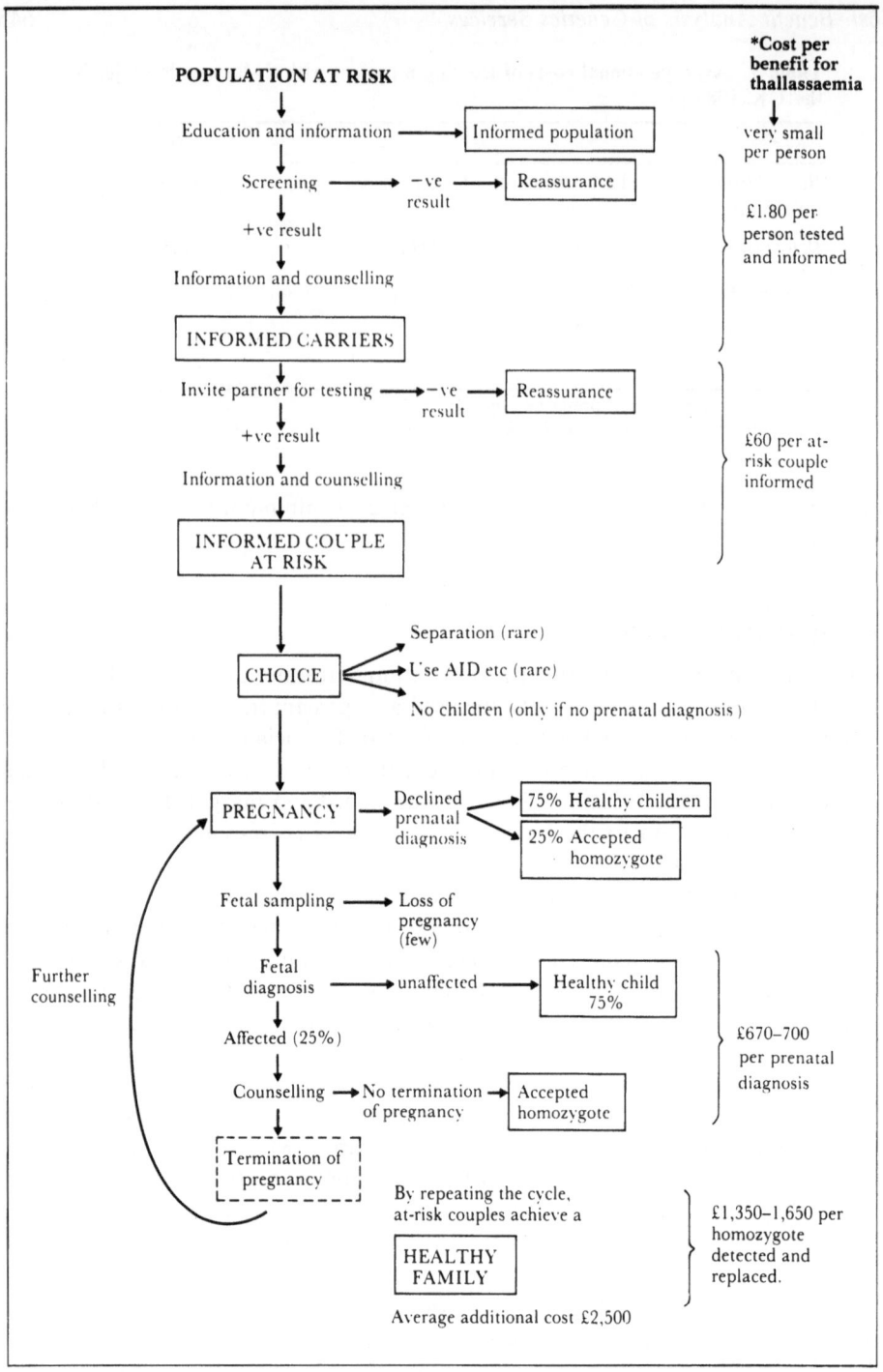

Figure 1 Flow-chart summarizing some of the real costs and benefits of screening for prenatal diagnosis. Benefits are framed. The main costs, termination of pregnancy and loss of a pregnancy as a complication of the obstetric procedure, are in broken frames. For the sake of clarity, costs such as the consequences of false positives and false negatives in screening tests have been omitted. The average cost per person for each step in screening for haemoglobin disorders in the UK (1987 prices) is indicated in the right-hand margin. (From Royal College of Physicians, 1989)

as congenital malformations and chromosomal anomalies that can be diagnosed only during pregnancy.

MEASURING THE EFFECTS OF DIFFERENT POLICIES IN TERMS OF PATIENT NUMBERS AND FINANCIAL COSTS

Costs, both non-financial and financial, depend primarily on patient numbers. However, no policy for thalassaemia completely prevents increases in costs, because some births still occur, and existing patients grow and need more blood, drugs, etc. Figure 2 shows the maximum possible effect of each policy on the number of affected thalassaemic children born. Policies 1–4 have relatively little effect: however, once population screening and prospective prenatal diagnosis become available, numbers may fall quite dramatically. In practice, prenatal diagnosis for thalassaemia is so acceptable that in parts of the Mediterranean the observed effect is now very near to the maximum theoretical figure (Figure 3) (Modell et al., 1990).

Figure 4 compares the total financial cost of each policy in the UK. It includes a single estimate for both thalassaemia and sickle-cell disease, using estimates of the numbers of births in the groups at risk and information on their relative interest in prenatal diagnosis (WHO, 1987). Since only about one-third of couples at risk for sickle-cell disease make use of prenatal diagnosis, total patient numbers and costs continue to rise steadily. However, the figure clearly shows the general point that

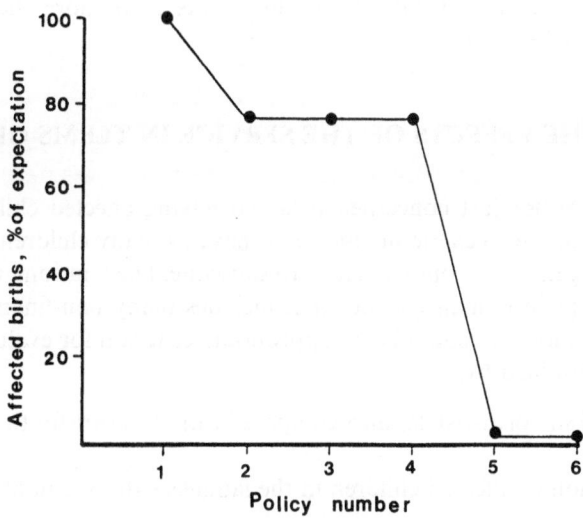

Figure 2 Maximum possible effect of the six different 'policies' listed in Table 1, on the birthrate of children with a recessively inherited disease. It is only prospective carrier diagnosis, included in Policies 5 and 6, that allows a really major reduction in births of affected children. (From WHO, 1987)

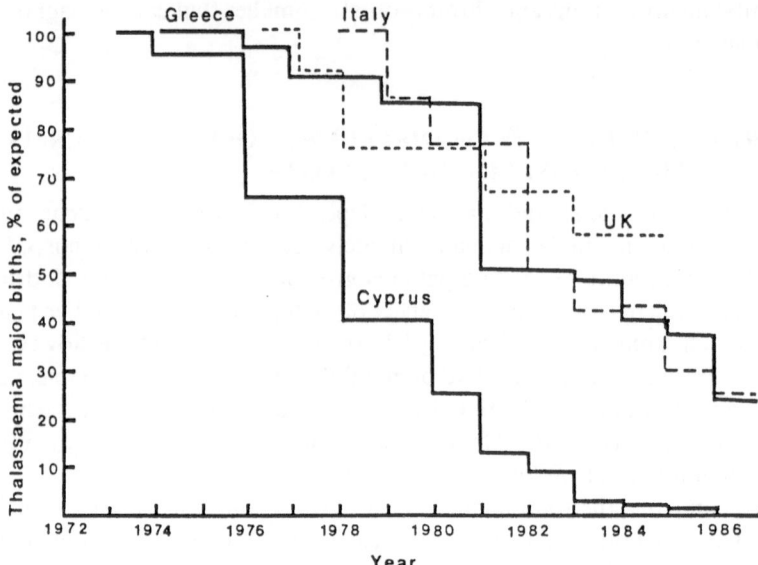

Figure 3 Summary of the results of monitoring thalassaemia control programmes in Europe: the fall in thalassaemia major births now approaches 100% in some national programmes. (From Modell *et al.*, 1990)

though Policy 6 (prospective community information, screening and counselling based in primary health care) is the most expensive to establish, it both provides the best medical service to the groups at risk and limits costs more effectively, in the short as well as the long term.

MEASURING THE EFFECTS OF THE SERVICE IN TERMS OF GENETIC FITNESS

At-risk couples are not just concerned to avoid having affected children. In most cases they are aiming for genetic fitness, i.e. to have as many children as their peers and to hand their genes on proportionately to subsequent generations. Genetic fitness is a central concept in human genetics that includes many non-financial costs and benefits for the family, and could be an appropriate criterion for evaluating genetics services. It is determined by:

(1) Average final size of at-risk families compared with the norm for their population-group.
(2) The proportion of affected children in the families (who are unlikely to pass on many genes).
(3) The proportion of unaffected children in the families (who are more likely to hand on their genes).
(4) The percentage of wanted pregnancies aborted, whether indiscriminately or selectively.

J. Inher. Metab. Dis. 14 (1991)

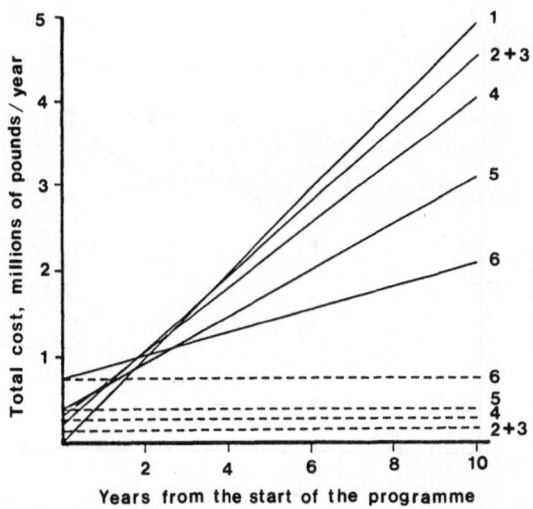

Years from the start of the programme

Figure 4 Estimated relative costs of the six different policies for haemoglobin disorders in the UK. Solid lines show projected cost of patient treatment and prevention with each policy. Broken lines show estimated cost of running the prevention component of each policy. Calculations are from the time of starting the programme, extrapolated over 10 years. A community-based programme including prospective carrier screening and counselling (Policy 6) is the most expensive option, but is rapidly the most effective in limiting costs

Figure 5 shows that using these criteria the genetic fitness of at-risk couples is about 75% of normal in the 'wild' state (Policy 1). (In this uninformed state, some families compensate for early childhood deaths by having more children than others, so their genetic fitness may be a bit higher than this.) With genetic counselling only (Policy 2), genetic fitness falls to less than half of the norm because so many at-risk couples refrain from reproducing (Modell *et al.*, 1980). Introducing retrospective prenatal diagnosis allows fitness to return to the original level of around 75%.

By contrast, prospective prenatal diagnosis (Policies 5 and 6) offers the possibility of near-normal genetic fitness for couples at risk — but at the price of terminating 25% of their wanted pregnancies. In practice, couples at risk for thalassaemia still have rather fewer children than others, because of the stresses associated with pregnancy (Angastiniotis *et al.*, 1986). Pre-implantation prenatal diagnosis may help to solve this problem, especially for couples who have had repeated abortions.

CONCLUSION

The majority of cost–benefit (or cost-effectiveness) analyses of specific genetic services consider only money, and therefore send out conflicting messages. A common framework is needed for describing the true costs and benefits of genetics services. Both treatment and prevention should be included, and costs and benefits should be expressed in language compatible with the caring objectives of medicine. We propose that the following are useful instruments for realistic analysis of costs and benefits:

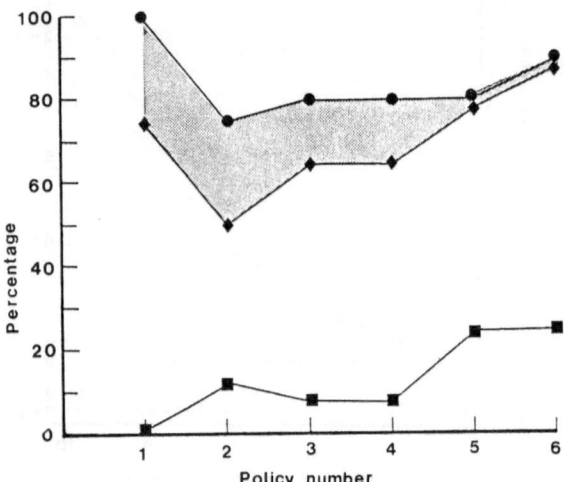

Figure 5 Effect of six different policies on the genetic fitness of families at risk for thalassaemia. The main effect of genetic counselling (every policy except No. 1) is to redue the total number of children in these families (●). The shaded area shows the proportion of affected children with the different policies. The proportion of healthy children (◆) is about 25% less than the norm in the baseline state (Policy 1, no treatment or counselling), and falls even further after genetic counselling without prenatal diagnosis becomes available (Policy 2), because so many couples then cease reproducing. Retrospective prenatal diagnosis (Policies 3 and 4) allows genetic fitness to return to the 75% level. Only prospective counselling (Policies 5 and 6) offers the possibility of equal genetic fitness. The main cost of counselling, terminations of wanted pregnancies (■), rises to a maximum of 25% when all at-risk pregnancies are detected prospectively. This explains why many families at risk still have fewer children than their peers

(1) A framework for describing services based on screening and the offer of prenatal diagnosis that clarifies the true costs and benefits of each step (Figure 1).

(2) A set of six 'policies' can be used to summarize the current possibilities for treatment of patients and identification of carriers and affected fetuses. These 'policies' determine the impact of a condition on patient, family and society.

(3) The concept of genetic fitness, which is central in genetic science, is an appropriate criterion for assessing genetics services.

ACKNOWLEDGEMENTS

This work formed part of a study of community genetics services in Europe carried out by the authors jointly for the European Regional Office of the World Health Organization, Maternal and Child Health Division. B. Modell is supported by a research grant from the Wellcome Trust.

REFERENCES

Angastiniotis, M. A., Kyriakidou, S. and Hadjiminas, M. How thalassaemia was controlled in Cyprus. *World Health Forum* 7 (1986) 291–297

Attanasio, E., Gallanello, R. and Rossi-Mori, A. Analisi costi-benefici di uno intervento preventivo per la talassemia. In: *La Preventione delle Malattie Microcitemice*. Editioni Minerva Medica, Roma, 1980, pp. 277–284

Chamberlain, J. Human benefits and costs of a national screening programme for neural tube defects. *Lancet* 2 (1978) 1293–1296

Drummond, M. F. *Principles of Economic Appraisal in Health Care*. Oxford Medical Publications, Oxford University Press, Oxford, 1980.

Fraser, G. R. The short-term reduction in birth incidence of recessive diseases as a result of genetic counselling after the birth of an affected child. *Hum. Hered.* 22 (1972) 1–6

Gill, M., Murday, V. and Slack, J. An economic appraisal of screening for Down's syndrome in pregnancy using maternal age and serum alpha fetoprotein concentration. *Soc. Sci. Med.* 24 (1986) 725–731.

Hagard, S. and Carter, F. A. Preventing the births of infants with Down's syndrome: a cost–benefit analysis. *Br. Med. J.* 1 (1976) 753–756

Henderson, J. B. Measuring the benefits of screening for neural tube defects. *J. Epidemiol. Commun. Health* 36 (1982) 214–219

Loukopolous, D. (ed.). *Prenatal Diagnosis of Thalassaemia and the Haemoglobinopathies*. CRC Press Inc., Boca Raton, Florida, 1988

Modell, B. and Berdoukas, V. *The Clinical Approach to Thalassaemia*. Grune and Stratton, New York, 1984

Modell, B. and Petrou, M. Comprehensive management of thalassaemia major. *Arch. Dis. Child.* 58 (1983) 1026–1030

Modell, B., Ward, R. H. T. and Fairweather, D. V. I. Effect of introducing antenatal diagnosis on the reproductive behaviour of families at risk for thalassaemia major. *Br. Med. J.* 2 (1980) 737

Modell, B., Kuliev, A. K. and Wagner, M. *Community Genetics Services in Europe*. WHO Regional Office for Europe, Public Health In Europe Series. (In press)

Old, J. M., Fitches, A., Heath, C., Thein, S. L., Weatherall, D. J., Warren, R., McKenzie, C., Rodeck, C. H., Modell, B., Petrou, M. and Ward, R. H. T. First trimester fetal diagnosis for the haemoglobinopathies: report on 200 cases. *Lancet* 2 (1986) 763–766

Ostrowsky, J. T., Lippman, A. and Scriver, C. R. Cost–benefit analysis of a thalassaemia disease prevention programme. *Am. J. Public Health* 75 (1985) 732–736

Royal College of Physicians. *Prenatal Diagnosis and Genetic Screening: Community and Service Implications*. The Royal College of Physicians of London, 1989

Sadovnik, A. D. and Baird, P. A. A cost–benefit analysis of prenatal diagnosis of Down syndrome and neural tube defects in older mothers. *Am. J. Med. Genet.* 10 (1981) 367–378

World Health Organization. Advisory Group on Hereditary Diseases. *Community Approaches to the Control of Hereditary Diseases*. Unpublished WHO document HMG/WG/85.4, 1985. [Can be obtained free of charge from, The Hereditary Diseases Programme, WHO, Geneva, Switzerland]

World Health Organization. *The Haemoglobinopathies in Europe*. WHO Regional Office for Europe, unpublished report IPC/MCH 110 (1987). (Can be obtained free of charge from: Maternal and Child Health Division, WHO Regional Office for Europe, 8 Scherfigsvej, DK-2100, Copenhagen, Denmark)

Journal of Inherited Metabolic Disease

Aims and Scope of the Journal

The *Journal of Inherited Metabolic Disease* is the official scientific and clinical journal of the Society for the Study of Inborn Errors of Metabolism. The aim of this international and multidisciplinary journal is to provide otherwise unavailable information on inherited metabolic disorders covering clinical (medical, dental and veterinary), biochemical (including molecular genetics), genetic, experimental (including cell biology), theoretical, epidemiological, ethical and counselling aspects. Widespread and efficient communication between professional workers should improve the handling and understanding of inherited disorders.

The journal publishes papers, case and short reports, short communications, invited articles which are generally reviews, and book reviews. *Papers for submission* and correspondence should be written in English and sent to:

Dr. R. A. Harkness
15 St Thomas' Drive, Hatch End, Pinner
Middlesex HA5 4SX, United Kingdom.

Acceptance of articles for publication is at the discretion of the editors. Authors are advised to consult a current issue of the journal before submission. It is a condition of acceptance that all articles have not been and will not be published elsewhere in substantially the same form. The submitting author must have circulated the article to and have secured agreement from all co-authors before submission of the article.

The *Journal of Inherited Metabolic Disease* is covered by *Current Contents/Life Sciences*, *ISI/Biomed*, *Science Citation Index*, *ASCA*, *SciSearch* database, *Index Medicus* and *MEDLINE*.

Detailed *Information for Authors* is published in issue no.1 of each volume of the journal, and in other issues as space permits, and is listed in the Contents.

Books for Review should be sent to Dr. Harkness at the above address.

Offprints. 25 offprints are provided free of charge. Authors will receive a form for ordering an extra 125 offprints with the proofs of their paper.

No page charges are levied on authors or their institutions.

Advertisements: As well as commercial advertisements, announcements of forthcoming scientific meetings and other material relevant to the journal can be included, at rates available from the publishers. All advertising is subject to the discretion of the editors.

Publication programme, 1991: Volume 14 (6 issues).
Subscriptions should be sent to: **Kluwer Academic Publishers Group, PO Box 322, 3300 AH Dordrecht, The Netherlands** or at **PO Box 358, Accord Station, Hingham, MA 02018-0358, USA**, or to any subscription agent.
Changes of mailing address should be notified together with your latest label.
Subscription prices, per volume (6 issues): Dfl 416.- plus postage: Dfl 32.- (Dfl 448.- per annum).
Subscription prices, per volume: US$254.50.
Second Class Postage paid at Rahway, NJ. USPS No. 757-750.
US Mailing Agent: Expediters of the Printed Word Inc., 2323 Randolph Ave., Avenel, NJ 07001, USA.
Published by Kluwer Academic Publishers, PO Box 55, Lancaster, LA1 1PE, UK.
Postmaster: please send all address corrections to: *Journal of Inherited Metabolic Disease*,
c/o Expediters of the Printed Word Inc., 2323 Randolph Ave, Avenel, NJ 07001, USA.

Contents (*continued from outside back cover*)